Molecular Oncology: Underlying Mechanisms and Translational Advancements

Ammad Ahmad Farooqi • Muhammad Ismail
Editors

Molecular Oncology: Underlying Mechanisms and Translational Advancements

Springer

Editors
Ammad Ahmad Farooqi
Institute of Biomedical
and Genetic Engineering (IBGE)
Islamabad, Pakistan

Muhammad Ismail
Institute of Biomedical
and Genetic Engineering (IBGE)
Islamabad, Pakistan

ISBN 978-3-319-53081-9 ISBN 978-3-319-53082-6 (eBook)
DOI 10.1007/978-3-319-53082-6

Library of Congress Control Number: 2017934477

Printed on acid-free paper

This Springer imprint is published by Springer Nature
The registered company is Springer International Publishing AG
The registered company address is: Gewerbestrasse 11, 6330 Cham, Switzerland

Preface

Cancer is a multifaceted and genomically complex disease and intriguingly not an unfamiliar term for clinicians over centuries. Earliest evidence of cancer was discovered in human mummies and Egyptian hieroglyphs (ancient manuscripts). Certain hints have emerged pinpointing towards the presence of tumors in fossilized bones in ancient Egypt era. Biologists and archaeological researchers have collaboratively unraveled different mysteries and collected clues of bone cancer (osteosarcoma) in mummies. Egyptian history is unique in the sense that it opened new horizons for clinicians because oldest cancer description was discovered in Egypt (even though the term "cancer" was not coined) and dates back to about 3000 BC. The Edwin Smith Papyrus is doubtlessly the oldest known document on the surgery of trauma. It contained descriptions of eight cases of ulcers or tumors of the breast that were removed by cauterization technique. "Fire drill" was used as a tool for cauterization. Mechanistically enigmatic and therapeutically challenging nature of cancer was also described as the writing says about the disease, "There is no treatment." Hippocrates (460–370 BC) was a Greek physician and considered as the "Father of Medicine." *Carcinos* and *carcinoma* were the terms coined by Hippocrates for description of non-ulcer forming and ulcer forming tumors. Carcinos was a giant crab in Greek mythology and the term was used because finger-like projections appeared like a moving crab or legs of a crab. Evolutionary phase continued and different distinguished medical experts of their times made efforts to make the terms more specific, descriptive, and understandable. Translation of the Greek term into *cancer* was done by the Roman physician, Celsus (28–50 BC), because it was the Latin equivalent of crab.

Another Greek physician who contributed to the development of terminologies was Galen (130–200 AD) who used the word *oncos* (Greek for swelling) for description or explanation of tumors. Interestingly, the crab analogy of Hippocrates and Celsus is still in use in modern cancer biology for description of malignant tumors. Galen's term has now become a part of the name for medical specialists who deal with cancer, "oncologists".

Contents

Substantial fraction of information has been added into the existing pool of information related to cancer biology and experimentally verified data is also shedding light on the involvement of different vitamins in modulation of cancers. 1α,25(OH)2 D3 has been shown to transcriptionally activate and repress target genes by binding to Vitamin D receptor (VDR). VDR belongs to a superfamily of steroid hormone receptors and reportedly involved in transcriptional regulation of different genes in a ligand dependent manner. N-terminal VDR variants are tissue-specifically expressed and required to differentially regulate network of genes by 1α,25(OH)2 D3. 1α,25(OH)2 D3–VDR-modulated transcriptional activity is triggered via structural interaction with RXR (retinoic X receptor). Mechanistically, 1α,25(OH)2 D3–VDR–RXR multi-component machinery is loaded at vitamin D response elements (VDREs), present within promoter region of target genes. VDR occupied the 3′ half-site whereas RXR interacted with 5′ half-site of VDRE for transcriptional modulation of different genes.

Transcriptional activation involved the co-activators, nuclear coactivator-62 kDa–Ski-interacting protein (NCoA62–SKIP), steroid receptor coactivators (SRCs), CREB binding protein (CBP)–p300 and polybromo- and SWI-2-related gene 1 associated factor (PBAF–SNF) and histone acetyltransferases (HATs). These proteins worked in a co-ordinated manner and regulated acetylation of histones to de-repress chromatin. Binding of the vitamin D receptor-interacting protein 205 (DRIP205) promoted assembly of different other DRIPs that structurally connected VDR–RXR–NCoA62–SKIP–DRIP205 complex with RNA Pol II and transcription factor 2B (TF2B) for transcriptional initialization. VDR-interacting repressor (VDIR) has an essential role in regulation of transcriptional repression of different genes. 1,25(OH)2D3-mediated transcriptional repression involved association of heterodimerically linked VDR and RXR with VDIR. Multi-protein complex occupied negative VDREs (nVDREs) and triggered removal of the co-activators and induced loading of co-repressors. Williams syndrome transcription factor (WSTF) potentiated transcriptional repression by interacting with ATP-dependent chromatin-remodeling complex (WINAC) and chromatin. Shown in Figs. 1 and 3.

This chapter is specifically focused on anticancer effects of vitamin D in gynecological cancers. We summarize most recent evidence of tumor suppressing role of vitamin D, how vitamin D bound receptor uniquely interacted with VDRE (Vitamin D response Element) in promoter regions of different genes to transcriptionally modulate their expression levels. We also discuss different nanotechnological strategies to enhance the delivery of vitamin D.

Ovarian Cancer

Despite the fact that ovarian cancer has been termed the ‘silent killer’, high percentage of patients are symptomatic, even when the disease is localized. Ovarian carcinoma arises from the epithelial lining of ovary or cortical inclusion cysts (CICs). Ovarian carcinoma directly spreads to adjacently located organs and normal

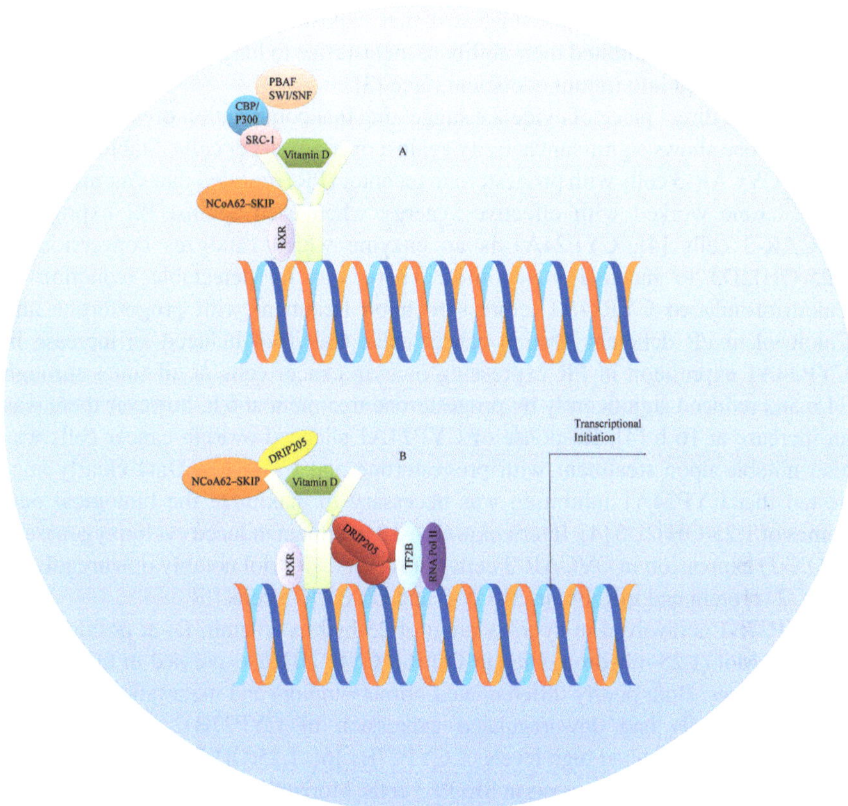

Fig. 1 Shows (**a**) loading of activator proteins to stimulate transcription of VDR target genes. (**b**) VDR–RXR–NCoA62–SKIP–DRIP205 complex interacted with RNA Pol II and TF2B to trigger expression of target genes (DDX5)

peritoneal fluid helps in the transportation of exfoliated tumor cells throughout the peritoneal cavity. This 'seeding' of the peritoneal cavity is frequently associated with formation of ASCITES. This mechanism has been extensively studied and considered as hallmark feature of ovarian carcinoma, particularly serous carcinoma.

1α,25-dihydroxyvitamin-D3 has been shown to suppress migratory potential of ovarian cancer SKOV-3 cells by inhibiting epithelial to mesenchymal transition [1]. Treatment of SKOV-3 with 10 ng/mL of TGF-β1 for 24 h induced morphological changes in the treated cells. Cellular morphology changed from pebble-like epithelial to spindle-like mesenchymal, and there was a gradual elongation in 72 h. TGF-β1 induced increase in cellular migration was considerably reduced after treatment with $1\alpha,25(OH)_2D_3$ [1].

1α,25 dihydroxyvitamin D_3 has also been reported to delay chemically induced malignant transformation of ovarian surface epithelial cells in mice. Vitamin D_3 administration considerably upregulated VDR and E-cadherin levels in treated mice [2].

Confluence of information suggested that exposure of A2780 ovarian cancer cells to vitamin D_3 inhibited their ability to metastasize to lung and liver when intravenously injected into immunodeficient mice [3].

There is a direct piece of evidence suggesting that combination of vitamin D and progesterone shows significant activity against ovarian cancer cells. Stable transfection of OVCAR-3 cells with progesterone receptor (PR) revealed that vitamin D and progesterone worked with effective synergy when used against PR expressing OVCAR-3 cells [4]. CYP24A1 is an enzyme which catalyzes conversion of 1,25(OH)2D3 to inactive metabolites. There was no detectable reduction in Calcitriol-induced CYP24A1 expression upon treatment with progesterone and Calcitriol in PR deficient ovarian cancer cells. Calcitriol induced an increase in CYP24A1 expression in PR expressing ovarian cancer cells at all times through 24 h and reduced significantly by progesterone treatment at 6 h, however there was an increase at 16 h [4]. Response of CYP24A1 silenced ovarian cancer cells was also notable upon treatment with progesterone and Calcitriol. Data clearly suggested that CYP24A1 inhibition was necessary to maximize the biological outcomes of 1,25(OH)2D3 [4]. Interleukin (IL)-1β treatment induced cyclooxygenase-2 (COX-2) expression in OVCAR-3 cells. However, calcitriol notably downregulated COX-2 (protein and mRNA) in SKOV-3 and OVCAR-3 cells [5].

CYP27B1 is involved in hydroxylation of 25-hydroxyvitamin D_3 at position C1α into calcitriol (1,25-dihydroxyvitamin D_3) [6]. CYP27B1 is expressed in tumors and normal tissues. Both poorly differentiated primary tumors and metastatically competent cancer cells had downregulated expression of CYP27B1. However, non-metastasizing tumors had high levels of CYP27B1 [6]. 1,25(OH)2D3 and carboplatin synergistically induced apoptosis in SKOV-3 cells. Moreover, generation of ROS (reactive oxygen species) was significantly higher in combinatorially treated cancer cells [7].

Omentum, a fold of peritoneum connecting or supporting abdominal structures is a potential site for spread of metastatically competent ovarian cancer cells. 1,25(OH)2D_3 (10^{-7} M) markedly impaired metastasizing capacity of OVCAR3 cells that consequently reduced colonization of ovarian cancer cells to mouse omenta in the *ex vivo* co-culture system [8]. 1,25(OH)2D_3 also remarkably reduced the ability of murine ovarian cancer cells (ID8-VEGF) to colonize omenta when injected intraperitoneally into mice. VDR has notable expression in different types of cells, including adipocytes, immune cells , fibroblasts and microvascular cells. These are important constituents of omental stroma. Metastasizing capacity of SKOV3 and OVCAR3 in terms of invasion of omenta isolated from VDR null and wild type VDR expressing mice was investigated. Colonization rate of ovarian cancer cells was considerably lower in wild type VDR expressing mice as compared to VDR null mice [8]. Seocalcitol (EB 1089), a vitamin D analogue, notably inhibited ID8-VEGF cells colonization to omenta in wild type mice. However, it was unable to exert inhibitory effects on the colonization of ID8-VEGF cells into omenta in VDR null mice [8].

PT19c, a non-hypercalcemic vitamin D derived agent has been noted to be effective against gynecological cancers. PT19c significantly inhibited tumor growth in mice xenografted with SKOV-3 cells [9].

EGFR/PI-3Kinase signaling axis is reportedly involved in modulation of different cellular activities. It also enhanced lipogenesis in cancer cells by activation of lipogenic fatty acid synthase (FASN) machinery [10]. MT19c time dependently downregulated expression levels of acetyl Co-A carboxylase (ACC) and FASN in SKOV-3 cells. Malonyl CoA is converted into palmitates by FASN. MT19c markedly decreased malonyl CoA levels in SKOV-3 cells [10].

Novel VDRE has previously been identified within intron 1 of EGFR gene. VDR protein was found to occupy intronic VDRE of EGFR in the presence of 1,25(OH)2D_3. VDR worked synchronously with repressor proteins to transcriptionally downregulate expression of EGFR in ovarian cancer cells (Fig. 3) [11].

Chemokine (C-X-C motif) ligand 1 (CXCL1) and CXCL2 are involved in cancer development and progression. Treatment of ovarian cancer cells with calcitriol and progesterone induced considerable downregulation of CXCL1 and CXCL2. CXCL1 and CXCL2 promoters have binding sites for NFKB (Nuclear Factor Kappa B) [12]. Expression levels of CXCL1 and CXCL2 were dramatically reduced in NFkB-silenced cells. Phosphorylation of IkBα at 32nd and 36th Serine residues sequestered it from NFKB for transcriptional modulation of CXCL1 and CXCL2 by NFKB. Calcitriol and progesterone rescued IkBα from phosphorylation and consequent degradation. Consequently IkBα bound NFKB was unable to trigger expression of CXCL1 and CXCL2 [12].

Human Studies

There is a recent report suggesting that 73% patients with recurrent ovarian cancer have insufficient levels of 25-OH vitamin D. Moreover, 47% patients with stable ovarian cancer have insufficiently low levels [13]. Higher 25(OH)D concentrations at diagnosis have been noted to be considerably linked with longer survival. However, PFS (progression-free survival) or 25(OH)D measured after primary treatment were not significantly associated [14]. The T helper cells (Th cells) are differentially modulated by low vitamin D levels. Low vitamin D levels inhibited Th2 activity and promoted Th1 activity in ovarian cancer patients [15]. In the upcoming section we discuss how vitamin D/VDR signaling axis efficiently modulates protein network in endometrial cancer cells.

Endometrial Cancer

Endometrial carcinomas are biologically and histopathologically classified into two types. Type I tumors are well-differentiated and endometrioid in histology. Type II endometrial cancers are poorly differentiated and non-endometrioid. This section mainly deals with the role of vitamin D/VDR signaling axis in inhibition of endometrial cancer.

PT19c, a non-hypercalcemic vitamin D derived agent has been noted to be effective against gynecological cancers. There was a reduction in tumor size during the last 15 days in the PT19c treatment group. Two of eight animals nearly completely responded and the remaining six animals partially responded to PT19c treatment. Calcitriol treatment although was effective against the endometrial tumor growth but size of the tumor increased continuously in mice xenografted with endometrial ECC-1 cells [9]. None of the animals either partially or completely responded to calcitriol. Furthermore, excessive hypercalcemia was noted in serum of calcitriol treated animals [9].

Class 3 semaphorins (SEMA3B and SEMA3F), are involved in regulation of tumor growth, metastasis and angiogenesis. These molecules transduced the signals through trans-membrane receptor complex consisted of plexins and neuropilins (NP) [16]. Expression levels of SEMA3F, SEMA3B and their receptor plexin A3 were notably downregulated in endometrial cancer cells. Treatment of endometrial cancer cells with progesterone (25 μmol/L) or 1,25(OH)2D3 (100 nmol/L) markedly upregulated SEMA3F and SEMA3B [16]. However, these effects were not observed in SEMA3B and SEMA3F silenced endometrial cancer cells. Endometrial cancer cells that ectopically expressed SEMA3B and SEMA3F had notably reduced proliferation and migration potential. Upregulation of SEMA3B and SEMA3F inhibited integrins and matrix metalloproteinases (MMPs) in endometrial cancer cells [16]. Shown in Fig. 2.

Progesterone considerably upregulated VDRs in endometrial cancer cells. Furthermore, Bax levels were notably enhanced in endometrial cancer cells combinatorially treated with Progesterone and calcitriol. Moreover, levels of Histone H1.4, histidine triad nucleotide-binding protein 2 (HINT2), Eukaryotic initiation-factor 2 α kinase family (EIF2AK2) were also noted to be enhanced in endometrial cancer cells after combinatorial treatment [17].

Calcitriol worked with effective synergy with carboplatin and inhibited the growth of RL95–2 endometrial cancer cells. Addition of 10–50 nM calcitriol to 5–20 μg/ml carboplatin increased growth inhibitory effects [18].

Icb-1 (C1orf38) is involved in differentiation processes of cancer cells. Upregulated level of icb-1 was noted in vitamin D_3 treated HEC-1B endometrial adenocarcinoma cells. E-cadherin level was markedly enhanced by 95% in vitamin D_3 treated HEC-1B cells. All-trans retinoic acid (ATRA), an inducer of differentiation also enhanced E-cadherin level in HEC-1B cells. However, ATRA mediated increase in the expression of E-cadherin was not noted in icb silenced cells [19].

Cervical Cancer

High-risk types of the human papilloma virus (hrHPV) infection triggered the development of cervical cancer and re-wired intracellular signaling cascades. Highly persistent hrHPV, hrHPV-induced epithelial transformation, development of precancerous lesions (cervical intraepithelial neoplasia graded 1–3 (CIN1–3)) and

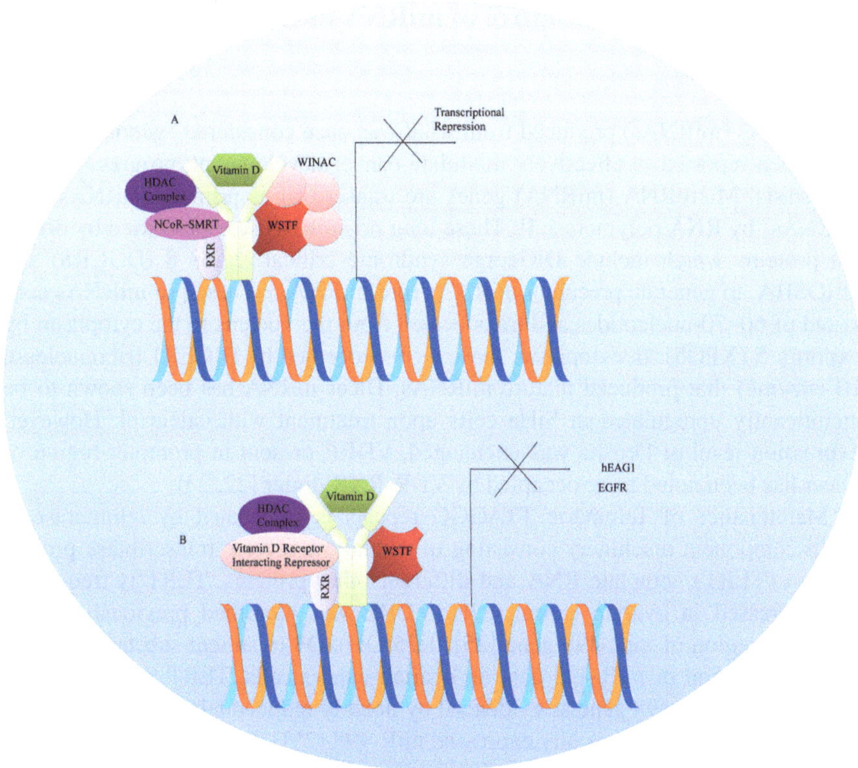

Fig. 2 Shows plexin and neuropilin mediated intracellular signaling. Integrins and MMPs were notably downregulated after semaphorin mediated signaling

consequently progresses to an invasive cervical cancer. Progression from pre-cancer to invasive cancer has been noted to take longer timespan in majority of the patients. It has been suggested that High-grade precancerous lesions (CIN2 and CIN3) developed within 3–5 years in hrHPV infected patients, while progression to an invasive phenotype can further require 20–30 years.

Human cervical cancer oncogene (HCCR-1) is frequently overexpressed in cervical cancer [20]. Calcitriol dose and time dependently downregulated expression level of HCCR-1 in HeLa cells [21]. DEAD box RNA helicase DDX5, an ATP-dependent RNA helicase was noted to be controlled by VDRE in its promoter region. Calcitriol treatment upregulated DDX5 (mRNA and protein) in SiHa cells. Complex consisting of VDR and RXR was noted to occupy most proximally located VDRE in promoter region of DDX5 [22, 23]. Negative VDRE have been reported in Human ether à go-go 1 potassium channel (hEAG1). hEAG1 is involved in proliferation of cervical cancer cells. VDR, RXR, VDR-interacting repressor and Williams syndrome transcription factor have been shown to transcriptionally repress hEAG1 by occupying nVDRE located within promoter region in the absence of ligand [24]. Shown in Fig. 3.

Vitamin D Mediated Control of miRNA in Gynecological Cancers

microRNAs (miRNAs) produced from what was once considered "genomic trash," have been reported to effectively modulate cancer development, progression, and metastasis. MicroRNA (miRNA) genes are transcribed as primary miRNAs (pri-miRNAs) by RNA polymerase II. These long pri-miRNAs are processed by different proteins which include DiGeorge syndrome critical region 8 (DGCR8) and DROSHA, to generate precursor miRNAs (pre-miRNAs). These pre-miRNAs consisted of 60–70-nucleotides and translocated from the nucleus to the cytoplasm by exportin 5 (XPO5). In cytoplasm, these were processed by DICER1 (ribonuclease III enzyme) that produced mature miRNAs. Dicer mRNA has been shown to be significantly upregulated in SiHa cells upon treatment with calcitriol. However, expression level of Drosha was unchanged. VDRE present in promoter region of Dicer has been noted to be occupied by VDR-RXR dimer [22, 23].

Maintenance of Telomeric TTAGGG repeats is modulated by telomerase, a multi-component machinery consisting of a catalytic reverse transcriptase protein subunit (TERT), template RNA and different other proteins. TERT is frequently overexpressed in ovarian cancer cells. VDRE was identified previously in the upstream region of miR-498 gene [25]. 1,25(OH)2D3 treatment substantially elevated expression of miR-498 gene in ovarian cancer cells. TERT was negatively regulated by miR-498 gene as evidenced by notably reduced telomerase activity in OVCAR3 cells that ectopically expressed miR-498 [25].

Nanotechnological Delivery of Vitamin D

Engineered nanoparticles have revolutionized the field of medicine and encouraging results obtained from studies of tumor retarding effects of efficiently delivered therapeutics using different nanotechnological strategies in xenografted mice have paved the way to clinical trials.

Poly(lactic-co-glycolic acid) (PLGA) nanoparticles (NPs) have been reported as potential drug delivery vehicles for calcitriol. Calcitriol loaded PLGA NPs were efficiently internalized by cancer cells and growth rates of cancer cells were significantly reduced [26]. Vitamin D_3 loaded Carboxymethyl chitosan-soy protein complex NPs are also remarkable delivery systems for encapsulation and controlled release of vitamin D based therapeutics [27]. Calcidiol/calcitriol loaded polymeric NPs showed higher encapsulation efficiencies, sustained releases over 7 days and enhanced stability [28]. Zein NPs coated with carboxymethyl chitosan (CMCS) have also been used for encapsulation of vitamin D_3. CMCS coated NPs were spherically structured having a particle size from 86 to 200 nm and displayed markedly increased encapsulation efficiency [29].

Vitamin D_3 loaded oleoyl alginate ester NPs have also shown efficiency in controlled release of payload to the target site [30].

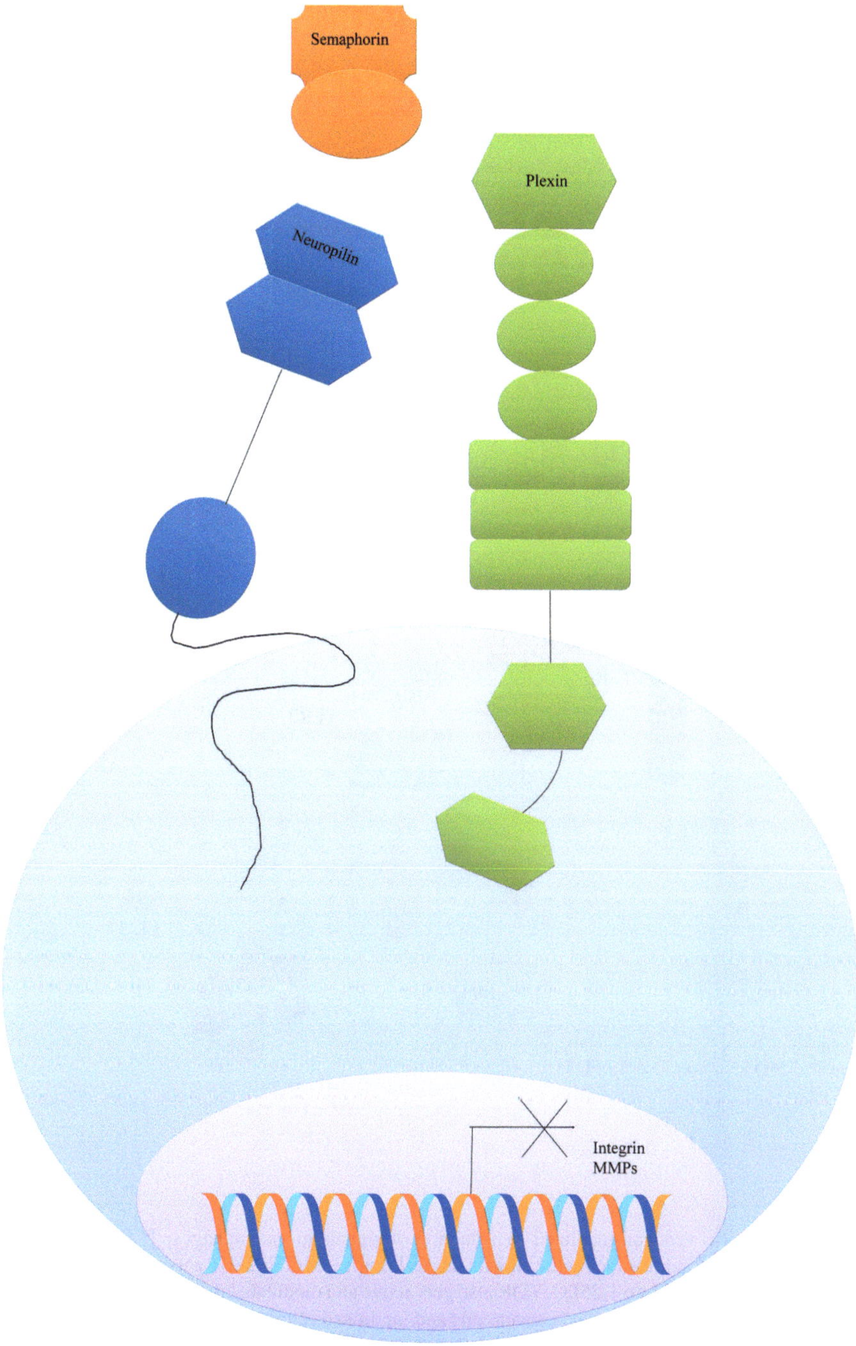

Fig. 3 Shows (**a**) loading of repressor proteins to inhibit transcription of target genes. (**b**) WSTF and VDR-interacting repressor downregulated hEAG1 and EGFR

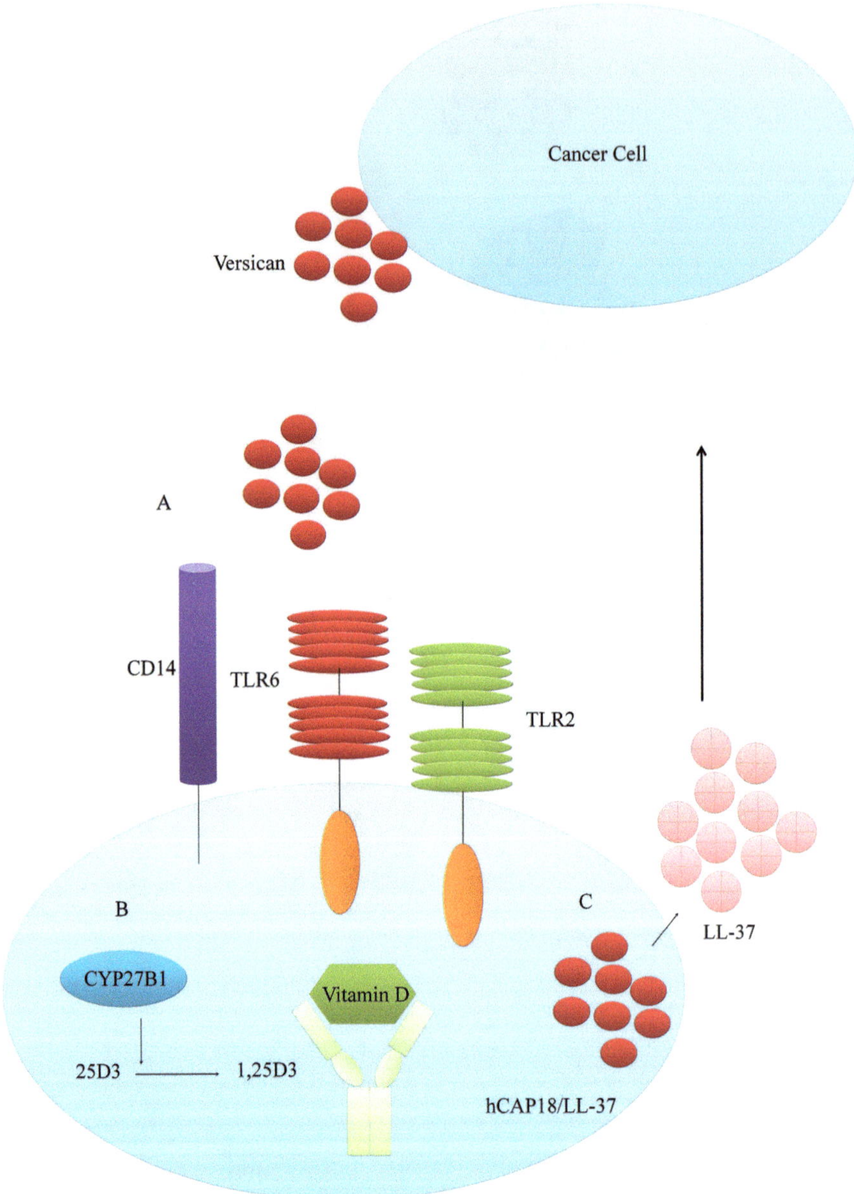

Fig. 4 Shows (**a**) versican mediated transduction of signals in macrophages. TLR2, TLR6 and CD14 are involved in transducing the signals intracellularly. (**b**) CYP27B1 gets active and triggers the conversion of 25D3 into 1,25D3. VDR also gets active and modulated the induction of hCAP18/LL-37. Processed LL-37 activated cancer cells and facilitated release of versican

As our concepts and knowledge of gynecological oncology become more complete, it is important for interdisciplinary researchers to discuss ideas for treatment of cancer with minimum off-target effects. Route of administration is also an essential requisite that still needs extensive research. Researchers are currently re-investigating underlying causes of the poor delivery efficiency from the perspectives of tumor biology (enhanced permeability and retention effect (EPR), inter-cellular versus trans-cellular transport, physico-chemically-dependent transport of nanoparticles through the tumor stroma) as well as competing organs which include renal and mononuclear phagocytic systems.

Cancer Promoting Role of Vitamin D/VDR Signaling Axis: Darker Side

Although tremendous research has been conducted in evaluating true potential of vitamin D induced signaling axis in suppression of cancer, however, certain clues have also emerged which warn us about cancer promoting role. In the following section, we draw attention to an incompletely studied mechanism exploited by cancers to promote their progression.

Human cationic antimicrobial protein-18 (hCAP18)/LL-37, a cathelicidin peptide is constitutively produced in different cell types. 1,25D_3 is involved in upregulation of hCAP18/LL-37 in macrophages, monocytes and epidermal kerationocytes. Co-incubation of ovarian cancer cells (OV-90, SKOV3, 3AO and HO-8910) with peripheral blood monocytes-derived macrophages markedly enhanced proliferation of the cells [31]. Detailed mechanistic insights revealed that co-culture of SKOV3 cells with macrophages considerably upregulated expression levels of VDR, Cyp24A1 (1,25 D3 catabolic enzyme) and Cyp27B1 which catalyzed the formation of bioactive vitamin D_3 in macrophages. Toll like receptors (TLR2, TLR6) and CD14 are present on surface of macrophages. Versican (V1), a macrophage activating factor transduced the signals through TLR2 and its co-receptors CD14 and TLR6 present on surface of macrophages. It is frequently overexpressed in ovarian cancer [31].TLR2, TLR6 and CD14 worked synchronously to transduce the signals to downstream effectors in macrophages. Shown in Fig. 2. Significant downregulation of hCAP18/LL-37 was noted in macrophages upon treatment with the TLR2 (Toll like receptor) neutralizing antibody [31]. Tumor-modulated upregulation of hCAP18/LL-37 required TLR2/6 induced signaling cascade in macrophage. VDR antagonist (ZK159222) treatment, notably downregulated hCAP18/LL-37 expression in treated cells. Addition of 25D3 dose dependently upregulated hCAP18/LL-37 in SKOV3-CM/macrophage co-culture experiments. Expression levels of CD14, TLR6, TLR2, VDR, Cyp27B1 and Cyp24 were remarkably downregulated when versican silenced SKOV3 cells were co-incubated with macrophages [31]. Shown Fig. 4.

Recent developments in molecular oncology require us to reconsider long-held assumptions about the context dependent biological effects exerted by vitamin D/VDR signaling axis. Ultimately, such a varied array of research directions will propel our understanding of VDR mediated crosstalk in gynecological cancers and the translation of these discoveries will be helpful in getting a step closer to personalized medicine.

Conclusion

Increasingly it is being realized that intracellular signaling cascades are hierarchically organized and modulated by a highly intricate and synchronized network of regulators and downstream effectors. These signaling cascades are spatio-temporally controlled and dysregulations of these cascades are contributory in cancer development and progression. It further needs to be seen how vitamin D/VDR signaling axis modulates different oncogenic and tumor suppressor miRNAs in gynecological cancers. Moreover, it will be exciting to see how natural products stimulate the expression of VDRs in different gynecological cancers and combination of vitamin D analogs with VDR stimulating natural products will be a very promising area of research.

References

1. Hou YF, Gao SH, Wang P, Zhang HM, Liu LZ, Ye MX, Zhou GM, Zhang ZL, Li BY (2016) $1\alpha,25(OH)_2D_3$ suppresses the migration of ovarian cancer SKOV-3 cells through the inhibition of epithelial-mesenchymal transition. Int J Mol Sci 17(8):1285. doi:10.3390/ijms17081285
2. Liu L, Hu Z, Zhang H, Hou Y, Zhang Z, Zhou G, Li B (2016) Vitamin D postpones the progression of epithelial ovarian cancer induced by 7, 12-dimethylbenz [a] anthracene both in vitro and in vivo. Onco Targets Ther 9:2365–2375. doi:10.2147/OTT.S100581
3. Abdelbaset-Ismail A, Pedziwiatr D, Suszyńska E, Sluczanowska-Glabowska S, Schneider G, Kakar SS, Ratajczak MZ (2016) Vitamin D3 stimulates embryonic stem cells but inhibits migration and growth of ovarian cancer and teratocarcinoma cell lines. J Ovarian Res 9:26. doi:10.1186/s13048-016-0235-x
4. Rodriguez GC, Turbov J, Rosales R, Yoo J, Hunn J, Zappia KJ, Lund K, Barry CP, Rodriguez IV, Pike JW, Conrads TP, Darcy KM, Maxwell GL, Hamilton CA, Syed V, Thaete LG (2016) Progestins inhibit calcitriol-induced CYP24A1 and synergistically inhibit ovarian cancer cell viability: an opportunity for chemoprevention. Gynecol Oncol 143(1):159–167. doi:10.1016/j.ygyno.2016.04.022
5. Thill M, Woeste A, Reichert K, Fischer D, Rody A, Friedrich M, Köster F (2015) Vitamin D inhibits ovarian cancer cell line proliferation in combination with celecoxib and suppresses cyclooxygenase-2 expression. Anticancer Res 35(2):1197–1203
6. Brożyna AA, Jóźwicki W, Jochymski C, Slominski AT (2015) Decreased expression of CYP27B1 correlates with the increased aggressiveness of ovarian carcinomas. Oncol Rep 33(2):599–606. doi:10.3892/or.2014.3666
7. Zhang Z, Zhang H, Hu Z, Wang P, Wan J, Li B (2014) Synergy of 1,25-dihydroxyvitamin D3 and carboplatin in growth suppression of SKOV-3 cells. Oncol Lett 8(3):1348–1354

8. Lungchukiet P, Sun Y, Kasiappan R, Quarni W, Nicosia SV, Zhang X, Bai W (2015) Suppression of epithelial ovarian cancer invasion into the omentum by 1α,25-dihydroxyvitamin D3 and its receptor. J Steroid Biochem Mol Biol 148:138–147. doi:10.1016/j.jsbmb.2014.11.005
9. Kawar N, Maclaughlan S, Horan TC, Uzun A, Lange TS, Kim KK, Hopson R, Singh AP, Sidhu PS, Glass KA, Shaw S, Padbury JF, Vorsa N, Arnold LA, Moore RG, Brard L, Singh RK (2013) PT19c, another nonhypercalcemic vitamin D2 derivative, demonstrates antitumor efficacy in epithelial ovarian and endometrial cancer models. Genes Cancer 4(11–12):524–534. doi:10.1177/1947601913507575
10. Moore RG, Lange TS, Robinson K, Kim KK, Uzun A, Horan TC, Kawar N, Yano N, Chu SR, Mao Q, Brard L, DePaepe ME, Padbury JF, Arnold LA, Brodsky A, Shen TL, Singh RK (2012) Efficacy of a non-hypercalcemic vitamin-D2 derived anti-cancer agent (MT19c) and inhibition of fatty acid synthesis in an ovarian cancer xenograft model. PLoS One 7(4):e34443. doi:10.1371/journal.pone.0034443
11. Shen Z, Zhang X, Tang J, Kasiappan R, Jinwal U, Li P, Hann S, Nicosia SV, Wu J, Zhang X, Bai W (2011) The coupling of epidermal growth factor receptor down regulation by 1alpha,25-dihydroxyvitamin D3 to the hormone-induced cell cycle arrest at the G1-S checkpoint in ovarian cancer cells. Mol Cell Endocrinol 338(1–2):58–67. doi:10.1016/j.mce.2011.02.023
12. Kavandi L, Collier MA, Nguyen H, Syed V (2012) Progesterone and calcitriol attenuate inflammatory cytokines CXCL1 and CXCL2 in ovarian and endometrial cancer cells. J Cell Biochem 113(10):3143–3152. doi:10.1002/jcb.24191
13. Granato T, Manganaro L, Petri L, Porpora MG, Viggiani V, Angeloni A, Anastasi E (2016) Low 25-OH vitamin D levels at time of diagnosis and recurrence of ovarian cancer. Tumour Biol 37(2):2177–2181. doi:10.1007/s13277-015-4055-1
14. Webb PM, de Fazio A, Protani MM, Ibiebele TI, Nagle CM, Brand AH, Blomfield PI, Grant P, Perrin LC, Neale RE, Australian Ovarian Cancer Study Group (2015) Circulating 25-hydroxyvitamin D and survival in women with ovarian cancer. Am J Clin Nutr 102(1):109–114. doi:10.3945/ajcn.114.102681
15. Mohapatra S, Saxena A, Gandhi G, Koner BC, Singh T, Ray PC (2015) Does vitamin D mediate inhibition of epithelial ovarian cancer by modulating cytokines? Clin Transl Oncol 17(8):590–595. doi:10.1007/s12094-015-1281-3
16. Nguyen H, Ivanova VS, Kavandi L, Rodriguez GC, Maxwell GL, Syed V (2011) Progesterone and 1,25-dihydroxyvitamin D_3 inhibit endometrial cancer cell growth by upregulating semaphorin 3B and semaphorin 3F. Mol Cancer Res 9(11):1479–1492. doi:10.1158/1541-7786.MCR-11-0213
17. Lee LR, Teng PN, Nguyen H, Hood BL, Kavandi L, Wang G, Turbov JM, Thaete LG, Hamilton CA, Maxwell GL, Rodriguez GC, Conrads TP, Syed V (2013) Progesterone enhances calcitriol antitumor activity by upregulating vitamin D receptor expression and promoting apoptosis in endometrial cancer cells. Cancer Prev Res (Phila) 6(7):731–743. doi:10.1158/1940-6207.CAPR-12-0493
18. Saunders DE, Christensen C, Wappler NL, Cho YL, Lawrence WD, Malone JM, Malviya VK, Deppe G (1993) Additive inhibition of RL95-2 endometrial carcinoma cell growth by carboplatin and 1,25 dihydroxyvitamin D3. Gynecol Oncol 51(2):155–159
19. Haselberger M, Springwald A, Konwisorz A, Lattrich C, Goerse R, Ortmann O, Treeck O (2011) Silencing of the icb-1 gene inhibits the induction of differentiation-associated genes by vitamin D3 and all-trans retinoic acid in gynecological cancer cells. Int J Mol Med 28(1):121–127
20. Ko J, Lee YH, Hwang SY, Lee YS, Shin SM, Hwang JH, Kim J, Kim YW, Jang SW, Ryoo ZY, Kim IK, Namkoong SE, Kim JW (2003) Identification and differential expression of novel human cervical cancer oncogene HCCR-2 in human cancers and its involvement in p53 stabilization. Oncogene 22(30):4679–4689
21. Wang G, Lei L, Zhao X, Zhang J, Zhou M, Nan K (2014) Calcitriol inhibits cervical cancer cell proliferation through downregulation of HCCR1 expression. Oncol Res 22(5–6):301–309. doi:10.3727/096504015X14424348425991

22. González-Duarte RJ, Cázares-Ordoñez V, Díaz L, Ortíz V, Larrea F, Avila E (2015) The expression of RNA helicase DDX5 is transcriptionally upregulated by calcitriol through a vitamin D response element in the proximal promoter in SiHa cervical cells. Mol Cell Biochem 410(1–2):65–73. doi:10.1007/s11010-015-2538-4
23. González-Duarte RJ, Cázares-Ordoñez V, Romero-Córdoba S, Díaz L, Ortíz V, Freyre-González JA, Hidalgo-Miranda A, Larrea F, Avila E (2015) Calcitriol increases Dicer expression and modifies the microRNAs signature in SiHa cervical cancer cells. Biochem Cell Biol 93(4):376–384. doi:10.1139/bcb-2015-0010
24. Cázares-Ordoñez V, González-Duarte RJ, Díaz L, Ishizawa M, Uno S, Ortíz V, Ordoñez-Sánchez ML, Makishima M, Larrea F, Avila E (2015) A cis-acting element in the promoter of human ether à go-go 1 potassium channel gene mediates repression by calcitriol in human cervical cancer cells. Biochem Cell Biol 93(1):94–101. doi:10.1139/bcb-2014-0073
25. Kasiappan R, Shen Z, Tse AK, Jinwal U, Tang J, Lungchukiet P, Sun Y, Kruk P, Nicosia SV, Zhang X, Bai W (2012) 1,25-Dihydroxyvitamin D3 suppresses telomerase expression and human cancer growth through microRNA-498. J Biol Chem 287(49):41297–41309. doi:10.1074/jbc.M112.407189
26. Ramalho MJ, Loureiro JA, Gomes B, Frasco MF, Coelho MA, Pereira MC (2015) PLGA nanoparticles as a platform for vitamin D-based cancer therapy. Beilstein J Nanotechnol 12(6):1306–1318. doi:10.3762/bjnano.6.135
27. Teng Z, Luo Y, Wang Q (2013) Carboxymethyl chitosan-soy protein complex nanoparticles for the encapsulation and controlled release of vitamin D_3. Food Chem 141(1):524–532. doi:10.1016/j.foodchem.2013.03.043
28. Almouazen E, Bourgeois S, Jordheim LP, Fessi H, Briançon S (2013) Nano-encapsulation of vitamin D3 active metabolites for application in chemotherapy: formulation study and in vitro evaluation. Pharm Res 30(4):1137–1146. doi:10.1007/s11095-012-0949-4
29. Luo Y, Teng Z, Wang Q (2012) Development of zein nanoparticles coated with carboxymethyl chitosan for encapsulation and controlled release of vitamin D3. J Agric Food Chem 60(3):836–843. doi:10.1021/jf204194z
30. Sun F, Ju C, Chen J, Liu S, Liu N, Wang K, Liu C (2012) Nanoparticles based on hydrophobic alginate derivative as nutraceutical delivery vehicle: vitamin D3 loading. Artif Cells Blood Substit Immobil Biotechnol 40(1–2):113–119. doi:10.3109/10731199.2011.597759
31. Li D, Wang X, Wu JL, Quan WQ, Ma L, Yang F, Wu KY, Wan HY (2013) Tumor-produced versican V1 enhances hCAP18/LL-37 expression in macrophages through activation of TLR2 and vitamin D3 signaling to promote ovarian cancer progression in vitro. PLoS One 8(2):e56616. doi:10.1371/journal.pone.0056616

Microtubule Targeting Agents in Cancer Therapy: Elucidating the Underlying Molecular Mechanisms

Mohadeseh Hasanpourghadi, Ashok Kumar Pandurangan, and Mohd. Rais Mustafa

Abstract Microtubules are intracellular components of cytoskeleton throughout the cytoplasm of all eukaryotic cells. Microtubules are dynamic polymers with continuous assembly and disassembly of tubulin dimers. This highly dynamic action of microtubule contributes to numerous cellular processes such as maintaining the structure of the cell, cell division and cell movement. For this reason, microtubule has become a notable target for chemotherapeutic achievements. Microtubule Targeting Agents (MTAs) that nowadays are used in chemotherapy, induce microtubule polymerization or depolymerization. They are categorized into two groups known as stabilizers such as texanes and destabilizers such as vincas. Either, stabilizing or destabilizing of microtubule polymer leads to spindle assembly poisoning, mitotic blockage and cell death. Yet, we are required to consider main forthcoming controversial difficulty which is resistance to MTAs. Clinical studies have documented different levels of resistance to MTAs with different durability among patients even within the same class of drugs. For instance, overexpression of P-glycoprotein (P-gp) is linked to resistance to taxanes, but not to ixabepilone, even though they have similar mechanism of action. Mutations in β-tubulin have been associated with resistance to taxanes but not to epithilones despite their mechanism of action being same. Also, there is association between poor response to taxanes and overexpression of βIII-tubulin. Either receiving benefit or harm from MTAs, depends on each individual patient considering their variable chemo-sensitivities to drugs. Therefore, it is crucial to understand the basic biology of microtubules and the molecular mechanisms by which MTAs exert their activity. This is especially important considering their current application in cancer therapy. In this chapter we discussed about MTAs in detail and illustrate their molecular mechanisms involved in various cancers.

Keywords Cancer therapy • Microtubules • Stabilizer • Destabilizer • Chemoresistance

---

M. Hasanpourghadi • A.K. Pandurangan (✉) • M.R. Mustafa, Ph.D. (✉)
Department of Pharmacology, Faculty of Medicine, University of Malaya,
50603 Kuala Lumpur, Malaysia
e-mail: panduashok@um.edu.my; rais@um.edu.my

A.A. Farooqi, M. Ismail (eds.), *Molecular Oncology: Underlying Mechanisms and Translational Advancements*, DOI 10.1007/978-3-319-53082-6_2

Cancer and Normal Cells Different Characteristics

Cancer is an ancient disease that afflicts about 40% of the global population despite improvement in the diagnosis and treatment to the disease. Rather more challenging when cancer become metastatic [1]. Surgery, chemotherapy and radiation therapy are the current strategies for cancer treatment. The conventional treatments failed achieving therapeutic selectivity to cancer cells, rather than non-specific targeting the normal cells, and this leaded to appearance of serious side effects. Therefore, the current target-based drug design and discovery requires new drugs with selectivity to cancer cells in molecular bases. Thus, differentiation of cancer cells from normal cells which includes their characteristics and behaviors, is a requirement. Based on the current knowledge of cancer cell characteristics, studies are directed to molecular–based paradigms. These paradigms are safe to say that increased drug efficacy with less side-effects [2]. In the last 25 years, countless researches have been done for understanding molecular-based strategies, which their discoveries have been improving diagnostic, prognostic and treatment of cancers [1]. In this chapter, we plan to discuss microtubule targeting and the list of microtubule targeting agents that have been reported so far (Table 1).

The hallmark characteristic attributed to cancer cells is their fast growth rate and their ability to proliferate indefinitely when compared to normal cells. To that, regulation of many key proteins involved in survival pathways and cell-cycle regulation are modified in cancer cells. In addition, apoptosis is suppressed in many of cancer cells through various pathways, and this adds to greater ability of cancer cells to survive [3]. Robust proliferative responses in normal cells, are actually sustained in cancer cells. The deregulation of Cyclin-Dependent Kinases (CDKs) that enable cell cycle progression [4] and the abnormal expression of Myc, a strategic controller of cell proliferation, are few prominent examples [5]. It is well known that occurrence of mutation is higher in cancer cells compared to normal cells. From carcinogen exposure to clinical detection, cancer cells require to grow, divide, invade and metastases. During this period, multiple mutations in genetic stability-genes are required that initiates cascade of other mutations in other genes. Many of those second group of genes are controller of key pathways [6]. In 2013, 140 genes were reported that if are altered by mutations, can "drive" to tumorigenesis. A typical cancer cell has two to eight of these driver genes mutations. Other mutations in these cells are "passenger" mutations that do not cause any specific proliferation advantages. Overall mutations cause cell-autonomous alterations which leads to different consequences such as dividing fast and going through different cell-cycle phases faster than normal cells. "Dividing rapidly" lowers balance between supply and consumption of nutrients and oxygen. Therefore, cancer cells acquire second set of mutations to provide an appropriate condition that endures nutrient and oxygen deficiency, like mutation in EGFR (Epidermal growth factor receptor), HER2 (Human epidermal growth factor receptor 2), RAS, RAF (rapidly accelerated fibrosarcoma), PTEN (Phosphatase and tensin homolog). Many of these new set of mutations cause abnormal vascularization with well-ordered net-

Table 1 Microtubule Targeting Agents (MTAs), and their mechanisms of action

Compound	Cancer type	Mechanisms of action	Reference
Paclitaxel (taxol)	Ovarian, breast, lung and pancreatic cancers	Natural stabilizer, stabilizes microtubule polymer, avoids microtubule disassembly Causes G2-M arrest Causes apoptosis	[202]
Docetaxel (taxotere)	Breast, head and neck, gastric, hormone-refractory prostate cancer and non-small-cell lung cancers	Natural stabilizer, stabilizes microtubule assembly, avoids microtubule disassembly in the absence of GTP Causes G2-M arrest	[36]
Epothilone	Breast, ovarian, prostate, lung, glioblastoma cancers and paclitaxel-resistant tumors	Natural stabilizer, stabilizes microtubule assembly, induce tubulin polymerization without the presence of GTP Causes G2-M arrest Causes apoptosis	[203, 204]
Peloruside A	Breast, ovarian, lung, head and neck cancers	Natural stabilizer Causes G2-M phase arrest Causes apoptosis Has synergistic effect with paclitaxel	[205]
Laulimalide	Cancer types that are resistant to paclitaxel and epothilones	Natural stabilizer Has synergistic effect with paclitaxel and epothilones	[47]
Taccalonolide	Cancer types that are resistant to paclitaxel and doxorubicin	Natural stabilizer Bind to β-tubulin covalently Causes microtubule bundles in interphase Causes mitotic arrest Causes apoptosis Has efficacy in cell with mutated paclitaxel-binding site Has efficacy in cells resistant to doxorubicin Escapes from P-gp and mutant β-tubulin-induced resistance	[51, 52]
Cyclostreptin	Cancer types that are resistant to paclitaxel	Natural stabilizer Induce and stabilizes microtubule polymerization by binding covalently 40-fold less toxic than paclitaxel Escapes from P-gp and mutant β-tubulin-induced resistance	[56]
Discodermolide	Ovarian cancer, Cancer types that are resistant to paclitaxel	Natural stabilizer Has efficacy in cell with mutated paclitaxel-binding site Escapes from P-gp and mutant β-tubulin-induced resistance Has synergistic effect with paclitaxel	[60, 206]

(continued)

Table 1 (continued)

Compound	Cancer type	Mechanisms of action	Reference
Dictyostatin	Cancer types that are resistant to paclitaxel	Natural stabilizer Stabilizes microtubule polymer by preventing depolymerisation Causes G2-M phase arrest Has efficacy in cell with mutated paclitaxel-binding site Escapes from P-gp -induced resistance Effective against MDR cancer cells	[62, 207]
Eleutheside		Natural stabilizer Inhibits microtubule dynamics Causes G2-M phase arrest	[79]
Discodermolide analogues		Synthetized stabilizer Causes G2-M phase arrest Has efficacy in paclitaxel-resistant cells and their own parental drug (discodermolide)	[59]
Discodermolide-dictyostatin hybrid	Breast, ovarian cancers	Synthetized stabilizer	[63]
Ixabepilone	Breast cancer	Synthetized stabilizer Inhibits microtubule dynamic instability Effective against MDR cancer cells Has synergistic effect with capecitabine	[45, 68]
Vinca alkaloid	Breast, head and neck cancer and Leukemia, lymphomas	Natural destabilizer Depolymerizes microtubule polymers Disrupt mitotic spindle at high dosage Blocks mitosis low clinically relevant dosage without depolymerizing mitotic spindle Causes apoptosis	[72, 204]
Estramustine	Prostate cancer	Natural destabilizer Inhibits microtubule dynamics Causes G2-M phase arrest	[79]
Dolastatin		Natural destabilizer Causes mitotic arrest Inhibit microtubule polymerization and dynamics Causes formation of non-microtubule structure assemblies of tubulin Causes multi-polarity Supressed naturally decay of tubulin	[80, 84]
Colchicine	Nonneoplastic diseases	Natural destabilizer Delays microtubule growth at low dosage and suppresses microtubule dynamic Depolymerizes microtubule at high dosage	[87, 204]

(continued)

Table 1 (continued)

Compound	Cancer type	Mechanisms of action	Reference
Nocodazole	Compound terminated from clinical trial Compound is used as a lead agent for design and discovery of analogues and also is used as a reference compound in cancer studies	Natural destabilizer Interferes with microtubules polymerization	[88]
Cryptophysin	Breast and lung cancer cell-lines	Natural destabilizer Suppress tubulin polymerization Effective against MDR cancer cells	[89, 208]
Halichondrin B	Breast cancer	Natural destabilizer Inhibits microtubule polymerization Inhibits tubulin-dependent GTP hydrolysis	[90]
Combretastatin	Lung and thyroid cancer	Natural destabilizer Potential VDR	[45, 204]
Hemiasterlin	Colon cancer, lung cancer and melanoma	Natural destabilizer Inhibits depolymerisation of existing microtubules Inhibits new microtubule assembly Effective against MDR cancer cells	[12, 94]
Podophyllotoxin	Lung, lymphomas and genital tumors	Natural destabilizer Inhibit microtubule polymerization Inhibit mitotic spindle assembly	[97, 209]
Curacin A	Renal, colon and breast cancer	Natural destabilizer	[88, 210]
2-Methoxyestradiol	Prostate cancer, myeloma and glioblastoma	Natural destabilizer Inhibit microtubule polymerization Suppresses tumor vascularization	[45, 88]
ENMD-1198		Synthetized destabilizer Stable analogues of 2-ME with improved properties	[88]
Eribulin (E7389)	Breast, prostate, head and neck, non-small cell lung cancer, pancreatic	Synthetized destabilizer Suppresses microtubule polymerization and dynamic instability, arrests mitosis Causes apoptosis Suppresses centromere dynamics at dosage that arrest mitosis	[14]
SMART	Prostate and melanoma cancer	Synthetized destabilizer Suppress microtubule polymerization Causes G2-M phase arrest Causes apoptosis Effective against MDR cancer cells	[99, 211]

(continued)

MCAK (Centromere-associated kinesin), EB1(End-binding protein 1) and FHIT (Fragile histidine triad protein).The importance of MAPs is their association with microtubules in formation of mitotic spindle apparatus which is the key requirement for rapidly dividing cells. The necessity of microtubule during mitosis is by means of separating the duplicate chromosomes of mother cell into two daughter cells and finally cell division. This virtue of microtubules took a lot of attention in cancer therapy as a target. Microtubules have known to be a target of many naturally occurring toxic yet self-protective molecules, extracted from microorganisms, sea flora and plants [7].

Microtubule Dynamic as a Target for Cancer Therapy

Microtubules are made of cellular components α- and β-tubulin heterodimers by polymerizing head to tail orientation of protofilaments. Protofilaments are around 12–13 in numbers that binds together and form microtubule, a dynamic structure that are principal member of mitosis, meiosis, cell movement, maintenance of cell structure and intracellular organelles movements. Hence they have become a target in cancer therapy [8]. The way of protofilament arrangement conveys the microtubule polarity. The α-tubulins are placed in the minus end while β-tubulins are placed in plus end. In the microtubule plus end, several proteins accumulate that are known as the microtubule plus end tracking proteins [9]. This group of proteins and their function will be elaborated further in this chapter. In mitosis, the microtubule-organizing center (MTOC or centrosome) binds to minus end of microtubules and cause microtubules accumulation. From there microtubule grows toward outside of MTOC [10]. γ-Tubulin in combination with other proteins forms γ-tubulin ring complex (γ-TuRC). γ-TuRC is the α- and β-tubulin scaffold before polymerization begins in MTOC. γ-Tubulin also protects the minus end from polymerization and/or depolymerization. GTP binds to β-tubulin and its hydrolyzation is necessary for further assembly. GTP-tubulin is stable while GDP-tubulin after losing a phosphate, is susceptible to depolymerization.

An important characteristic of microtubule is the dynamic instability which is considered as nature of microtubule to switch rapidly between growth and shrinkage. Microtubule dynamicity is highly regulated via different post-translational modifications and by some MAPs that bind to tubulin dimers or at poles of microtubules. This dynamicity provides cell living-needs such as cell movement, migration and division. Prior to mitosis, the whole structure of microtubule rearranges from the interphase microtubule architecture to specialized rapidly dynamic mitotic spindle assembly. These specialized microtubule spindles direct sister chromatids toward either poles of the cell. This responsibility ultimately ensures each new daughter cell receive correct and complete genetic content [11].

In the beginning of mitosis, at prophase, microtubule grows out from the centrosome, and in case the microtubule plus end meets the chromosome, it becomes stabilized, and otherwise disassembly is initiated. These disassembled free tubulins would be available for other microtubule growths. However these events are not happening just by interaction between microtubule and chromosomes. There are different ways to achieve functional diversity of microtubule: (i) through the expression of various tubulin isotypes which each having different functions, (ii) through post-translational modifications on tubulin and (iii) through binding of numerous regulatory proteins such as MAPs. These proteins interact with soluble tubulin and/or microtubule's surface and ends. Human tubulin isotypes include 7 forms of β-tubulin and 6 forms of α-tubulin. Their expression varies in different cell types. The post-translational modification of tubulin includes polyglutamylation, polyglycylation, acetylation, phosphorylation, tyrosination/detyrosination and removal of some residues such as the penultimate glutamic-acid from α-tubulin. Among MAPs, the motor proteins such as kinesin and dynein. Microtubule regulatory proteins include stathmin, survivin, MCAK, TOG, EB1, MAP4, dynactin 1, PAC1. Some of these proteins are associated with resistance of the cell to certain drugs [7]. Many proteins are involved in the microtubule dynamics. Stathmin is an endogenous depolimerizer/destabilizer that attaches to free tubulin dimers and avoids their bindings, therefore inhibits formation of protofilaments and microtubules. In contrary, some other proteins attach to polymerized microtubule and protect their stability or decreasing the duration and speed of depolymerization. The activity of these native stabilizers and destabilizers are regulated (phosphorylated/dephosphorylated) by cell cycle-dependent kinases.

Mutations in α- and β-tubulins affects the microtubule polymer mass and more or less effect on drug binding sites. As expected, this matter is contributing in resistance to MTAs which will be discussed broadly in this chapter. On the other hand, abnormal expression of some of β-tubulin isotypes, such as βIII-tubulin, or aberrant expressions of MAPs are also reported to be associated to resistance to MTAs. Cells survive optimally within a certain range of tubulin polymerization, about 22–58% of intracellular tubulin. Cells with lower levels of polymerized tubulin are resistant to tubulin-stabilizers such as epothilones and taxanes, but at the same time they are more sensitive to microtubule-destabilizers such as vinca alkaloids. Opposed to that, cells with increased levels of microtubules, are more resistant to microtubule-destabilizers but more sensitive to microtubule-stabilizers [12, 13].

Microtubules are playing a critical role in the mitosis. In the process of mitosis, duplicated chromosomes of mother cells are divided into two identical chromosomes before division of the cell into daughter cells. Since, cancer cells divide rapidly compared to the normal cells, therefore this made microtubule a noticeable target in anticancer researches. Various MTAs through different binding sites bind to tubulin and target microtubule structure which more or less affects microtubule dynamics. Microtubule has two types of dynamic behaviors. First type is called as "dynamic instability" which is a process wherein each microtubule ends switch between two phases of growing and shrinkage (shortening). The two ends of microtubule are not equivalent. Growing and/or shortening of plus end are much faster than minus end. Dynamic instability is characterized by four key factors: by the rate of microtubule growth; by the rate of microtubule shrinkage; the frequency of transition from the growth to shrinkage which this transition is called "catastrophe"; and

subsequently causes high affinity of phospho-survivin for caspases and therefore inhibits caspase-dependent apoptosis [21, 22].

To know MTAs we listed out some of the natural/synthetic stabilizers and destabilizers below in detail.

Natural Stabilizers

Taxanes

Taxanes include paclitaxel and its semi-synthetized analogue docetaxel were the most significant additions to the chemotherapeutic industry in late twentieth century especially in the treatment of breast cancer [23]. Monroe Wall in 1967 extracted a compound from the bark of yew tree (*Taxusbrevifolia*) and named it "Taxol" which is known as Paclitaxel. Wall and his colleagues began the journey of introducing microtubule stabilizers to cancer therapy. In 1979, Peter Schiff and Susan Horwitz discovered that paclitaxel induces microtubule polymerization. By that time the development of this drug was limited due to limited storage of natural compound. Until drug discovery and developments outgrowed to introduce semi-synthetized analogues of paclitaxel. Paclitaxel discovery and development as the first known stabilizer have taken almost 30 years [24]. It was reported that HeLa cells treated with paclitaxel is blocked in metaphase but unlike vinca alkaloid- and colchicine-induced metaphase blockage, microtubules mass are not disrupted and destabilized into tubulin dimers, but microtubule polymers are organized. Nowadays, we know this reorganization of microtubule as "microtubule stabilization". They suggested paclitaxel induces microtubule assembly and stabilizes the formation of those microtubules that already been assembled before applying the drug. The confirmation of this idea was through preparation of cold- and Ca^{+2}-induced depolymerization condition without applying MAPs and GTP. Then paclitaxel was applied and the result was increase of microtubule assembly by increase of tubulin polymerization and continues elongation of already polymerized microtubules [25]. Taxanes bind weakly to soluble tubulin but binds tightly to tubulins that are embedded along the length of microtubule. Taxane-binding site is on β-subunit located in inner side of microtubule lumen. The exact binding site of this drug was found by electron crystallography of tubulin bound to paclitaxel [26]. It is suggested that the way paclitaxel accesses its binding site inside the microtubule lumen is by diffusion mechanism or by fluctuations of the microtubule lattice. The exact mechanism of action is after binding to its binding site, paclitaxel changes the conformation of tubulin by an unknown mechanism which increases tubulin's affinity for neighbor tubulins therefore stabilizes the microtubule and causes increase of polymerization [27]. Exact binding site of paclitaxel is on β-tubulin [28]. Development of various photoactive group conjugated-paclitaxel analogues, revealed more details of paclitaxel binding site on β-tubulin until eventually by electron crystallography they determined the exact binding site [29]. Each tubulin has one paclitaxel binding site. Paclitaxel at high dosage (>10 nM) stabilizes microtubule dynamics with few paclitaxel molecules without increasing microtubule polymerization. In this scenario, just one paclitaxel molecule is required to bound to microtubule per hundreds of tubulin molecules and this paclitaxel molecule can reduce extend and rate of microtubule shrinkage around 50% [30]. Paclitaxel was approved for clinical use by 1995, and nowadays it is used to treat ovarian, breast, non-small-cell lung cancers and kaposi's sarcoma. The side effects of paclitaxel are neurotoxicity and myelosuppression [31].

Another interesting fact about paclitaxel's efficacy is paclitaxel-induced reduction of protofilaments that form the microtubule from 13 to 12 [32]. However exposure of microtubule to high dosage of paclitaxel, increases microtubule polymer mass but researches showed at the dosage of below 10 nM, there is no significant effect on microtubule polymerization and stabilization [30, 33]. There are other class of stabilizers such as epothilones, sarcodictyins, discodermolide and eleutherobin that compete with paclitaxel to bind to taxane-binding site or nearby [34]. Another advantage of stabilizers in regard of avoid cancer cell proliferation is causing multipolar spindle assembly formation [35].

Docetaxel (Taxotere)

Docetaxel was discovered after paclitaxel. Docetaxel is actually semi-synthesis from 10-deacetyl baccatin III which is an inactive taxoid precursor isolated from needles of European yew *Taxusbaccata*. Docetaxel promotes tubulin assembly in microtubule polymer and suppresses their depolymerization [36]. This discovery prompted scientists to discover more stabilizers. Years of research resulted in approaching several other natural stabilizers which were not related to taxanes [37].

Epothilones

The Epothilones are natural macrolides, considered as non-taxane microtubule stabilizers including epothilone A and epothilone B. This family of stabilizers are secondary metabolites isolated from myxobacterium *Sorangiumcellulpsum* in the 1990s [38]. The myxobacterial source of epothilones causes easy culture and isolation of this compound. Epothilones are classified into two groups, epoxides and olefins based on the absence or presence of epoxide group in their C-12 to C-13 position on macrolide. Examples include epoxides such as epothilones A, B, E and F and olefins such as epothilones C and D [39]. Epothiones may target taxanes binding site or a region near that because studies showed, epothilone competes with paclitaxel in binding to tubulin. Epotilone causes tubulin polymerization, induces microtubule elongation and stabilizes microtubule polymer [40]. Two main advantages of epothilones are: unlike paclitaxel it can overcome resistance caused by P-gp, therefore compared to taxanes, epothilones are improved MTA. Another advantage of epothilone is chemically offers a unique chemotype that makes it available for fermentation-based semi-synthetic approach to synthesiszing its analogues [41]. Currently several members of epothilone family are under clinical trials, such as patupilone a natural epothilone B (EPO906), a second generation epothilone B (BMS-310705), a third generation epothilone B (ZK-EPO), an epothilone D (KOS-862) and a second generation epothilone D (KOS-1584) [42].

Peloruside A

Peloruside A is a macrolide MTA that was isolated from a New Zealand marine sponge called *Mycale hentscheli* by West and Northcote. Peloruside A shows microtubule stabilizing activity and mitotic blockage at dosage of 10 nM and it has shown a synergistic effect with paclitaxel, even though its binding site is not taxane-binding site. Peloruside is a rare natural product and contains an intriguing structural feature, therefore became attractive for synthetic studies [43].

Laulimalides

Laulimalides are extracted from marine sponge *Cacospongiamycofijiensis* [44] and this compound also displays microtubule stabilizing activity, binding to microtubule in a non-texane site [45]. The compound actually binds to α-tubulin [46]. This compound is reported to exhibit a synergistic stabilizing activity in combination with paclitaxel or epothilones [47]. These properties make laulimalides considered for next generation of stabilizers in combination therapy. But the mechanistic action of this compound and how they have synergism with taxane-site binding drugs is not completely understood.

Prota et al. [48] have showed laulimalides and peloruside A stabilize β-tubulin M-loop without forming any secondary structure plus causing formation of a bridging between two tubulin dimers across protofilaments in structure of microtubule. Also in same study they reported that there is an allosteric crosstalk activity between laulimalide/peloruside and taxane-binding site in either assembled or unassembled tubulins [48]. Ligand that binds to laulimalide/peloruside-binding site, stabilizes the conformation of the taxane site, including the M-loop [49]. On the contrary, ligands which binding to taxane-binding site, stabilize the elements that form laulimalide/peloruside-binding site in microtubule [49]. This study is the first study that showed the structural framework for this crosstalk and therefore they proposed the synergistic effect of laulimalide/pelorusideand taxane-binding site ligands on tubulin [48].

Taccalonolide

Taccalonolides are isolated from roots and rhizomes of *Taccachantrieri* species. They are another class of microtubule stabilizers that do not bind to taxane-binding site. The uniqueness of taccalonolides is that they do not bind directly to tubulin or microtubule and also do not induce polymerization of purified tubulin. They are able to bind to β-tubulin covalently and this is how they contribute considerable efficacy at low concentrations [50]. Taccalonolide causes bundling of microtubules in interphase. There is a group of this compound include at least 25 members. Among them taccalonolide A and E are the most rare naturally occurring secondary metabolite. The greatly acetylated pentacyclic skeleton in taccalonolides structure makes them distinct from other stabilizers. Taccalonolides A and E specifically cause bundling of microtubules in interphase and mitotic arrest of cancer cells which includes multiple aberrant spindles that is able to initiate apoptosis in same manner as paclitaxel. However, taccalonolides keep their efficacy in cells that are mutated in paclitaxel-binding site [51] as well as those cells that overexpress P-gp [52], or cells that show resistance due to expression of βIII-isotype of tubulin. Taccalonolides A and E showed excellent efficacy in paclitaxel and doxorubicin resistant mammary tumor model in vivo [53].

Cyclostreptin

Cyclostreptin is a bacterial product that was reported to have a weak paclitaxel-like activity on tubulin and exhibited anticancer activity in vivo [54]. Cyclostreptin is noteworthy for its characteristic feature of not being a taxane-binding compound but displaces taxane-binding ligands from their binding sites. Cyclostreptin poorly induces microtubule polymerization [55]. Buey et al. [56] reported that cyclostreptin binds to microtubule covalently. Mass spectrometry (MS) results showed cyclostreptin covalently binds to microtubule with either Thr^{220} or Asn^{228}. With the preference for Thr^{220} in case of binding to the free tubulin dimer. This was the first MTA agent that has been shown to bind to microtubule in such particular way. This covalent type of binding explains unusual properties of cyclostreptin including requirement for higher temperature for polymerization induction. Cyclostreptin binds to microtubules irreversibly and is thought to be much more stable in complex compared to unbound microtubules and even more stable than paclitaxel-induced microtubule. Cyclostreptin's activity retains in paclitaxel-resistant cancer cells. The cells that overexpression of P-gp or the expression of mutant β-tubulin is thought to be responsible for resistance to paclitaxel. It was suggested the covalent binding of cyclostreptin to microtubules could be one of the reasons for overcoming resistance as observed with paclitaxel. It is interesting that cyclostreptin is 40-fold less toxic than paclitaxel [56]. However, we must consider the fact that drugs that react covalently with any specific target, could be extremely toxic for humans [57].

Discodermolide

Discodermolide, is a polyketide natural product extracted from Caribbean marine sponge *Discodermia dissolute*, that was initially reported to be an immunosuppressive and an antifungal agent [58]. Later discodermolide was reported to be a potential microtubule stabilizer. Recent studies reported this stabilizer or its analogues may have advantages compared to other class of microtubule stabilizers [59]. Discodermolide has demonstrated its potent effects against those cancer cells that express P-gp and the cells that exhibit resistance to taxanes via incorporating mutated tubulins. Discodermolide also has been shown to have a synergistic effect with paclitaxel [60].

Dictyostatin

Macrolactone (-)-dictyostatin first was isolated from a Maldives marine sponge *Sponqia sp.*[61]. Dictyostatin stabilizes microtubule polymer by preventing depolymerization of tubulin dimers in the same way as discodermolide does. Dictyostatin provcd to be effective against multidrug-resistant (MDR) cancer cells. In spite of this interesting result, further study of dictyostatin was not undertaken due to rarity of this natural agent and its unknown structure. Eventually, researchers elucidated its structure to be related to discodermolide [62]. In 2002, Shin and his colleagues reported the synthesis of first discodermolide-dictyostatin hybrid [63].

Eleutheside

Sarcodictyin and eleutherobin are two members of diterpene glycosides that belong to eleutheside family. They are natural microtubule stabilizers with the activity profiles different from paclitaxel [64]. Sarcodictyin was first extracted from Mediterranean stolonifer *Sarcodictyonroseum.* Later, it was isolated from the South African soft coral *Eleutherobiaaurea* along with isolation of two glycosidated congeners, eleuthosides A and B. Sarcodictyin was reported to stabilize microtubule and compete with paclitaxel in binding to taxane-binding sites [65]. Sarcodictyin and eleutherobin are active against paclitaxel-resistant human cancer cells therefore are classified as second generation of natural microtubule stabilizers. Eleuthesides are marine products therefore their isolation is difficult and obtained compound is in a very limited quantities. Therefore, once again, the synthesis of these natural products analogues are required for further studies [66].

Synthetized Stabilizers

Discodermolide Analogues

Minguez et al. [59] produced analogues of discodermolide in simplest synthetic steps wherein they described it as simplified discodermolide analogues. By that time synthesize of analogues have not been reported in simpler production steps (30 or more steps starting from commercial material to the final product). All of the analogues kept the C8-C14 core of discodermolide because three stereocenters and two alkenes of this core form a characteristic shape for the molecule. These analogues have been tested beside discodermolide and paclitaxel for their cytotoxic effects. The result showed even drastic structural simplification has microtubule targeting activity. Six novel derivatives of discodermolide were produced. Here we mention the cytotoxic activity of few of these analogues.

Analogue 1 was tested on microtubule assembly assay in isolated bovine brain tubulin and the results showed that this agent caused very low tubulin nucleation in vitro. Moreover, this agent caused displacement of (3H) paclitaxel bound to microtubules. High content multi-parameter fluorescent cell profile displayed disruption of microtubule assembly by this discodermolide analogue and blocked the cell in G2-M cell cycle phase. Analogue 6 showed targeted multiple cellular survival patterns in cells that are resistance to paclitaxel and its own parental agent, discodermolide [59].

Discodermolide-Dictyostatin Hybrid

Shin et al. [63] reported the first series of discodermolide-dictyostatin hybrid agents by inverting the absolute configuration of dictyostatin, therefore this way it resembles discodermolide. Some of these new hybrids showed 50% anti-proliferation activity against human breast cancer cell-line MDA-MB-231 and human ovarian cancer cell-line 2008 at 1 μM. Further study showed this hybrid displaced (3H) paclitaxel bound in microtubules [63].

Ixabepilone

The Ixabepilone (aza-epothilone B, BMS-247550, trade name: Ixempra®) is a microtubule stabilizer and it is semi-synthetized analogue of epothilone B by exchange of an azide group with oxygen at position 16 on the macrolide ring. Ixabepilone is one of latest epothilones being approved by FDA for clinical treatment in 2007. Ixabepilone binds to taxane-binding site but its interaction with tubulin is different than that by paclitaxel. Once it binds to β-tubulin subunit, it suppresses the dynamic instability of microtubules.

Ixabepilone exhibited activity against cells that show multiple drug-resistance such as that induced by P-gp [67]. A phase III randomized study compared ixabepilone plus capecitabine v against capecitabine alone in advanced or metastatic breast cancer patients who showed resistant to taxanes and anthracyclins. Ixabepilone in combination with capecitabine resulted in a 25% reduction in the disease progression compared with capecitabine alone [68]. It is also recommended for treatment in the cancers of bladder, colon, pancreatic, breast, kidney etc. It is noteworthy to mention that Ixabepilone side effects are low and manageable [67].

Natural Destabilizers

Vinca Alkaloids

The Vinca alkaloids are successful MTAs from their introduction to clinical trials. Vinblastine and vincristine are two well-known members of vinca alkaloid family. They are extracted from leaves of the periwinkle plant *Catharanthusroseus* (L) G. Don. Periwinkle plant leaves were used for their traditional medicinal properties from the seventieth century. But in late 1950s, their anti-mitotic property was discovered by Eli Lily Research Laboratories and at the University of Western Ontario [69, 70]. Initially, vinca alkaloids were used for treatment of haematological malignancies. They were called "wonder drugs" for their successful outcome, and their efficacy in several combination therapies was also remarkable. The success of vinca alkaloids persuaded development of numerous semi-synthetic analogues such as vinflunine, vindesine and vinorelbine. Myelosuppression and peripheral neuropathy are the major side effects of vinca alkaloids [71]. Especially, myelosuppression occurs due to the mitotic blockage of rapidly dividing bone-marrow cells. Vinca alkaloids depolymerize microtubule polymers and disrupt mitotic spindle at high dosage (10–100 nM in HeLa cell-line) [72]. But at low clinically relevant dosage (0.8 nM in HeLa cell-line), vinblastine blocks mitosis without depolymerizing microtubules involved in spindle assembly and cells finally die by apoptosis [72]. This mitotic blockage happens due to inhibition of microtubule dynamics rather than depolymerization. Vinblastine is a dimeric alkaloid extracted from the genus Vinca [73]. In 2005, the exact mechanisms by which vinblastine exerts its action structurally have been characterized. Its major effect is the ability to induce formation of spiral-like tubulin accumulation by interacting with both α-tubulin and β-tubulin. This type of contacts would form and stabilize a curved proto-filament. Vinblastine also induces accumulation of ternary complex of two tubulin dimers which are helical assemblies of complexes in which vinblastine act like a bridge between them. This bridge is formed by the interaction of vinblastine with α-tubulin of the first dimer and β-tubulin of the second dimer. Electron micrographs revealed long proto-filament curls upon vinblastine treatment. These curls are shorter and more flexible than those formed under colchicine treatment under the same condition. Vinblastine at its low dosage suppresses microtubules plus (+) end's dynamic instability. Therefore, cells that are under clinically relevant dosage of vinblastine, encounter mitotic blockage. But by increasing its dosage, vinblastine depolymerizes the microtubule by increasing the proto-filaments spiral-like structures and curls. Gigant et al. [74] was the first study that introduced curvature into tubulin and tubulin assemblies. Compared to colchicne, another natural destabilizer, vinblastine binds in different binding sites. Vinblastine acts at the inter-dimer interface of tubulin while colchicine acts at the intra-dimer interface of tubulin. Compare to other MTAs such as paclitaxel and colchicine, vinca-binding site is equally shared between two tubulin dimers [74]. Variety of other drugs such as vincristine, vinorelbine, viinfluine, cryptophysin 52, halichondrins, doolastatins and hemiasterline also bind at vinca-binding site [7]. Vinblastine binds to soluble tubulin rapidly and it is reversible [75]. Binding of vinblastine to tubulin enhances a conformational change in connection with tubulin self-association [76], meaning vinblastine increases the affinity of tubulin for itself. In already polymerized microtubules, vinblastine binds to last tubulin at the far ends of microtubule with high affinity but it binds with very low affinity to those tubulins which are localized deep in the microtubule lattice [77]. One or two vinblastine molecules are enough for each microtubule to lose both dynamic instability and treadmilling without going through any microtubule depolymerization. To be more specific, vinblastine causes reduction of extent and rate of microtubule growth and shrinkage but causes increase of microtubule pause state with neither grow nor shrinkage. Reduction of dynamic instability and treadmilling causes mitotic blockage by reducing normal mitotic spindle assembly and reducing the tension at the kinetochore of chromosomes. Cells in this step are stuck in metaphase-like state, chromosomes are stuck at the spindle poles, unable to move to spindle equator. Also in this step the signal to anaphase-promoting complex/cyclosome (APC/C) is blocked therefore cell is unable to transit from metaphase to anaphase. These cells eventually will die through apoptosis [7]. One significant property of vincristine and vinblastine is they bind to tubulin in lower than 5 min, while colchicine binding takes over 4 h [78].

Estramustine

Estramustine is a nitrogen mustard derivative of estradiol-17β-phosphate that is currently used alone or in combination with other anticancer drugs for prostate cancer treatment. Estramustine inhibits the microtubule dynamics and arrests the cells in G_2-M phase. The Considerable side effects of estramustine exist and include the development of anaemia [79].

Dolastatin

Dolastatin is a natural peptide and it was originally found in Indian Ocean sea hare, *Dolabellaauricu-laria.* A variety of dolastatin analogues have been reported to disrupt microtubules and therefore induce mitotic arrest [80]. Some of dolastatin analogues

Hemiasterlins

Hemiasterlin was isolated from sponge *Hemiasterella minor* in Sodwana Bay, South Africa. It displays anticancer activity against human colon carcinoma, lung carcinoma and melanoma in vivo [94]. This compound inhibits depolymerization of existing microtubules and inhibits new microtubule assembly. Hemiasterlins are poor substrates for P-gp, therefore they are interesting candidates for cancer therapy and they are under clinical trials [12]. Hemiasterlin efficacy is banned by overexpressed P-gp mouse tumor xenograft models. But synthesis of several analogues of hemiasterlin, their in vitro and in vivo anticancer activities and their indifference reaction to P-gp-mediated drug efflux, could overcome the flaw [95].

Podophyllotoxin

Podophyllotoxinalso known as podofilox and it is a toxic lignin isolated from rhizomes and root of *Podophyllumpeltatum*. This agent compete with colchicine in colchicine-binding site and it binds to tubulin faster than colchicine [88]. Podophyllotoxin semi-synthetic derivatives teniposide, etoposide andetopophos (etoposide phosphate) are used for therapy of numerous malignant conditions [96]. Podophyllotoxin mechanism of action is through the inhibition of tubulin polymerization and inhibition of microtubule assembly in the mitotic spindle apparatus. However, its two derivatives, etoposide and teniposide were reported not to follow same mechanism of action as parent compound but their efficacy is through interaction with DNA and suppressing DNA topoisomerase II [97].

Curacin A

Curacin A is a lipid component isolated from a strain of the cyano bacterium *Lyngbyamajuscule*. Curacin A binds tightly and rapidly to colchicine-binding site on tubulin. It is not developed in clinical trials owing to its poor water-solubility and lack of stability, however development of its synthetic analogues with improved water-solubility and bioavailability may provide new hopes [88].

2-Methoxyestradiol (2-ME)

2-Methoxyestradiol is an endogenous estrogen metabolite, formed by hepatic cytochrome P450 2-hydroxylation of β-estradiol and 2-*O*-methylation. 2-ME targets tubulin polymerization by binding to colchicine-binding site and suppresses tumor vascularization in vivo. Its main side effects are nausea, fatigue, edema, diarrhea, neuropathy and dyspnea. Therefore, the development of metabolically stable analogues of 2-ME has started with the aim of improved properties. In this regard, ENMD-1198 was generated through the chemical modifications at 3 and 17 position of 2-ME [88].

Synthetized Destabilizers

Eribulin (E7389)

Eribulin is a synthetized analogue of halichondrin B already it is in phase III clinical trial for breast cancer treatment. At low dose, it binds to tubulin dimer and suppresses the polymerization of microtubule and microtubule dynamic instability in interphase, arrests mitosis and causes apoptosis. In one study they measured the effects of eribulin on centromere dynamics and the microtubules that attached to centromere and kinetochore by time-lapse confocal microscopy in U-2 OS human osteosarcoma cell-line. Eribulin suppressed centromere dynamics at dosage that arrest mitosis (60 nmol/L). The result showed that dynamicity decreased 35% without centromere separation. This indicated that eribulin decreased microtubule-dependent spindle tension at the kinetochores, preventing the signal for mitotic checkpoint passage [14]. A study in 2009, in order to understand the exact molecular interaction between halichondrin B and tubulin, investigated the binding of two halichondrin B analogues, eribulin and ER-076349 to tubulin by quantitative analytical ultracentrifugation. Under critical dosage of tubulin for microtubule assembly and in the presence of GDP, tubulin undergoes weak self-association into short curved oligomers. In the presence of eribulin, this oligomer formation is suppressed 4–6-fold, while ER-076349 slightly induces oligomer formation by 2-fold. This is exactly opposite of the vinblastine effect. Vinblastine strongly induces large spiral polymers around 1000-fold under same condition. Vinblastine-induced spiral formation is suppressed by both eribulin and ER-076349. Colchicine does not have any significant effect on small oligomer formation or does not undergo inhibitory effect of eribulin. These results suggest that halichondrin B analogues bind to the interdimer interface of tubulin or to the β-tubulin alone, disrupt polymer stability, and compete with vinblastine-induced spiral formation. Eribulin is a comprehensive inhibitor of tubulin polymer formation while ER-076349 also perturbs tubulin-tubulin contacts, but in more polymer formation. These results suggested that halichondrin B analogues show unique tubulin-based activities [98].

SMART

Among synthetized destabilizers, a class of 4-substituted methoxybenzoylaryl-thiazoles (SMART) including 3 compounds known as SMART-H (H), SMART-F (F) and SMART-OH (OH) were recently reported. These compounds are with varying substituents at the 4-position of aryl ring, showed their potency to colchicine-binding site on tubulin, which causes suppression of tubulin polymerization, arrest cancer cells in G_2-M phase and induce apoptosis. A remarkable characteristic of SMART compounds is that they can inhibit the growth of MDR overexpressing cells in vitro. This potency indicates that they can overcome MDR. SMART compounds suppressed the growth of 4 human prostate cancer cell-lines, and 2 melanoma cell-lines at a nanomolar range. In human prostate (PC-3) and melanoma (A375) cancer xenograft models, SMART-H and SMART-F treatments resulted in G_2-M arrest and induced apoptosis. Incubating SMART compounds with bovine brain tubulin (>97% pure) showed effect of SMART compounds on tubulin polymerization. SMART-H and SMART-F suppressed tubulin polymerization by 90%, SMART-OH inhibited the polymerization by only 55%. In vivo treatment of SMART-H for 21 days at the higher dosage (15 mg/kg) failed to produce any apparent neurotoxicity. In the same study under same experimental conditions, the IC_{50} for SMART-H (4.23 mmol/L) was close to colchicine's IC_{50} (4.91 mmol/L). Also by using novel MS competitive binding assay which corresponding to the 3 binding sites on tubulin, colchicine, vinca alkaloid and paclitaxel, they found out that SMART-H specifically competed for colchicine-binding site on tubulin, but it did not compete for either vinca alkaloid-or paclitaxel-binding sites. Among them, SMART-OH had the least potent anti-proliferative effects [99].

Methyl 2-(5-Fluoro-2-Hydroxyphenyl)-1H-Benzo (d) Imidazole-5-Carboxylate (MBIC)

A recent study in 2016, a benzimidazole-derivative, Methyl 2-(5-fluoro-2-hydroxyphenyl)-1H-benzo (d) imidazole-5-carboxylate known as MBIC was introduced as a potential MTA more specifically a tubulin destabilizer. Tubulin polymerization assay demonstrated MBIC disrupted tubulin nucleation and polymerization at similar dosage as nocodazole, colchicine and paclitaxel. The maximal velocity (Vmax) for MBIC was 2.45mOD/min which was more close to colchicine (Vmax: 2.25 mOD/min) rather than nocodazole (Vmax: 3 mOD/min), in contrast with paclitaxel (Vmax: 33 mOD/min) and untreated cells (Vmax: 12 mOD/min). This result indicated the resemblance of MBIC to colchicine. Also in this study, live-cell imaging result showed untreated HeLa cells formed bipolar spindle assembly but MBIC-treated cells did not form proper mitotic spindle and stayed in mitotic arrest for long time until cells undergo apoptosis. A remarkable characteristic of MBIC is the cytotoxic effect of this novel drug against HeLa cancer cell-lines is about 0.02 μM while its toxicity against normal cell WRL-68 is around 10.09 μM. Another considerable characteristics of MBIC is its synergistic effect with conventional drugs such as colchicine, nocodazole, doxorubicin and even paclitaxel (due to overall mutual interruption of microtubule dynamics) [100].

N-Acetylcolchinol O-Methyl Ether and Thiocolchicine

N-Acetylcolchinol O-Methyl Ether (NCME) and Thiocolchicine are two colchicine analogues with modification only in C ring that are reported to be a better destabilizer than colchicine. Radio-labelled thio colchicine (with a thiomethyl instead of a methoxy group at position C-10) and NCME (with amethoxy-substituted benzenoid instead of the methoxy-substituted tropone C ring) were produced to be compared with colchicine. The result showed that, NCME and thiocolchicine bind to tubulin much faster than colchicine even though there is differences between these two analogues and colchicine. The binding of thiocolchicine to tubulin is temperature-dependent but thiocolchicine has similar rate of binding to tubulin with colchicine so as a function of temperature, almost there are no differences in activation energy of thiocolchicine and colchicine binding reaction. In a contrary, NCME binds to tubulin at low temperatures and reaction is done at low tubulin and drug dosage. The binding rate of NCME to tubulin is 16 times faster than colchicine binding and it is constant from 10C to 37C. The high binding rate is constant therefore the reaction eventually increases relatively while temperature rises. On the other hand the activation energy is only 40% of colchicine activation energy [101].

ZD6126

ZD6126 is a synthetic form of a water-soluble phosphate prodrug *N*-acetylcolchinol. In vitro studies have shown appearance of pronounced and reversible changes in the morphology of endothelial cells that being treated with ZD6126 compared to those being treated with *N*-acetylcolchinol, at sub-cytotoxic dosage. None of ZD6126 nor *N*-acetylcolchinol have induced changes in growth of human umbilical vein endothelial cells at dosages below 100 μM. But, changes in endothelial cell morphology were detectable at 0.1 μM of ZD6126. In vivo studies using a murine tumor model (CaNT) with dosage below the maximum tolerated dosage have showed a significant reduction in vascularization volume and induction of extreme necrosis in the tumor. Another in vivo study in the human xenograft FaDu, paclitaxel stabilizing activity was enhanced by adding a single dose of ZD6126 in the combination. This overall pronounced growth delay given by paclitaxel and ZD6126 combination was much higher than the effect of each individual drug alone. These finding offers ZD6126 as a promising anti-vascular agent for the treatment of solid tumors.

E7974

E7974 is a synthetic analogue of hemiasterlin and the benefit of E7974 over hemiasterlin is exhibition of same efficacy against numerous human cancer cell-lines at nanomolar dosage. A significant in vivo anticancer activity of E7974 in numerous human tumor

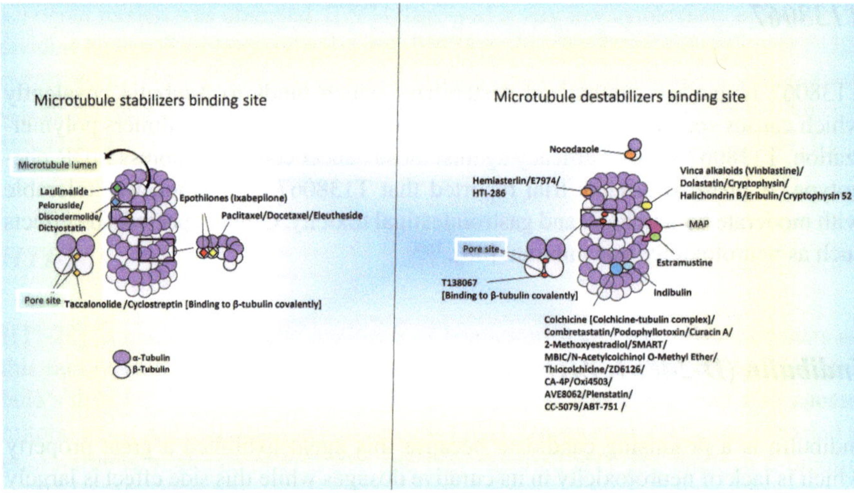

Fig. 2 Microtubule stabilizers and destabilizers binding sites in microtubule

End-Binding Proteins; MTAs Assistants

Despite the fact, MTAs are widely used, still researches continue to find more effective and less toxic agents to substitute and/or combine with conventional MTAs. Some MTAs at low concentrations interact with microtubule ends [7]. As we explained earlier in this chapter, the plus (+) end of growing microtubule has a stabilizing GTP-bound tubulin cap which if is lost, microtubule depolymerizes (catastrophe). In fact catastrophe depends on microtubule age and happens after several steps [109]. There are several endogenous microtubule destabilizing proteins that increase the speed of microtubule ageing or decrease the number of steps leading to catastrophe [110]. At plus end of microtubule a group of proteins known as microtubule plus end-tracking proteins (+TIPs) are accumulated which regulate dynamics and function of microtubule [111]. +TIP includes end-binding proteins (EB) in the core of +TIP. EB proteins recognize a stabilizing cap at microtubule growing end [112]. EBs affect microtubule dynamics therefore it has been suggested that EBs might affect MTAs efficacies. Maurer et al. [113] reported that EBs effecting the interfilaments contacts and/or alter the rate of GTP hydrolysis in the microtubule stabilizing cap [113]. In 2013, a group of researchers investigated the EB proteins effect on various types of MTAs and its function on microtubule dynamics. They found out in the absence of EBs, destabilizer agents suppress elongation of microtubules by delaying the polymerization. In contrast, in the presence of EBs, the elongation was inhibited due to highly increased rate of catastrophe at a dosage of destabilizer which is insufficient to effect the microtubule growth. On the other hand, in the EBs supporting stabilizer side, to inhibit the catastrophe stabilizer agents do not require any EBs' existence but they mildly increase the catastrophe rate when EBs are added. Regardless MTAs mechanism of action and their binding site, they increase the frequency of catastrophe if EBs are bound to microtubules. In the presence of EBs, stabilizers and destabilizers could be applied in lower dosage, yet exhibit the promoted catastrophe [9]. Analyzing microtubule growth times proved that destabilizer agents increased the frequency of catastrophe in a dose-dependent manner by increasing the occurrence rate, not by number of intermediate-catastrophe-promoting steps. This result suggests that these destabilizer agents do not alter the microtubule aging mechanism but in interaction with EBs, destabilizer agents accelerate microtubule aging progression. Moreover stabilizing agents increase rate of both catastrophe and rescue in EBs presence [9]. In the presence of EBs, both stabilizers and destabilizers induce the formation or increase of microtubule lattice defects for example by altering the protofilaments structure [114]. The EB proteins are extensive and ubiquitous in the cells, the MTAs and EBs synergism in induction of catastrophe has important consequences for the final MTAs effect in the treated cells. For example in the interphase, increased catastrophe causes decrease of effective microtubule penetration into lamellae or into actin-rich cortex of cell-cell junctions, which defect cell migration and adhesion (final defect on cancer cell metastasis) [115]. At mitosis, highly increased catastrophe effects the mitotic spindle organization, microtubule attachment to kinetochore and manipulation of spindle assembly checkpoint [116].

MTAs Extra Tasks in Interphase

Since mitotic kinases have fundamental roles in mitosis, they became noticeable as targets in anticancer studies. There was idea of developing MTAs that co-target mitotic kinases as well, to achieve greater result. However, until today, many non-tubulin targeting mitotic inhibitors exhibited unsuccessful results in clinical trials [117]. Since microtubules are always present in the cells, both in interphase and mitosis, but mitotic kinases are only present in M-phase of the cell cycle, therefore they can be suppressed by desired drug about 10% of the whole cell cycling [118]. On the other hand cancer cell-lines have flaw of overexpression of some certain proteins which may involve some of mitotic kinases. If a protein is overexpressed, the chance of being more effected by a certain potential drug is much more. Aurora kinases and polo-like kinases are part of mitosis regulatory system, at the same time they are overexpressed in numerous human cancer cell-lines. This fact validating them as anticancer drug target [119, 120]. The Aurora kinase and Polo-like kinase inhibitors have been developed and introduced; nonetheless they have shown infrequent clinical results with limited efficacies [118].

The main problem may be the fact that mitotic kinases are involved in different cellular pathways therefore, even if they totally are inhibited by a certain drug, their inhibition may remain only for a period of time. While an alternative pathway may carry out the rest of cell cycle regulation and tumor is likely to return. To explain it better at molecular base, drug that causes defect in one signal-transduction pathway, may up-regulate other signaling pathways that could lead to raise of resistance against same drug [121]. Therefore, worth to mention besides MTAs there is no other cellular structure that can compensate mitotic blockage and cell division interruption therefore, there is no back-up signaling pathway to retreat MTA induced-defects of cell division. Thus, safe to say that effects of MTAs are potential to cover both microtubules disruption and mitotic regulatory system alteration. The MTAs success does not stop here. Since there are microtubules in interphase, these groups of drugs are also alters interphase events. Paclitaxel has been reported to correlate with apoptotic events more than mitotic blockage [122]. Several studies reported MTAs alter mitotic signaling pathway by manipulating mitotic proteins in expression levels and/or in post-translational modification levels [123]. MTAs were believed for long time, to prolong spindle assembly checkpoint activation which resulted in incomplete mitosis [124].

MTAs even impair non-mitotic proteins. There are studies that reported paclitaxel effects on bcl-2 protein level and subsequently causes apoptosis [125]. Microtubule network provided an extreme delicate surface area for protein-protein contact and with polarity of microtubule it allows various proteins and organelles movement throughout the cell by the help of motor proteins such as dynein and kinesin. Moreover, microtubule is required for cell migration, cytokines secretions and vascularization.

MTAs neurotoxicity characteristics proved the efficacy of MTAs in interphase. Because neurons are not dividing rapidly unlike cancer cells, therefore they enter mitosis so rarely, but yet the effect of MTAs were detected [124]. The evidence of MTAs on cellular secretion came from studies that have been conducted on impairment of T-cells with disrupted microtubules. This disruption in T-cells effected on antigen presenting cells during immune response [126]. In addition, in interphase microtubules track transportation of numerous proteins and transcription factors such as p53, androgen receptor and hypoxia inducible factor-1 (HIF-1) [127–129]. Pathways that are controlled by microtubules in interphase are complex and poorly understood. Many studies reported the transportation of oncogenic proteins by interphase microtubules. This emphasizes the role of interphase microtubule in cancer cell survival, therefore efficacy of MTAs on interphase microtubules are undeniable. The tumor suppressor p53 is transported into nucleus by microtubules when DNA is damaged. Even low dosage of MTAs changes nuclear accumulation of p53 and consequently activates target genes that cause apoptosis [127]. Another example is the effect of taxane on interphase microtubule dynamics which prevents dynein-mediated nuclear accumulation of androgen receptor, therefore suppresses transcriptional activation of genes that are involved in prostate cancer [128].

MTAs target cancer cells vascularization and this is a remarkable approach given to cancer cells accessibility to blood, the source of oxygen and nutrients, while they typically go through lack of these vital materials due to their fast division. Hence, the development of blood vessels is crucial for cancer growth and metastasis. MTAs are reported to suppress endothelial cell angiogenic function including cell proliferation, migration and vascular tubes formation [130]. Disruption of cytoskeletal tubulin in vascular cells causes vascular permeability and stops blood supply for tumors [131]. The importance of MTAs effect against tumor vascularization is clearer when we understand blood vessels in tumors are much more than in normal tissues due to endothelial cells high proliferation and their elevated vascular permeability. To be more sensitive to MTAs is associated to increase of vascular permeability [131]. For instance, opaxio™ (paclitaxel bound to biodegradable polyglutamate polymer) has anticancer advantages for highly permeable (leaky) vessels. When paclitaxel is bound to this polymer, it is inactive, thus it does not affect normal tissues. Meanwhile tumor blood vessels are highly penetrable for macromolecules, allowing opaxio™ to pass through tumor tissues. When opaxio™ penetrated into tumor, it is cleaved by lysosomal enzymes, therefore it lets paclitaxel to stabilize the microtubules. Opaxio™ is currently in phase II of clinical trial of glioblastoma and in phase III of clinical trial for ovarian cancer [132].

It is well-known that cancer cells are potential to be metastatic and this requires newly formed blood vessels which are made by angiogenic proliferation and migration of endothelial cells. During cell migration, there is cell to cell connection and cell to extracellular matrix connection. These processes have been reported to be suppressed by MTAs [133]. For example effect of taxanes on HUVEC cells migration has been reported much more than effect of this drug on HUVEC mitosis [134]. Focal adhesion of cell is necessary for migration. Focal adhesion to be formed requires Rho GTPase activity which microtubule disruption can affect them negatively [130].

HIF-1α activates tumor angiogenesis therefore it causes cancer cell survival. HIF-1α is overexpressed in most of the solid tumors. MTAs inhibits HIF-1α activity by disrupting HIF-1α mRNA trafficking on altered microtubules [129]. Also in protein level, those HIF-1α proteins that already have been expressed and exist in the cells, are supposed to be transferred into nucleus via microtubule by the aid of dynein. Therefore, MTAs inhibit HIF-1α transcriptional activity as well [135]. Hence, MTAs are involved in anti-angiogenic activity. There are other evidences that prove "MTAs effect on interphase microtubules" are important as well as their effect on mitosis. For example renal cell carcinomas shows resistance to MTA in interphase and it might be due to this cell-lines microtubule-independent trafficking [45].

Compretatins are vascular disrupting agents (VDAs) that disrupt cytoskeletal tubulin. Several of this class of agents are in clinical trials now to serve as an anticancer drugs [131].

MTAs Against Actin and Intermediate Filaments

For successful spindle positioning and suppression of cytokinesis, tubulin and actin interaction is important. In addition, there are numerous non-mitotic functions that require microtubule and microfilaments interactions such as cell migration [136], or microtubule and actin interactions, such as wound healing [137]. MTAs have been reported to disrupt intermediate filaments and actin in addition to their effect on microtubules [138]. However, actin and microtubule interaction are needed for neuronal growth cones which are highly mobile [139], therefore, disruption of microtubule impairs axon path-finding [140].

MTAs Against Mitotic Kinases

It has been reported that there are variety of cell responses against anti-mitotic drugs even among cells from same cell-line [141]. To know this fact, preserve us to expect that each individual tumor may response differently to different MTAs. This understanding is helpful in the design and development of the future new MTAs. As mitosis has been identified further, mitotic mediators have being known and classified. Targeting these proteins in virtue of their significant responsibility in controlling, guarding and processing mitosis is a rational extension to successful attempts of targeting microtubules. For instance, Polo-like kinase 1 is part of centrosome maturation and construction of mitotic spindle apparatus. This protein is also required for pass the mitosis and for separation of sister chromatids [142]. Aurora family members are required for occurrence of multiple events in mitosis. Aurora A is required for spindle assembly, Aurora B is required to phosphorylate histone H3, chromosome segregation and cytokinesis [119]. Kinesin spindles are motor proteins which are required for the formation of spindle apparatus in the beginning of mitosis [143]. Focusing on these mediators and their roles broadened the efforts of targeting cancer cell division in other ways besides microtubule disruption.

Some of agents that target these proteins happened to have synergistic effects with MTAs. For instance, AZD1152 is an Aurora B inhibitor and synergically enhances the anti-proliferative activity of vincristine in human acute leukemia cells in vitro and in vivo [144].

As we mentioned earlier, BubR1 is a tension-sensing protein. If kinetochores and microtubules are not attached together correctly, the lack of sufficient tension causes BubR1 accumulation in kinetochore and causes mitotic arrest until all kinetochore-microtubule attachments are correct. A study was done in absence and presence of DL15 in two groups of cells and they were incubated for one cell cycle. Later cells were stained by anti-BubR1 antibody. The result showed DL15 promoted BubR1 accumulation, caused loss of tension all across the kinetochores and subsequently caused mitotic arrest [84].

MBIC a synthetic destabilizer class of MTAs is also reported to alter some of mitotic kinases such as Aurora-B, BubR1, Cyclin B1 and CDK1 in human cervical cancer cell-line (HeLa) which along with disruption of tubulin polymerization, caused mitotic arrest and finally apoptosis [100].

Resemblance Between Stabilizers and Destabilizers

MTAs are divided into two classes and characteristics of these agents as stabilizers and destabilizers refer to their efficacy when drugs dosages are high and tubulin concentration is high. Nevertheless the main resemblance between these two classes of drugs is that they suppress microtubule dynamic (grow and shrinkage) instability.

This resemblance is central in all MTAs [145]. That is why in some drug combination among combined stabilizer and destabilizer we can see great synergism. Each individual MTA may regulate different mechanism or mode of action but together in combination they increase the efficacy of treatment. For example the roots and rhizomes of *Tacca species* have a stabilizer compound named Taccalonolide and a destabilizer compound named Taccabulin A. These two compounds with their two opposite actions on microtubule polymerization, together they interfere with microtubule dynamics and overall effect is interrupting the proliferation of cancer cells. During mitosis separation of two sister chromatids are necessary and their separation requires mitotic spindles grow and shrink fast (3.6-fold more rapid than interphase). Therefore combination of stabilizer and destabilizer interferes with microtubule overall dynamics. This ability is considerable in cancer cells because of their rapid cell division compared to normal cells [146]. Moreover, in a recent study synergism between paclitaxel (stabilizer) and a newly introduced MTA, MBIC which acts as a destabilizer, was reported in treatment of cervical cancer cells in vitro [100].

Abnormal Genetic Expression and Genetic Mutations: Basic Crisis in Resistance to MTAs

α-Tubulin Mutation

There are two paclitaxel-resistant A549 cell-lines namely: A549-T12 and A549-T24. For normal growth these two cell-lines require low dose of paclitaxel [60]. In lack of paclitaxel, A549-T24 showed a most dramatic increase of microtubule dynamic and A549-T12 showed increase of dynamics in lesser degree both compared with their parental A549 cell-line. Therefore, these cell-lines are paclitaxel resistant/dependent [147]. The studies revealed that mutations on α-tubulin gene can modulate the sensitivity to agents that interact with β-tubulin. The mutation that was identified at Ser^{379} in A549-T12 cells corresponds to α-tubulin Ser 380 in the yeast which is located between resistant and sensitive loci in yeast genes [148]. Hence, mutation of α-tubulin in the yeast alters the binding site. In the α-tubulin gene region, mutation at α 379 in the paclitaxel-resistant cells is located between helix 10 (that contains stathmin gene [149]) and helix 11 (that is inside a domain containing MAPs genes). Therefore a mutation at α 379 cause changes in stathmin and MAPs genes leading to alter the microtubule stability and dynamics [150]. Curmi et al. [151] evaluated the expression levels of stathmin and MAP4 and they found stathmin is up-regulated in aggressive breast cancer patients [151]. It was same increase as in paclitaxel-resistant cell-lines. Thus, one suggestion is α-tubulin mutation may cause altered binding position of stathmin to β-tubulin combined with elevated protein expression level of stathmin [150].

β-Tubulin Mutations

Since β-tubulin is a target of many MTAs, several studies have investigated the DNA sequences of this protein. Reports indicated β-tubulin mutations and mutation-related clinical observations resulted from non-functional β-tubulin pseudo genes. All these known pseudo-genes, share substantial sequence homology with β-tubulin functional gene. β-Tubulin includes six isotypes. It is very well-conserved between species with similar amino-acid sequences. β-Tubulin isotypes differences are in regions of sequences that can be used for classifications between different species. In human cancer cells, class I β-tubulin is most commonly expressed β-tubulin isotype [152]. Each six isotypes has their own gene plus β-tubulin family includes pseudo-genes. Pseudo-gene sequences are not functional and probably are generated from mutations on duplicated functional β-tubulin genes [153]. Many studies have been conducted to investigate association between resistance to MTAs and changes in β-tubulin isotypes expressions and mutations [18].

Giannakakou et al. [154] performed in vitro tubulin polymerization assay and they have shown paclitaxel caused microtubule polymerization of wild-type tubulin but it did not show same efficacy in mutant tubulin purified from paclitaxel-resistant cells [154]. A study was done in 1A9 cell-line which is a paclitaxel-resistant ovarian cancer cell-line, and this cell-line carries functionally inactive mutant p53. Cells that carry p53 mutations are more likely to have additional mutations due to increase of genome instability. Among various studies that investigated this theory, one study identified presence of p53 response element in promoter region of human MSH2 gene in human ovarian cancer cell-line (A2780) which carries mutated p53. Apparently, this element is required for expression of hMSH2, Therefore non-functional p53 prevents expression of hMSH2 [155]. MSH2 is member of human mismatch repair (MMR) gene, therefore hMSH2 (human mutS homolog-2) is a DNA repair gene [156]. This study proved the role of P53 in genomic stability. Therefore, p53 mutation itself accelerates acquisition of more mutations within the cells. Giannakakou et al. [127, 157] selected several clones which were isolated from 1A9 human ovarian cell-line (PTX10 and PTA22). DNA sequencing experiment revealed that PTX22 included both mutated and wild-type p53. Silencing of P53 caused accumulation of mutated β-tubulin. Once mutation in β-tubulin genes occurred, even restoring wild-type p53 could not return the cells back to paclitaxel-sensitive state. Therefore p53 silenced cells had better chance to confer paclitaxel-resistance [157]. Although, another study in 2000 reported patients with ovarian cancer who are carriers of mut-P53 gene, had better sensitivity to paclitaxel (86%) than those patients with wt-p53 gene (47%) [158].

Investigation of connection between β-tubulin gene mutation and resistant to MTA also is done for vinca alkaloids. Kavallaris et al. [159] found point mutation of β-tubulin gene in leukemia cell-lines resistant to vinblastine (CEM/VLB 100) and to vincristine (CEM/VCR R). However both cell-lines contained elevated level of drug efflux pump P-gp but overexpression of this protein did not match the whole drug resistant phenotype [159], therefore, we can conclude β-tubulin mutation can confer resistance to MTAs.

Alteration in Class III β-Tubulin Isotype Expression

The class III β-tubulin overexpression is correlated to resistant to MTAs such as paclitaxel and vinorelbine in vitro and in vivo for various cancers especially for breast cancer. Alteration in tubulin isoform expression is associated to resistance to taxanes. Although identifying the connection of class III β-tubulin and drug resistance is complicated due to complexity of tubulin auto-regulation systems, but there are studies that investigated effects of changes in tubulin isoform expressions on efficacy of several new tubulin-binding agents. For instance, Suzuki et al. [160] reported that STX140 is able to suppress proliferation of resistant MCF-7 dox cell-line with overexpressed P-gp [160]. When the level of soluble tubulin increases, β-tubulin mRNA degrades through a co-translational degradation that also regulates the expression of β-tubulin isotypes [161]. In a study, Hari et al. [162] overexpressed the class III β-tubulin in CHO cell-line. This experiment increased resistance to paclitaxel by decrease of paclitaxel suppression on microtubule dynamics [162]. Data showed breast cancer patients with resistance to docetaxel, had five-fold increase of class III β-tubulin [163]. Joe et al. [164] transfected class III β-tubulin in cervical carcinoma HeLa cell-line and tested taccalonolides efficacy. It was reported there is no evidence of resistance against this drug in cells with overexpressed class III β-tubulin [53], however, overexpression of class III β-tubulin caused resistance to paclitaxel [164]. Gan et al. [165] investigated the effect of class III β-tubulin expression in different pattern. They silenced class III β-tubulin and observed that this experiment induced resistance to vincristine, paclitaxel and DNA-damaging agents in non-small cell lung carcinoma [165]. Stengel et al. [166] have shown that alteration in class III β-tubulin expression (both silencing and overexpression) in two breast cancer cell-lines, MCF-7 and MDA-MB-231 did not affect the efficacies of STX140, STX243, ENMD1198, 2-MeOE2 and colchicine. While efficacies of paclitaxel and vinorelbine have changed [166]. Small difference between class I and III of β-tubulin is one amino-acid which causes different final three dimensional formations. Class III β-tubulin carries Arg 277 instead of Ser 277 which exist in class I. Ser^{277} and Arg^{278} are key amino-acid for stable binding of tubulin to paclitaxel in its binding site at class I β-tubulin [167], but in class III β-tubulin structure changed and lost its stable taxane-binding site [168]. Class III β-tubulin is correlated with increased microtubule dynamics which is opposite of assembling activity of paclitaxel at microtubules plus (+) end [169]. The reason that high contained class III β-tubulin cancer cells are not resistant to STX140, STX243, ENMD1198, 2-MeOE2 and colchicine, but are resistant to paclitaxel, is these agents bind to colchicine-binding site which includes a different conformation and leads to formation of a stable complex containing class III β-tubulin. Besides, these agents are destabilizers, therefore overexpression of class III β-tubulin is even an advantage for this class of drugs due to class III β-tubulin increases microtubule dynamics. Although, vinorelbine which binds to vinca-binding site appeared to have less efficacy in cancer cells with class III β-tubulin overexpression in small lung cancer cell-line [165], breast cancer cell-line [166] and *in vivo* [170]. These observations suggest that resistant cancer cells with overexpressed class III β-tubulin is related to drug binding-site. This idea is supported by study of Stengel et al. [166], wherein they showed those MTAs that binds to colchicine-binding site in cells which contain altered class III β-tubulin, do not exhibit resistance to these drugs, but those MTAs binding to taxane- and vinca-binding sites, alteration in class III β-tubulin, affected their efficacies. A satisfactory conclusion here could be the importance of design and development of new agents that bind to colchicine-binding site as taxanes alternatives for resistant cancers [166].

Alteration in Class VI β-Tubulin Isotype Expression

Lack of β-tubulin VI in non-hematopoietic tissues confirmed that β-tubulin VI is a hematology-specific isotype and consequently it is a marker that mediates hematologic toxicity of β-tubulin binding drugs. These cells express a specific variant of β-tubulin VI named β-tubulin VI 274 M variant. This variant is less sensitive to paclitaxel compared to other variants and compared to β-tubulin VI wild-type [171]. Within paclitaxel-binding site of all human β-tubulin isotypes, there is a conserved residue (residue 274) [172]. This residue is necessary for binding of paclitaxel to tubulin. Mutation in this residue (T274 M) leads to resistance to paclitaxel [173], therefore patients who carrying this mutation could be resistant to myelosuppressive effects of MTAs. Leandro-Garcia et al. [171] for first time showed β-tubulin class VI is a hematology-specific isotype which differentiates from other β-tubulin genes by few genetic and expression variability. Also they have shown patients who are carriers of TUBB1 T274 M in their β-tubulin class VI gene, had protection against paclitaxel effect [171].

P-Glycoprotein Overexpression

One of the major current problem in chemotherapy is efflux of drugs into extracellular matrix. This occurs by activity of ATP-binding cassette protein known as P-gp product of MDR1 gene and it is part of MDR mechanism [174]. The main natural positive role of P-gp is pumping the toxic substances out of cells in brain and gastrointestinal tracts [175]. In many cancer types, overexpression of P-gp seemed to be related to resistance to taxanes [176], but in same cancers ixabepilone a class of epothilone, showed cytotoxicity [40]. A meta-analysis of 31 breast cancer trials showed that the P-gp was overexpressed in 41% of patients after treatment and interestingly, there was 3-fold reduction of response to paclitaxel in same patients. This result suggested chemotherapy induces P-gp expression [177]. Investigation on connection between other taxanes such as docetaxel and expression of P-gp in breast cancer were done and no significant correlation has been reported [178].

Epothilones and taxanes bind to same tubulin binding site but they are functioning differently. The main advance of epothilones is that unlike taxanes they are not P-gp substrate [179]. In this regard, epothilones are active in models that are taxane resistance because epothilones tolerance is provided. As an example, epothilone B causes much higher levels of tubulin polymerization when it is compared with equimolar dosages of paclitaxel in vitro [180]. Other experiments showed almost all models that are resistant to paclitaxel display sensitivity to epothilone A and epothilone B. Recent studies have reported that, α-tubulin mutations in cells that are resistant to microtubule-depolymerizing agents, causes decreased drug accumulation even when P-gp overexpression is not present [181]. If P-gp causes resistance to certain drugs therefore those agents that inhibit P-gp activity, are able to bring back the sensitivity of the cell to those certain drugs [174]. A recent drug, tariquidar is a P-gp inhibitor which showed an ability to bring back the sensitivity to paclitaxel in 17 women with stage III-IV breast cancer but final result was lack of efficacy [182]. Therapeutic industry needs more offer on P-gp inhibitors more specific those drugs that increase the efficacy of taxanes. Also more MTAs are required to be introduced with less susceptibility to P-gp-mediated resistance.

Tau: Intracellular Competitor of Paclitaxel

Tau protein was first time described in 1975 to be a product of a gene located in chromosome 17 (17q21) [183]. Tau is one of microtubule-associated proteins (MAPs) and attaches to tubulin both exterior and interior surfaces of microtubule and also it binds in paclitaxel-binding site therefore practically tau competes with paclitaxel. When tau attaches to paclitaxel-binding site, in the same way stabilizes the microtubule as paclitaxel does but with much more reversibility [184]. Studies revealed that those breast cancer patients that have genetically low tau expression, benefit more from paclitaxel treatment due to competition of paclitaxel and tau in attaching to microtubule. One study was experimented with paclitaxel-based neoadjuvant chemotherapy on 82 breast cancer patients. Those patients with low tau mRNA expression level, succeeded to achieve total pathologic response ($P < 0.001$) [185]. Furthermore, there is a correlation between tau and ER in breast cancer patients. Those with high tau expression were reported to be more among ER-positive patients (57%) than those with ER-negative (15%) [186] and this is due to oestrogen regulation of tau gene. Oestrogen induces tau expression. Therefore co-expression of ER and tau is considered a good sign for prognosis in the breast cancer therapy and it is related to better overall survival. ER-positive patients with high tau expression are more sensitive to hormone therapy than paclitaxel therapy. On the other hand, ER-negative patients had better response to paclitaxel therapy [187]. In 2005 a group of researchers silenced tau protein in breast cancer cells and they achieved higher sensitivity to taxanes [188]. Thus, tau expression level could be an important biomarker of resistance to paclitaxel [187].

HER2 Overexpression

HER2 is a transmembrane receptor and it has a tyrosine kinase activity [189]. HER2 belongs to a family with four members namely: EGFR/HER1, HER2, HER3 and HER4 receptors that are involved in cell growth regulation, differentiation and survival through interlink with some of survival pathways including PI3K/AKT pathway and Ras/Raf/MEK/MAPK pathway. Therefore, when HER2 is expressed, there is signaling to downstream pathways [190]. HER2 is always in active form and ready to interact with its ligands [191]. Amplification and/or overexpression of HER2 were detected in 20% of early stage breast cancer patients [192]. Breast cancer patients with HER2-negative ER-positive, had no significant benefit from paclitaxel treatment while patients with HER2-positive whether ER-positive or ER-negative showed significant improved response to therapy including 5 years of disease-free survival. Also patients with overexpressed HER2 seemed to receive even better benefit compared to HER2-negative. Therefore, HER2 amplification and overexpression is a marker of potential to emerge better response to taxane therapy. Interestingly, overexpression of HER2 is associated with lower expression of tau protein which is somehow a brief explanation for increased sensitivity to taxane therapy [193].

Determinants of Sensitivity and Resistance to MTAs

The major logic behind continuous production of MTAs is their lack of tissue selectivity and perpetual drug resistance against these drugs. For instance paclitaxel and vinca alkaloid are active against breast, ovarian and lung cancers but inactive against colon and kidney cancers and many sarcomas. Seems these drugs are more effective against haematological type of cancers rather than solid ones. The determinants of being sensitive or resistance to specific drug is inside the cell and their level of access to drugs pharmacological benefits [15]. Different levels of resistance were reported against MTAs. Those cells that ultimately resist against MTAs, oftentimes display overexpression of a class of a membrane transporter named ABC-transporters (ATP-dependent drug efflux pumps or ATP-binding cassettes). These pumps reduce intracellular drug accumulation by pumping them out of cell. Since, they may pump various drugs at the same time, they cause cross-resistance or MDR. Many of these transmembrane pumps have been identified such as P-gp which is explained earlier in this chapter [194]. To remove this obstacle considerable efforts are in the way to produce MTAs which are not removed by transmembrane pumps [195]. However, the cell's host factors are also determine to pose the cell as sensitive or resistance to drugs. Such as abnormal expression of regulatory proteins, the different level of expression of tubulin isotypes and their post-translational modifications. There are various studies reported the correlation between high level of a specific tubulin isotype and resistance to a specific MTA [15, 19, 159, 196]. The cellular host determinants can be divided into two groups. Those that affect microtubule polymer level and therefore they also affect microtubule dynamics. Microtubule polymer level is a significant host determinant considering most organelles and components move inside the cell by attaching and moving along microtubules. Therefore, those cells that have the ability of preserve their microtubule mass in required level for organelles and components to move, survive longer under treatment of destabilizers such as vinca alkaloids. On the other hand, under paclitaxel treatment and consequently appearance of increased microtubule polymers, motor-proteins such as dynein and kinesin are not able to support the transportations anymore. Certain cancer cells that overexpress endogenous microtubule-depolymerizing factors, develop resistance against stabilizers like paclitaxel.

The importance of microtubule dynamics as host determinant was showed that those MTAs that suppress microtubule dynamics without any significant change in microtubule-polymer level, prevent metaphase to anaphase transition, such as in paclitaxel-resistance/dependent A549 lung cancer cell-line. After omitting paclitaxel in these cells, results show 57% to 167% faster microtubule dynamics compared to paclitaxel-sensitive A549 cells [147]. Fast microtubule dynamics behavior cost this group of cells disrupted spindle assembly and they were unable to transit from metaphase to anaphase. Addition of paclitaxel to this group of cells caused microtubule dynamics slow down and they went through successful mitosis. This shows their resistance and at the same time dependence to paclitaxel. This group of A549 cells undergo several endogenous changes such as overexpression of βIII-tubulin isotype, As mutated α-tubulin, overexpression of endogenous microtubule-destabilizer protein stathmin and inactivation of endogenous microtubule-stabilizer protein MAP4 [150, 197]. The point that we can understand here is microtubules destiny is affected by many endogenous determinants. Therefore, there are many undiscovered potential determinants which could be targets of chemotherapeutic drug design.

Natural or Synthetized MTAs? Which Are More Beneficial?

As early as discovery of natural products, they provided a rich source of compounds that were applicable in many fields of medical researches. Above half of currently used drugs in chemotherapy are natural products. Synthetized or semi-synthetized agents are either obtained from natural sources with few structural modifications (semi-synthetized), or they are totally new compounds which are designed according to a natural compound structure as a model (synthetized) [198]. The main aim of synthetizing a drug is to establish a relationship between pharmacological advantages and structure of the compound, therefore the aim is obtaining a new drug which is better than "prototype" with a view of collecting advantages from potency, less toxicity and more selectivity. Natural products which are extracted from marine products, plants and microorganisms are considered as prototype, origin, template or lead compounds [199].

To answer the question of "which one is better", we must consider natural products provide major structural diversity which some of them have sufficient biological potency in some aspect, but some disadvantages in another aspect. For example taxanes which are great stabilizers, on the other hand they are also great substrate for plasma membrane drug-efflux pump [200]. The search for natural products is necessary and will continue to provide greater range of template [201]. These prototypes are modified to produce more improved semi-synthetized agents with better therapeutic potential by molecular modifications. Or they are template for entirely new synthetized agents as their analogues, which contain greater pharmacological activity, magnificent therapeutic possibilities and less side effects. Nowadays, drug synthesis provides huge range of improved drugs in regard of both structure and activity [198]. According to data, we can conclude both natural and synthetized drugs have different range of advantages that must be considered.

Conclusion

Critical obstacle in current cancer therapy is low selectivity of anticancer drugs against cancer cells. To differentiate between cancer and normal cells, the knowledge of cancer-specific characteristics, origin and differences of these characteristics is required. This aim directed researchers to develop molecular-based strategies. One of the main different characteristics is rapid mitosis of cancer cells. Microtubules, the main component of mitosis have two types of dynamic behaviors. The duration of each and switch rate between these two behaviors caused microtubule interesting as a potential target. MTAs are class of anticancer drugs which effect mitosis by targeting microtubules. This paradigm makes MTAs applicable to rapidly dividing cancer cells, compared to slowly dividing normal cells. Proliferation mechanisms are tightly under control in normal cells while these mechanisms are manipulated in cancer cells, due to continuous mutations. Mutations in cancer cells alter microtubule dynamic behaviors. Studying different characteristics in molecular level also clarified that mutations such as α- and β-tubulin mutations and abnormal expression of β-tubulin isotypes are associated with resistance to some of MTAs. MTAs are verity of small molecules either from natural sources or synthetized/semi-synthetized as improved analogues of natural agents, interrupt microtubule dynamic behaviors with either stabilizing or destabilizing activities. Studies showed some of MTAs beside their main task, manipulate mitotic kinases as well, or manipulate some other specific proteins that directly or indirectly boost MTAs' main task. Moreover, MTAs suppress tumor vascularization, which avoid tumor accessibility to source of oxygen and nutrients "the blood". No matter stabilizer or destabilizer, MTAs' main resemblance is their final task which is suppressing microtubule dynamic behaviors. That is why more drug combination strategies were successful in emerge of synergism between different MTAs. Natural MTAs always have been main source of applicable drugs or great template in the view of structure or bioactivity. Synthetized/semi-synthetized MTAs have been improved drugs to associate between structure and bioactivity with lesser side effects and resistance to MTAs.

Acknowledgement The first author (Mohadeseh Hasanpourghadi) thanks University of Malaya, Kuala Lumpur, Malaysia, for providing financial support through Postgraduate grant (PG) (PG048-2015A). This study was also supported by a High-Impact Research grant from the University of Malaya (E00002–20001).

References

1. Livingston DM, Shivdasani R (2001) Toward mechanism-based cancer care. JAMA 285(5):588–593
2. Pecorino L (2012) Molecular biology of cancer: mechanisms, targets, and therapeutics. Oxford University Press, Oxford
3. Evan GI, Vousden KH (2001) Proliferation, cell cycle and apoptosis in cancer. Nature 411(6835):342–348
4. Sherr CJ (1996) Cancer cell cycles. Science 274(5293):1672–1677
5. Stocker H, Hafen E (2000) Genetic control of cell size. Curr Opin Genet Dev 10(5):529–535
6. Loeb LA, Loeb KR, Anderson JP (2003) Multiple mutations and cancer. Proc Natl Acad Sci 100(3):776–781
7. Jordan MA, Wilson L (2004) Microtubules as a target for anticancer drugs. Nat Rev Cancer 4(4):253–265
8. Sharp DJ, Rogers GC, Scholey JM (2000) Microtubule motors in mitosis. Nature 407(6800): 41–47
9. Mohan R, Katrukha EA, Doodhi H, Smal I, Meijering E, Kapitein LC et al (2013) End-binding proteins sensitize microtubules to the action of microtubule-targeting agents. Proc Natl Acad Sci 110(22):8900–8905
10. Oakley BR (2000) An abundance of tubulins. Trends Cell Biol 10(12):537–542
11. Rohena CC, Mooberry SL (2014) Recent progress with microtubule stabilizers: new compounds, binding modes and cellular activities. Nat Prod Rep 31(3):335–355
12. Poruchynsky MS, Kim J-H, Nogales E, Annable T, Loganzo F, Greenberger LM et al (2004) Tumor cells resistant to a microtubule-depolymerizing hemiasterlin analogue, HTI-286, have mutations in α-or β-tubulin and increased microtubule stability. Biochemistry 43(44): 13944–13954
13. Barlow SB, Gonzalez-Garay ML, Cabral F (2002) Paclitaxel dependent mutants have severely reduced microtubule assembly and reduced tubulin synthesis. J Cell Sci 115(17):3469–3478
14. Amos LA (2011) What tubulin drugs tell us about microtubule structure and dynamics. Semin Cell Dev Biol 22(9):916–926
15. Dumontet C, Sikic BI (1999) Mechanisms of action of and resistance to antitubulin agents: microtubule dynamics, drug transport, and cell death. J Clin Oncol 17(3):1061
16. Downing KH, Nogales E (1999) Crystallographic Structure of Tubulin. Implications for Dynamics and Drug Binding. Cell Struct Funct 24(5):269–275
17. Snyder JP, Nettles JH, Cornett B, Downing KH, Nogales E (2001) The binding conformation of Taxol in β-tubulin: A model based on electron crystallographic density. Proc Natl Acad Sci 98(9):5312–5316
18. Berrieman HK, Lind MJ, Cawkwell L (2004) Do β-tubulin mutations have a role in resistance to chemotherapy? Lancet Oncol 5(3):158–164
19. Burkhart CA, Kavallaris M, Horwitz SB (2001) The role of β-tubulin isotypes in resistance to antimitotic drugs. Biochim Biophys Acta 1471(2):O1–O9
20. Igney FH, Krammer PH (2002) Death and anti-death: tumour resistance to apoptosis. Nat Rev Cancer 2(4):277–288

21. Zaffaroni N, Pennati M, Colella G, Perego P, Supino R, Gatti L et al (2002) Expression of the anti-apoptotic gene survivin correlates with taxol resistance in human ovarian cancer. Cell Mol Life Sci 59(8):1406–1412
22. O'Connor DS, Grossman D, Plescia J, Li F, Zhang H, Villa A et al (2000) Regulation of apoptosis at cell division by p34cdc2 phosphorylation of survivin. Proc Natl Acad Sci 97(24):13103–13107
23. Sparano JA (2000) Taxanes for breast cancer: an evidence-based review of randomized phase II and phase III trials. Clin Breast Cancer 1(1):32–40
24. Horwitz SB (1994) How to make taxol from scratch. Nature 367(6464):593
25. Schiff PB, Horwitz SB (1981) Taxol assembles tubulin in the absence of exogenous guanosine 5'-triphosphate or microtubule-associated proteins. Biochemistry 20(11):3247–3252
26. Nogales E, Wolf SG, Khan IA, Ludueña RF, Downing KH (1995) Structure of tubulin at 6.5 Å and location of the taxol-binding site. Nature 375(6530):424–427
27. Nogales E (2001) Structural insights into microtubule function. Annu Rev Biophys Biomol Struct 30(1):397–420
28. Rao S, Krauss NE, Heerding JM, Swindell CS, Ringel I, Orr GA et al (1994) 3'-(p-azidobenzamido) taxol photolabels the N-terminal 31 amino acids of beta-tubulin. J Biol Chem 269(5):3132–3134
29. Nogales E, Wolf SG, Downing KH (1998) Structure of the αβ tubulin dimer by electron crystallography. Nature 391(6663):199–203
30. Derry WB, Wilson L, Jordan MA (1995) Substoichiometric binding of taxol suppresses microtubule dynamics. Biochemistry 34(7):2203–2211
31. Von Hoff D (1997) The taxoids: same roots, different drugs. Semin Oncol 24(4 Suppl 13):S13-3–S13-10
32. Díaz JF, Valpuesta JM, Chacón P, Diakun G, Andreu JM (1998) Changes in Microtubule Protofilament Number Induced by Taxol Binding to an easily accessible site. Internal microtubule dynamics. J Biol Chem 273(50):33803–33810
33. Jordan MA, Toso RJ, Thrower D, Wilson L (1993) Mechanism of mitotic block and inhibition of cell proliferation by taxol at low concentrations. Proc Natl Acad Sci 90(20):9552–9556
34. Pryor DE, O'Brate A, Bilcer G, Díaz JF, Wang Y, Wang Y et al (2002) The microtubule stabilizing agent laulimalide does not bind in the taxoid site, kills cells resistant to paclitaxel and epothilones, and may not require its epoxide moiety for activity. Biochemistry 41(29): 9109–9115
35. Chen J-G, Horwitz SB (2002) Differential mitotic responses to microtubule-stabilizing and-destabilizing drugs. Cancer Res 62(7):1935–1938
36. Lavelle F, Bissery M, Combeau C, Riou J, Vrignaud P, Andre S (1995) Preclinical evaluation of docetaxel (Taxotere). Semin Oncol 22(2 Suppl 4):3–16
37. He L, Orr GA, Horwitz SB (2001) Novel molecules that interact with microtubules and have functional activity similar to Taxol™. Drug Discov Today 6(22):1153–1164
38. Gerth K, Bedorf N, Höfle G, Irschik H, Reichenbach H (1996) Epothilons A and B: antifungal and cytotoxic compounds from Sorangium cellulosum (Myxobacteria). Production, physico-chemical and biological properties. J Antibiot 49(6):560–563
39. Goodin S (2008) Novel cytotoxic agents: epothilones. Am J Health Syst Pharm 65(10 Suppl 3):S10–S15
40. Bollag DM, McQueney PA, Zhu J, Hensens O, Koupal L, Liesch J et al (1995) Epothilones, a new class of microtubule-stabilizing agents with a taxol-like mechanism of action. Cancer Res 55(11):2325–2333
41. Lee FY, Borzilleri R, Fairchild CR, Kim S-H, Long BH, Reventos-Suarez C et al (2001) BMS-247550 a novel epothilone analog with a mode of action similar to paclitaxel but possessing superior antitumor efficacy. Clin Cancer Res 7(5):1429–1437
42. Villanueva C, Vuillemin AT, Demarchi M, Bazan F, Chaigneau L, Pivot X (2009) Ixabepilone: a new active chemotherapy in the treatment of breast cancer. Womens Health (Lond) 5(2):115–121

43. Ghosh AK, Xu X, Kim J-H, Xu C-X (2008) Enantioselective total synthesis of peloruside A: a potent microtubule stabilizer. Org Lett 10(5):1001–1004
44. Hamel E, Sackett DL, Vourloumis D, Nicolaou K (1999) The coral-derived natural products eleutherobin and sarcodictyins A and B: effects on the assembly of purified tubulin with and without microtubule-associated proteins and binding at the polymer taxoid site. Biochemistry 38(17):5490–5498
45. Dumontet C, Jordan MA (2010) Microtubule-binding agents: a dynamic field of cancer therapeutics. Nat Rev Drug Discov 9(10):790–803
46. Pineda O, Farràs J, Maccari L, Manetti F, Botta M, Vilarrasa J (2004) Computational comparison of microtubule-stabilising agents laulimalide and peloruside with taxol and colchicine. Bioorg Med Chem Lett 14(19):4825–4829
47. Hamel E, Day BW, Miller JH, Jung MK, Northcote PT, Ghosh AK et al (2006) Synergistic effects of peloruside A and laulimalide with taxoid site drugs, but not with each other, on tubulin assembly. Mol Pharmacol 70(5):1555–1564
48. Prota AE, Bargsten K, Northcote PT, Marsh M, Altmann KH, Miller JH et al (2014) Structural basis of microtubule stabilization by laulimalide and peloruside A. Angew Chem Int Ed Engl 53(6):1621–1625
49. Khrapunovich-Baine M, Menon V, Yang C-PH, Northcote PT, Miller JH, Angeletti RH et al (2011) Hallmarks of molecular action of microtubule stabilizing agents effects of epothilone b, ixabepilone, peloruside a, and laulimalide on microtubule conformation. J Biol Chem 286(13):11765–11778
50. Li J, Risinger AL, Mooberry SL (2014) Taccalonolide microtubule stabilizers. Bioorg Med Chem 22(18):5091–5096
51. Tinley TL, Randall-Hlubek DA, Leal RM, Jackson EM, Cessac JW, Quada JC et al (2003) Taccalonolides E and A plant-derived steroids with microtubule-stabilizing activity. Cancer Res 63(12):3211–3220
52. Fojo T, Menefee M (2007) Mechanisms of multidrug resistance: the potential role of microtubule-stabilizing agents. Ann Oncol 18(suppl 5):v3–v8
53. Risinger AL, Jackson EM, Polin LA, Helms GL, LeBoeuf DA, Joe PA et al (2008) The taccalonolides: microtubule stabilizers that circumvent clinically relevant taxane resistance mechanisms. Cancer Res 68(21):8881–8888
54. Edler MC, Buey RM, Gussio R, Marcus AI, Vanderwal CD, Sorensen EJ et al (2005) Cyclostreptin (FR182877), an antitumor tubulin-polymerizing agent deficient in enhancing tubulin assembly despite its high affinity for the taxoid site. Biochemistry 44(34): 11525–11538
55. Buey RM, Barasoain I, Jackson E, Meyer A, Giannakakou P, Paterson I et al (2005) Microtubule interactions with chemically diverse stabilizing agents: thermodynamics of binding to the paclitaxel site predicts cytotoxicity. Chem Biol 12(12):1269–1279
56. Buey RM, Calvo E, Barasoain I, Pineda O, Edler MC, Matesanz R et al (2007) Cyclostreptin binds covalently to microtubule pores and lumenal taxoid binding sites. Nat Chem Biol 3(2):117–125
57. Evans DC, Watt AP, Nicoll Griffith DA, Baillie TA (2004) Drug-protein adducts: an industry perspective on minimizing the potential for drug bioactivation in drug discovery and development. Chem Res Toxicol 17(1):3–16
58. Mínguez JM, Kim S-Y, Giuliano KA, Balachandran R, Madiraju C, Day BW et al (2003) Synthesis and biological assessment of simplified analogues of the potent microtubule stabilizer (+)-discodermolide. Bioorg Med Chem 11(15):3335–3357
59. Minguez JM, Giuliano KA, Balachandran R, Madiraju C, Curran DP, Day BW (2002) Synthesis and High Content Cell-based Profiling of Simplified Analogues of the Microtubule Stabilizer (+)-Discodermolide 1 Supported by National Cancer Institute Grant CA78039. 1. Mol Cancer Ther 1(14):1305–1313
60. Martello LA, McDaid HM, Regl DL, Yang C-PH, Meng D, Pettus TR et al (2000) Taxol and discodermolide represent a synergistic drug combination in human carcinoma cell lines. Clin Cancer Res 6(5):1978–1987

61. Pettit GR, Cichacz ZA, Gao F, Boyd MR, Schmidt JM (1994) Isolation and structure of the cancer cell growth inhibitor dictyostatin 1. J Chem Soc Chem Commun 9:1111–1112
62. Kalesse M (2000) The chemistry and biology of discodermolide. ChemBioChem 1(3): 171–175
63. Shin Y, Choy N, Balachandran R, Madiraju C, Day BW, Curran DP (2002) Discodermolide/dictyostatin hybrids: synthesis and biological evaluation. Org Lett 4(25):4443–4446
64. Telser J, Beumer R, Bell AA, Ceccarelli SM, Monti D, Gennari C (2001) Synthesis of a simplified sarcodictyin analogue which retains microtubule stabilising properties. Tetrahedron Lett 42(52):9187–9190
65. Nakao Y, Yoshida S, Matsunaga S, Fusetani N (2003) (Z)-Sarcodictyin A, a new highly cytotoxic diterpenoid from the soft coral Bellonella a lbiflora. J Nat Prod 66(4):524–527
66. Brocksom TJ, de Oliveira KT, Ferreira MA, Servilha BM (2015) Essential oils as raw materials in the synthesis of anticancer drugs. In: Bioactive essential oils and cancer. Springer, New York, pp 81–109
67. Mandhare A, Biradar S, Gurule A (2016) Azaepothilone B and its derivatives: a patent review. Expert Opin Ther Pat 26(8):891–905
68. Thomas ES, Gomez HL, Li RK, Chung H-C, Fein LE, Chan VF et al (2007) Ixabepilone plus capecitabine for metastatic breast cancer progressing after anthracycline and taxane treatment. J Clin Oncol 25(33):5210–5217
69. Noble R, Beer C, Cutts J (1959) Further biological activities of vincaleukoblastine—an alkaloid isolated from *Vinca rosea* (L.). Biochem Pharmacol 1(4):347–348
70. Johnson I, Wright H, Svoboda G 1959 Experimental basis for clinical evaluation of anti tumor principles derived from Vinca-Rosea Linn. J Lab Clin Med 54:830. Mosby-Year Book Inc 11830 Westline Industrial Dr, St Louis, MO 63146–3318
71. Gidding C, Kellie S, Kamps W, De Graaf S (1999) Vincristine revisited. Crit Rev Oncol Hematol 29(3):267–287
72. Jordan MA, Thrower D, Wilson L (1991) Mechanism of inhibition of cell proliferation by Vinca alkaloids. Cancer Res 51(8):2212–2222
73. Bryan J (1971) Vinblastine and microtubules: I. Induction and isolation of crystals from sea urchin oocytes. Exp Cell Res 66(1):129–136
74. Gigant B, Wang C, Ravelli RB, Roussi F, Steinmetz MO, Curmi PA et al (2005) Structural basis for the regulation of tubulin by vinblastine. Nature 435(7041):519–522
75. Jordan MA, Wilson L (1990) Kinetic analysis of tubulin exchange at microtubule ends at low vinblastine concentrations. Biochemistry 29(11):2730–2739
76. Na GC, Timasheff SN (1980) Stoichiometry of the vinblastine-induced self-association of calf brain tubulin. Biochemistry 19(7):1347–1354
77. Singer WD, Jordan M, Wilson L, Himes RH (1989) Binding of vinblastine to stabilized microtubules. Mol Pharmacol 36(3):366–370
78. Owellen RJ, Owens AH, Donigian DW (1972) The binding of vincristine, vinblastine and colchicine to tubulin. Biochem Biophys Res Commun 47(4):685–691
79. Bissinger R, Modicano P, Frauenfeld L, Lang E, Jacobi J, Faggio C et al (2013) Estramustine-induced suicidal erythrocyte death. Cell Physiol Biochem 32(5):1426–1436
80. Hu Z-B, Gignac SM, Quentmeier H, Pettit GR, Drexler HG (1993) Effects of dolastatins on human B-lymphocytic leukemia cell lines. Leuk Res 17(4):333–339
81. Ebbinghaus S, Rubin E, Hersh E, Cranmer LD, Bonate PL, Fram RJ et al (2005) A phase I study of the dolastatin-15 analogue tasidotin (ILX651) administered intravenously daily for 5 consecutive days every 3 weeks in patients with advanced solid tumors. Clin Cancer Res 11(21):7807–7816
82. Mitra A, Sept D (2004) Localization of the antimitotic peptide and depsipeptide binding site on β-tubulin. Biochemistry 43(44):13955–13962
83. Cruz-Monserrate Z, Mullaney JT, Harran PG, Pettit GR, Hamel E (2003) Dolastatin 15 binds in the vinca domain of tubulin as demonstrated by Hummel–Dreyer chromatography. Eur J Biochem 270(18):3822–3828

84. Lopus M (2013) Mechanism of mitotic arrest induced by dolastatin 15 involves loss of tension across kinetochore pairs. Mol Cell Biochem 382(1–2):93–102
85. Yue Q-X, Liu X, Guo D-A (2010) Microtubule-binding natural products for cancer therapy. Planta Med 76(11):1037
86. Niel E, Scherrmann J-M (2006) Colchicine today. Joint Bone Spine 73(6):672–678
87. Ravelli RB, Gigant B, Curmi PA, Jourdain I, Lachkar S, Sobel A et al (2004) Insight into tubulin regulation from a complex with colchicine and a stathmin-like domain. Nature 428(6979):198–202
88. Lu Y, Chen J, Xiao M, Li W, Miller DD (2012) An overview of tubulin inhibitors that interact with the colchicine binding site. Pharm Res 29(11):2943–2971
89. Weiss C, Sammet B, Sewald N (2013) Recent approaches for the synthesis of modified cryptophycins. Nat Prod Rep 30(7):924–940
90. Hu Y (2013) Halichondrin B analogs. Google Patents
91. Pettit GR, Cragg GM, Herald DL, Schmidt JM, Lohavanijaya P (1982) Isolation and structure of combretastatin. Can J Chem 60(11):1374–1376
92. Kanthou C, Tozer GM (2002) The tumor vascular targeting agent combretastatin A–4-phosphate induces reorganization of the actin cytoskeleton and early membrane blebbing in human endothelial cells. Blood 99(6):2060–2069
93. Anderson HL, Yap JT, Miller MP, Robbins A, Jones T, Price PM (2003) Assessment of pharmacodynamic vascular response in a phase I trial of combretastatin A4 phosphate. J Clin Oncol 21(15):2823–2830
94. Kowalczyk JJ, Kuznetsov G, Schiller S, Seletsky BM, Spyvee M, Yang H (2006) Hemiasterlin derivatives and uses thereof. Google Patents
95. Kowalczyk JJ, Schiller SE, Spyvee M, Yang H, Seletsky BM, Shaffer CJ et al (2005) Synthetic analogs of the marine natural product hemiasterlin: optimization and discovery of E7974, a novel and potent antitumor agent. Cancer Res 65(9 Supplement):282
96. Canel C, Moraes RM, Dayan FE, Ferreira D (2000) Podophyllotoxin. Phytochemistry 54(2):115–120
97. Gordaliza M, Md C, Miguel del Corral J, Feliciano AS (2000) Antitumor properties of podophyllotoxin and related compounds. Curr Pharm Des 6(18):1811–1839
98. Alday PH, Correia JJ (2009) Macromolecular interaction of halichondrin B analogues eribulin (E7389) and ER-076349 with tubulin by analytical ultracentrifugation. Biochemistry 48(33):7927–7938
99. Li C-M, Wang Z, Lu Y, Ahn S, Narayanan R, Kearbey JD et al (2011) Biological activity of 4-substituted methoxybenzoyl-aryl-thiazole: an active microtubule inhibitor. Cancer Res 71(1):216–224
100. Hasanpourghadi M, Karthikeyan C, Pandurangan AK, Looi CY, Trivedi P, Kobayashi K et al (2016) Targeting of tubulin polymerization and induction of mitotic blockage by Methyl 2-(5-fluoro-2-hydroxyphenyl)-1 H-benzo [d] imidazole-5-carboxylate (MBIC) in human cervical cancer HeLa cell. J Exp Clin Cancer Res 35(1):1
101. Kang G-J, Getahun Z, Muzaffar A, Brossi A, Hamel E (1990) N-acetylcolchinol O-methyl ether and thiocolchicine, potent analogs of colchicine modified in the C ring. Evaluation of the mechanistic basis for their enhanced biological properties. J Biol Chem 265(18):10255–10259
102. Kuznetsov G, Tendyke K, Towle MJ, Cheng H, Liu D, Rowell C et al (2005) In vitro and in vivo antitumor activities of novel hemiasterlin analog E7974. Cancer Res 65(9 Supplement):809
103. Krishnamurthy G, Cheng W, Lo M-C, Aulabaugh A, Razinkov V, Ding W et al (2003) Biophysical characterization of the interactions of HTI-286 with tubulin heterodimer and microtubules. Biochemistry 42(46):13484–13495
104. Rowinsky EK, Calvo E (2006) Novel agents that target tublin and related elements. Semin Oncol 33(4):421–435
105. Nunes M, Kaplan J, Loganzo F, Zask A, Ayral-Kaloustian S, Greenberger L (2002) Two photoaffinity analogs of HTI-286, a synthetic analog of hemiasterlin, interact with alpha-

tubulin. Eur J Cancer 38:S119. Pergamon-Elsevier Science Ltd The Boulevard, Langford Lane, Kidlington, Oxford OX5 1GB, England
106. Loganzo F, Discafani C, Annable T, Beyer C, Musto S, Hardy C et al (2002) HTI-286, a synthetic analog of the antimicrotubule tripeptide hemiasterlin, potently inhibits growth of cultured tumor cells, overcomes resistance to paclitaxel mediated by various mechanisms, and demonstrates intravenous and oral in vivo efficacy. 93rd annual meeting of American Association for Cancer Research. San Francisco, USA
107. Jordan MA, Wendell K, Gardiner S, Derry WB, Copp H, Wilson L (1996) Mitotic block induced in HeLa cells by low concentrations of paclitaxel (Taxol) results in abnormal mitotic exit and apoptotic cell death. Cancer Res 56(4):816–825
108. Panda D, DeLuca K, Williams D, Jordan MA, Wilson L (1998) Antiproliferative mechanism of action of cryptophycin-52: kinetic stabilization of microtubule dynamics by high-affinity binding to microtubule ends. Proc Natl Acad Sci 95(16):9313–9318
109. Gardner MK, Zanic M, Howard J (2013) Microtubule catastrophe and rescue. Curr Opin Cell Biol 25(1):14–22
110. Gardner M, Zanic M, Gell C, Bormuth V, Howard J (2011) The depolymerizing kinesins Kip3 (kinesin-8) and MCAK (kinesin-13) are catastrophe factors that destabilize microtubules by different mechanisms. Cell 147(5):1092–1103
111. Howard J, Hyman AA (2003) Dynamics and mechanics of the microtubule plus end. Nature 422(6933):753–758
112. Maurer SP, Fourniol FJ, Bohner G, Moores CA, Surrey T (2012) EBs recognize a nucleotide-dependent structural cap at growing microtubule ends. Cell 149(2):371–382
113. Maurer SP, Bieling P, Cope J, Hoenger A, Surrey T (2011) GTPγS microtubules mimic the growing microtubule end structure recognized by end-binding proteins (EBs). Proc Natl Acad Sci 108(10):3988–3993
114. Elie-Caille C, Severin F, Helenius J, Howard J, Muller DJ, Hyman A (2007) Straight GDP-tubulin protofilaments form in the presence of taxol. Curr Biol 17(20):1765–1770
115. Brieher WM, Yap AS (2013) Cadherin junctions and their cytoskeleton (s). Curr Opin Cell Biol 25(1):39–46
116. Bakhoum SF, Compton DA (2012) Kinetochores and disease: keeping microtubule dynamics in check! Curr Opin Cell Biol 24(1):64–70
117. Komlodi-Pasztor E, Sackett DL, Fojo AT (2012) Inhibitors targeting mitosis: tales of how great drugs against a promising target were brought down by a flawed rationale. Clin Cancer Res 18(1):51–63
118. Komlodi-Pasztor E, Sackett D, Wilkerson J, Fojo T (2011) Mitosis is not a key target of microtubule agents in patient tumors. Nat Rev Clin Oncol 8(4):244–250
119. Keen N, Taylor S (2004) Aurora-kinase inhibitors as anticancer agents. Nat Rev Cancer 4(12):927–936
120. Strebhardt K (2010) Multifaceted polo-like kinases: drug targets and antitargets for cancer therapy. Nat Rev Drug Discov 9(8):643–660
121. Melnikova I, Golden J (2004) Targeting protein kinases. Nat Rev Drug Discov 3(12): 993–994
122. Milross CG, Mason KA, Hunter NR, Chung W-K, Peters LJ, Milas L (1996) Relationship of mitotic arrest and apoptosis to antitumor effect of paclitaxel. J Natl Cancer Inst 88(18): 1308–1314
123. Rohena CC, Peng J, Johnson TA, Crews P, Mooberry SL (2013) Chemically diverse microtubule stabilizing agents initiate distinct mitotic defects and dysregulated expression of key mitotic kinases. Biochem Pharmacol 85(8):1104–1114
124. Gornstein E, Schwarz TL (2014) The paradox of paclitaxel neurotoxicity: mechanisms and unanswered questions. Neuropharmacology 76:175–183
125. Ferlini C, Cicchillitti L, Raspaglio G, Bartollino S, Cimitan S, Bertucci C et al (2009) Paclitaxel directly binds to Bcl-2 and functionally mimics activity of Nur77. Cancer Res 69(17):6906–6914

126. Gomez TS, Billadeau DD (2008) T cell activation and the cytoskeleton: you can't have one without the other. Adv Immunol 97:1–64
127. Giannakakou P, Sackett DL, Ward Y, Webster KR, Blagosklonny MV, Fojo T (2000) p53 is associated with cellular microtubules and is transported to the nucleus by dynein. Nat Cell Biol 2(10):709–717
128. Darshan MS, Loftus MS, Thadani-Mulero M, Levy BP, Escuin D, Zhou XK et al (2011) Taxane-induced blockade to nuclear accumulation of the androgen receptor predicts clinical responses in metastatic prostate cancer. Cancer Res 71(18):6019–6029
129. Carbonaro M, O'Brate A, Giannakakou P (2011) Microtubule disruption targets HIF-1α mRNA to cytoplasmic P-bodies for translational repression. J Cell Biol 192(1):83–99
130. Schwartz EL (2009) Antivascular actions of microtubule-binding drugs. Clin Cancer Res 15(8):2594–2601
131. Tozer GM, Kanthou C, Baguley BC (2005) Disrupting tumour blood vessels. Nat Rev Cancer 5(6):423–435
132. Lippert JW (2007) Vascular disrupting agents. Bioorg Med Chem 15(2):605–615
133. Lu H, Murtagh J, Schwartz EL (2006) The microtubule binding drug laulimalide inhibits vascular endothelial growth factor-induced human endothelial cell migration and is synergistic when combined with docetaxel (taxotere). Mol Pharmacol 69(4):1207–1215
134. Kamath K, Smiyun G, Wilson L, Jordan MA (2014) Mechanisms of inhibition of endothelial cell migration by taxanes. Cytoskeleton 71(1):46–60
135. Carbonaro M, Escuin D, O'Brate A, Thadani-Mulero M, Giannakakou P (2012) Microtubules regulate hypoxia-inducible factor-1α protein trafficking and activity implications for taxane therapy. J Biol Chem 287(15):11859–11869
136. Goode BL, Drubin DG, Barnes G (2000) Functional cooperation between the microtubule and actin cytoskeletons. Curr Opin Cell Biol 12(1):63–71
137. Mandato CA, Bement WM (2003) Actomyosin transports microtubules and microtubules control actomyosin recruitment during Xenopus oocyte wound healing. Curr Biol 13(13):1096–1105
138. Kanakkanthara A, Teesdale-Spittle PH, Miller JH (2013) Cytoskeletal alterations that confer resistance to anti-tubulin chemotherapeutics. Anticancer Agents Med Chem 13(1):147–158
139. Geraldo S, Gordon-Weeks PR (2009) Cytoskeletal dynamics in growth-cone steering. J Cell Sci 122(20):3595–3604
140. Tanaka E, Ho T, Kirschner MW (1995) The role of microtubule dynamics in growth cone motility and axonal growth. J Cell Biol 128(1):139–155
141. Gascoigne KE, Taylor SS (2008) Cancer cells display profound intra-and interline variation following prolonged exposure to antimitotic drugs. Cancer Cell 14(2):111–122
142. Strebhardt K, Ullrich A (2006) Targeting polo-like kinase 1 for cancer therapy. Nat Rev Cancer 6(4):321–330
143. Slangy A, Lane HA, d'Hérin P, Harper M, Kress M, Niggt EA (1995) Phosphorylation by p34 cdc2 regulates spindle association of human Eg5, a kinesin-related motor essential for bipolar spindle formation in vivo. Cell 83(7):1159–1169
144. Yang J, Ikezoe T, Nishioka C, Tasaka T, Taniguchi A, Kuwayama Y et al (2007) AZD1152, a novel and selective aurora B kinase inhibitor, induces growth arrest, apoptosis, and sensitization for tubulin depolymerizing agent or topoisomerase II inhibitor in human acute leukemia cells in vitro and in vivo. Blood 110(6):2034–2040
145. Fojo AT, Adelberg DE (2010) Microtubule Targeting Agents. In: Drug Management of Prostate Cancer. Springer, New York, pp 179–194
146. Risinger AL, Peng J, Rohena CC, Aguilar HR, Frantz DE, Mooberry SL (2013) The bat flower: a source of microtubule-destabilizing and-stabilizing compounds with synergistic antiproliferative actions. J Nat Prod 76(10):1923–1929
147. Goncalves A, Braguer D, Kamath K, Martello L, Briand C, Horwitz S et al (2001) Resistance to Taxol in lung cancer cells associated with increased microtubule dynamics. Proc Natl Acad Sci 98(20):11737–11742

148. Richards KL, Anders KR, Nogales E, Schwartz K, Downing KH, Botstein D (2000) Structure–function relationships in yeast tubulins. Mol Biol Cell 11(5):1887–1903
149. Müller D, Schindler P, Towbin H, Wirth U, Voshol H, Hoving S et al (2001) Isotope-tagged cross-linking reagents. A new tool in mass spectrometric protein interaction analysis. Anal Chem 73(9):1927–1934
150. Martello LA, Verdier-Pinard P, Shen H-J, He L, Torres K, Orr GA et al (2003) Elevated levels of microtubule destabilizing factors in a Taxol-resistant/dependent A549 cell line with an α-tubulin mutation. Cancer Res 63(6):1207–1213
151. Curmi P, Nogues C, Lachkar S, Carelle N, Gonthier M, Sobel A et al (2000) Overexpression of stathmin in breast carcinomas points out to highly proliferative tumours. Br J Cancer 82(1):142
152. Nicoletti MI, Valoti G, Giannakakou P, Zhan Z, Kim J-H, Lucchini V et al (2001) Expression of β-Tubulin Isotypes in Human Ovarian Carcinoma Xenografts and in a Sub-Panel of Human Cancer Cell Lines from the NCI-Anticancer Drug Screen Correlation with Sensitivity to Microtubule Active Agents. Clin Cancer Res 7(9):2912–2922
153. Wilde C, Crowther C, Cowan N (1982) Diverse mechanisms in the generation of human beta-tubulin pseudogenes. Science 217(4559):549–552
154. Giannakakou P, Sackett DL, Kang Y-K, Zhan Z, Buters JT, Fojo T et al (1997) Paclitaxel-resistant human ovarian cancer cells have mutant β-tubulins that exhibit impaired paclitaxel-driven polymerization. J Biol Chem 272(27):17118–17125
155. Warnick CT, Dabbas B, Ford CD, Strait KA (2001) Identification of a p53 response element in the promoter region of the hMSH2 gene required for expression in A2780 ovarian cancer cells. J Biol Chem 276(29):27363–27370
156. Leach FS, Hsieh JT, Molberg K, Saboorian MH, McConnell JD, Sagalowsky AI (2000) Expression of the human mismatch repair gene hMSH2. Cancer 88(10):2333–2341
157. Giannakakou P, Poy G, Zhan Z, Knutsen T, Blagosklonny MV, Fojo T (2000) Paclitaxel selects for mutant or pseudo-null p53 in drug resistance associated with tubulin mutations in human cancer. Oncogene 19(27):3078–3085
158. Lavarino C, Pilotti S, Oggionni M, Gatti L, Perego P, Bresciani G et al (2000) p53 gene status and response to platinum/paclitaxel-based chemotherapy in advanced ovarian carcinoma. J Clin Oncol 18(23):3936–3945
159. Kavallaris M, Tait AS, Walsh BJ, He L, Horwitz SB, Norris MD et al (2001) Multiple micro-tubule alterations are associated with Vinca alkaloid resistance in human leukemia cells. Cancer Res 61(15):5803–5809
160. Suzuki R, Newman S, Purohit A, Leese M, Potter B, Reed M (2003) Growth inhibition of multi-drug-resistant breast cancer cells by 2-methoxyoestradiol-bis-sulphamate and 2-ethylo estradiol-bis-sulphamate. J Steroid Biochem Mol Biol 84(2):269–278
161. Yen TJ, Gay DA, Pachter JS, Cleveland D (1988) Autoregulated changes in stability of polyribosome-bound beta-tubulin mRNAs are specified by the first 13 translated nucleotides. Mol Cell Biol 8(3):1224–1235
162. Hari M, Yang H, Zeng C, Canizales M, Cabral F (2003) Expression of class III β-tubulin reduces microtubule assembly and confers resistance to paclitaxel. Cell Motil Cytoskeleton 56(1):45–56
163. Hasegawa S, Miyoshi Y, Egawa C, Ishitobi M, Taguchi T, Tamaki Y et al (2003) Prediction of response to docetaxel by quantitative analysis of class I and III β-tubulin isotype mRNA expression in human breast cancers. Clin Cancer Res 9(8):2992–2997
164. Joe PA, Banerjee A, Ludueña RF (2008) The roles of Cys124 and Ser239 in the functional properties of human βIII tubulin. Cell Motil Cytoskeleton 65(6):476–486
165. Gan PP, Pasquier E, Kavallaris M (2007) Class III β-Tubulin Mediates Sensitivity to Chemotherapeutic Drugs in Non–Small Cell Lung Cancer. Cancer Res 67(19):9356–9363
166. Stengel C, Newman S, Leese M, Potter B, Reed M, Purohit A (2010) Class III β-tubulin expression and in vitro resistance to microtubule targeting agents. Br J Cancer 102(2):316–324

167. Löwe J, Li H, Downing K, Nogales E (2001) Refined structure of αβ-tubulin at 3.5 Å resolution. J Mol Biol 313(5):1045–1057
168. Ferlini C, Raspaglio G, Mozzetti S, Cicchillitti L, Filippetti F, Gallo D et al (2005) The secotaxane IDN5390 is able to target class III β-tubulin and to overcome paclitaxel resistance. Cancer Res 65(6):2397–2405
169. Kamath K, Wilson L, Cabral F, Jordan MA (2005) βIII-tubulin induces paclitaxel resistance in association with reduced effects on microtubule dynamic instability. J Biol Chem 280(13):12902–12907
170. Sève P, Isaac S, Trédan O, Souquet P-J, Pachéco Y, Pérol M et al (2005) Expression of Class III β-Tubulin Is Predictive of Patient Outcome in Patients with Non–Small Cell Lung Cancer Receiving Vinorelbine-Based Chemotherapy. Clin Cancer Res 11(15):5481–5486
171. Leandro-García LJ, Leskelä S, Inglada-Pérez L, Landa I, de Cubas AA, Maliszewska A et al (2012) Hematologic β-tubulin VI isoform exhibits genetic variability that influences paclitaxel toxicity. Cancer Res 72(18):4744–4752
172. Huzil JT, Ludueña RF, Tuszynski J (2006) Comparative modelling of human β tubulin isotypes and implications for drug binding. Nanotechnology 17(4):S90
173. Huzil JT, Chen K, Kurgan L, Tuszynski JA (2007) The roles of [beta]^2-tubulin mutations and isotype expression in acquired drug resistance. Cancer Informat 3:159–181
174. Szakács G, Paterson JK, Ludwig JA, Booth-Genthe C, Gottesman MM (2006) Targeting multidrug resistance in cancer. Nat Rev Drug Discov 5(3):219–234
175. Leonard GD, Fojo T, Bates SE (2003) The role of ABC transporters in clinical practice. Oncologist 8(5):411–424
176. Fojo AT, Menefee M (2005) editors. Microtubule targeting agents: basic mechanisms of multidrug resistance (MDR). Semin Oncol 32(6 Suppl 7):S3–S8
177. Trock BJ, Leonessa F, Clarke R (1997) Multidrug resistance in breast cancer: a meta-analysis of MDR1/gp170 expression and its possible functional significance. J Natl Cancer Inst 89(13):917–931
178. Noguchi S (2006) Predictive factors for response to docetaxel in human breast cancers. Cancer Sci 97(9):813–820
179. Bode CJ, Gupta ML, Reiff EA, Suprenant KA, Georg GI, Himes RH (2002) Epothilone and paclitaxel: unexpected differences in promoting the assembly and stabilization of yeast microtubules. Biochemistry 41(12):3870–3874
180. Agrawal M, Abraham J, Balis FM, Edgerly M, Stein WD, Bates S et al (2003) Increased 99mTc-sestamibi accumulation in normal liver and drug-resistant tumors after the administration of the glycoprotein inhibitor, XR9576. Clin Cancer Res 9(2):650–656
181. Loganzo F, Hari M, Annable T, Tan X, Morilla DB, Musto S et al (2004) Cells resistant to HTI-286 do not overexpress P-glycoprotein but have reduced drug accumulation and a point mutation in α-tubulin. Mol Cancer Ther 3(10):1319–1327
182. Pusztai L, Wagner P, Ibrahim N, Rivera E, Theriault R, Booser D et al (2005) Phase II study of tariquidar, a selective P-glycoprotein inhibitor, in patients with chemotherapy-resistant, advanced breast carcinoma. Cancer 104(4):682–691
183. Weingarten MD, Lockwood AH, Hwo S-Y, Kirschner MW (1975) A protein factor essential for microtubule assembly. Proc Natl Acad Sci 72(5):1858–1862
184. Kar S, Fan J, Smith MJ, Goedert M, Amos LA (2003) Repeat motifs of tau bind to the insides of microtubules in the absence of taxol. EMBO J 22(1):70–77
185. Andre F, Hatzis C, Anderson K, Sotiriou C, Mazouni C, Mejia J et al (2007) Microtubule-associated protein-tau is a bifunctional predictor of endocrine sensitivity and chemotherapy resistance in estrogen receptor–positive breast cancer. Clin Cancer Res 13(7):2061–2067
186. Pusztai L, Jeong J-H, Gong Y, Ross JS, Kim C, Paik S et al (2009) Evaluation of microtubule-associated protein-Tau expression as a prognostic and predictive marker in the NSABP-B 28 randomized clinical trial. J Clin Oncol 27(26):4287–4292
187. Smoter M, Bodnar L, Duchnowska R, Stec R, Grala B, Szczylik C (2011) The role of Tau protein in resistance to paclitaxel. Cancer Chemother Pharmacol 68(3):553–557

188. Rouzier R, Rajan R, Wagner P, Hess KR, Gold DL, Stec J et al (2005) Microtubule-associated protein tau: a marker of paclitaxel sensitivity in breast cancer. Proc Natl Acad Sci U S A 102(23):8315–8320
189. Gschwind A, Fischer OM, Ullrich A (2004) The discovery of receptor tyrosine kinases: targets for cancer therapy. Nat Rev Cancer 4(5):361–370
190. Yarden Y, Sliwkowski MX (2001) Untangling the ErbB signalling network. Nat Rev Mol Cell Biol 2(2):127–137
191. Graus-Porta D, Beerli RR, Daly JM, Hynes NE (1997) ErbB-2, the preferred heterodimerization partner of all ErbB receptors, is a mediator of lateral signaling. EMBO J 16(7): 1647–1655
192. Ross JS, Slodkowska EA, Symmans WF, Pusztai L, Ravdin PM, Hortobagyi GN (2009) The HER-2 receptor and breast cancer: ten years of targeted anti–HER-2 therapy and personalized medicine. Oncologist 14(4):320–368
193. Pusztai L (2007) Markers predicting clinical benefit in breast cancer from microtubule-targeting agents. Ann Oncol 18(suppl 12):xii15–xii20
194. Ambudkar SV, Kimchi-Sarfaty C, Sauna ZE, Gottesman MM (2003) P-glycoprotein: from genomics to mechanism. Oncogene 22(47):7468–7485
195. Geney R, Ungureanu IM, Li D, Ojima I (2002) Overcoming multidrug resistance in taxane chemotherapy. Clin Chem Lab Med 40(9):918–925
196. Galmarini C, Kamath K, Vanier-Viornery A, Hervieu V, Peiller E, Falette N et al (2003) Drug resistance associated with loss of p53 involves extensive alterations in microtubule composition and dynamics. Br J Cancer 88(11):1793–1799
197. Kavallaris M, Burkhart C, Horwitz S (1999) Antisense oligonucleotides to class III β-tubulin sensitize drug-resistant cells to Taxol. Br J Cancer 80(7):1020
198. Gordaliza M (2007) Natural products as leads to anticancer drugs. Clin Transl Oncol 9(12):767–776
199. Newman DJ, Cragg GM, Snader KM (2003) Natural products as sources of new drugs over the period 1981-2002. J Nat Prod 66(7):1022–1037
200. Clardy J, Walsh C (2004) Lessons from natural molecules. Nature 432(7019):829–837
201. Glaser KB (2007) HDAC inhibitors: clinical update and mechanism-based potential. Biochem Pharmacol 74(5):659–671
202. Brito DA, Yang Z, Rieder CL (2008) Microtubules do not promote mitotic slippage when the spindle assembly checkpoint cannot be satisfied. J Cell Biol 182(4):623–629
203. Ganguly A, Yang H, Cabral F (2010) Paclitaxel-dependent cell lines reveal a novel drug activity. Mol Cancer Ther 9(11):2914–2923
204. Mukhtar E, Adhami VM, Mukhtar H (2014) Targeting microtubules by natural agents for cancer therapy. Mol Cancer Ther 13(2):275–284
205. Hood KA, West LM, Rouwé B, Northcote PT, Berridge MV, Miller JH (2002) Peloruside A, a novel antimitotic agent with paclitaxel-like microtubule-stabilizing activity. Cancer Res 62(12):3356–3360
206. Huang GS, Lopez-Barcons L, Freeze BS, Smith AB, Goldberg GL, Horwitz SB et al (2006) Potentiation of taxol efficacy by discodermolide in ovarian carcinoma xenograft-bearing mice. Clin Cancer Res 12(1):298–304
207. Isbrucker RA, Cummins J, Pomponi SA, Longley RE, Wright AE (2003) Tubulin polymerizing activity of dictyostatin-1, a polyketide of marine sponge origin. Biochem Pharmacol 66(1):75–82
208. Vijayakumar S, Menakha M (2015) Pharmaceutical applications of cyanobacteria—A review. JACME 5(1):15–23
209. Gordaliza M, Garcıa P, Del Corral JM, Castro M, Gómez-Zurita M (2004) Podophyllotoxin: distribution, sources, applications and new cytotoxic derivatives. Toxicon 44(4):441–459
210. Verdier-Pinard P, Lai J-Y, Yoo H-D, Yu J, Marquez B, Nagle DG et al (1998) Structure-activity analysis of the interaction of curacin A, the potent colchicine site antimitotic agent, with tubulin and effects of analogs on the growth of MCF-7 breast cancer cells. Mol Pharmacol 53(1):62–76

211. Lu Y, Li C-M, Wang Z, Ross CR, Chen J, Dalton JT et al (2009) Discovery of 4-substituted methoxybenzoyl-aryl-thiazole as Novel Anticancer Agents: Synthesis, biological evaluation, and structure – activity relationships. J Med Chem 52(6):1701–1711
212. Hadaschik BA, Ettinger S, Sowery RD, Zoubeidi A, Andersen RJ, Roberge M et al (2008) Targeting prostate cancer with HTI-286, a synthetic analog of the marine sponge product hemiasterlin. Int J Cancer 122(10):2368–2376
213. Salmon HW, Siemann DW (2006) Effect of the second-generation vascular disrupting agent OXi4503 on tumor vascularity. Clin Cancer Res 12(13):4090–4094
214. Eskens F, Tresca P, Tosi D, Van Doorn L, Fontaine H, Van der Gaast A et al (2014) A phase I pharmacokinetic study of the vascular disrupting agent ombrabulin (AVE8062) and docetaxel in advanced solid tumours. Br J Cancer 110(9):2170–2177
215. Rudek MA, Dasari A, Laheru D, He P, Jin R, Walker R et al (2016) Phase 1 Study of ABT-751 in Combination With CAPIRI (Capecitabine and Irinotecan) and Bevacizumab in Patients With Advanced Colorectal Cancer. J Clin Pharmacol 56(8):966–973
216. Ma T, Fuld AD, Rigas JR, Hagey AE, Gordon GB, Dmitrovsky E et al (2012) A phase I trial and in vitro studies combining ABT-751 with carboplatin in previously treated non-small cell lung cancer patients. Chemotherapy 58(4):321–329
217. Traina T, Hudis C, Seidman A, Gajria D, Gonzalez J, Anthony S et al (2012) Abstract P6-11-10: IBL2001: Phase I/II study of a novel dose-dense schedule of oral indibulin for the treatment of metastastic breast cancer. Cancer Res 72(24 Supplement):P6-11-0-P6--0
218. Nahrwold M, Weiß C, Bogner T, Mertink F, Conradi J, Sammet B et al (2013) Conjugates of modified cryptophycins and RGD-peptides enter target cells by endocytosis. J Med Chem 56(5):1853–1864

New Challenges in Cancer Therapy: MAPK Inhibitors from Bench to Bedside

Catherine Ropert and Hugo W. Huth

Abstract The mitogen-activated protein kinases (MAPKs) belong to a family of serine/threonine kinases which transduce the signals by post-translational modifications of different downstream effectors and transcription factors involved in different aspects of the cell life, such as proliferation, migration, differentiation and death. The deregulation of MAPK pathways is well correlated with cancer development. Recent advancements made in genetics, genomics and proteomics have provided a better understanding of the mechanisms involved in tumor progression and have confirmed the relevance of aiming MAPKs as novel therapeutic targets in cancer. Indeed, different MAPK inhibitors are currently under investigation demonstrating the potential of such compounds in cancer therapy. Here, we present the latest advances involving MAPK inhibitors in clinical trials, and we summarize key parameters for the translation of results from bench to bedside.

Keywords Cancer therapy • MAPK • MAPK inhibitor • Signaling pathway • Tumor heterogeneity

Introduction

Cancer is a multifaceted and genomically complex disease and rapidly expanding information related to subtype-specific molecular abnormalities has revolutionized the development of molecular diagnostics for cancer subtypes and rationally designed therapeutics tailored to patients based on the molecular profiles of their tumors [1, 2]. Recent breakthroughs in unbiased genome wide association studies

C. Ropert (✉)
Departamento de Bioquímica e Imunologia, Instituto de Ciências Biológicas, Universidade Federal de Minas Gerais, Belo Horizonte, Minas Gerais 31270-910, Brazil

Departamento de Morfologia, Instituto de Ciências Biológicas, Universidade Federal de Minas Gerais, Belo Horizonte, Minas Gerais 31270-910, Brazil
e-mail: ropertcatherine@gmail.com

H.W. Huth
Departamento de Morfologia, Universidade Federal de Minas Gerais, Belo Horizonte, Minas Gerais 31270-910, Brazil

A.A. Farooqi, M. Ismail (eds.), *Molecular Oncology: Underlying Mechanisms and Translational Advancements*, DOI 10.1007/978-3-319-53082-6_3

have helped in the identification of previously unrecognized genetic predisposing factors which are contributory to an individual's risk of developing cancer [2, 3]. Furthermore, over the past several years, analyses of data from high-throughput studies of somatic alterations of the genomic and transcriptomic landscapes in tumors have provided convincing evidence related to intracellular signaling cascades which are characteristically dysregulated in cancer subtypes [4, 5]. Tumor cells have evolved different mechanisms to escape from apoptosis. Imbalance of pro-apoptotic and anti-apoptotic proteins also plays instrumental role in cancer development [4, 6–8]. p53 protein is involved in positive regulation of apoptotic pathway [9–11]. Substantial fraction of information has been added into the pre-existing pool of knowledge and it is now more understandable that dysregulations of spatio-temporally controlled signaling cascades, existence of significant inter-tumoral and intra-tumoral heterogeneity,genetic/epigenetic mutations are some of the most widely studied mechanisms which underlie cancer development. Moreover, different mechanisms including loss of apoptosis, Darwinian evolution in response to therapeutic pressures and highly intricate multi-directional spread of metastatically competent cancer cells from primary site to the metastatic sites are also being widely studied.

Many of the signals transduced intracellularly through different receptors and environmental cues converge on mitogen-activated protein kinases (MAPKs), which phosphorylate and activate different downstream effectors and transcription factors. MAPKs are members of a dynamic and hierarchially organized protein kinase network through which signals from the respective MAPK are transduced to the specific spatio-temporal cellular loci.

In this context, a growing interest in a better understanding of the signaling pathways involved in cancer has created new avenues for the identification and development of new anticancer drugs at molecular level. Here, we present challenges and opportunities in the targeting of MAPKs in cancer.

MAPK Signaling Pathway in Cancer

Mitogen Protein Activated-Kinases (MAPKs), that comprise a serine/threonine kinase group, are among most deeply studied signal transduction pathways. The MAPK pathways present in all eukaryotic cells respond to a plethora of extracellular stimuli and control many biological activities like gene expression, mitosis, metabolism, migration, survival, apoptosis, and differentiation [12–14]. A canonical MAPK pathway consists of a three-kinase module in which a MAPK is activated upon phosphorylation on threonine and tyrosine residues by a mitogen-activated protein kinase kinase (MAPKK), when phosphorylated by a MAPKKK (Fig. 1). Once activated, the MAPK may translocate to the nucleus to activate transcription factors and induce a biological response [15]. This assembly of MAPK pathways in a three-component module has been conserved from yeast to humans. The MAPK network includes extracellular signal-regulated kinase (ERK), p38 mitogen-activated protein kinase (p38), c-Jun N-terminal kinase (JNK). MAPK pathways play

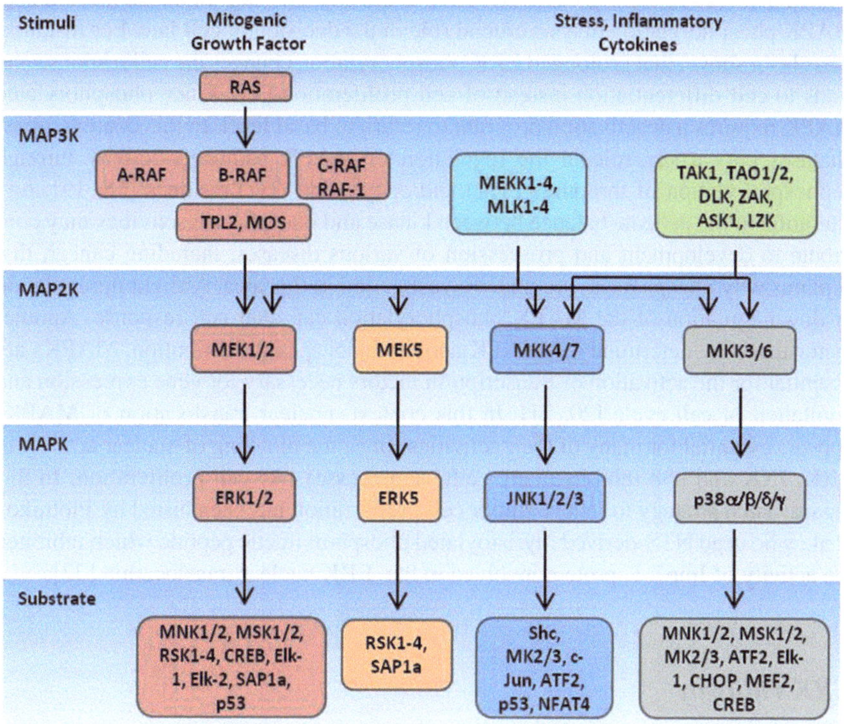

Fig. 1 Schematic representation of the different MAPK signaling pathway. The various upstream activators of ERKs, JNKs and p38 MAPKs, such as MAP2K and MAP3K family members, are depicted in the figure. ERK pathway is mainly activated through growth factors while p38 and JNK pathways are defined as stress pathways and consequently activated by environmental stress and inflammatory cytokines. The phosphorylation of MAPK leads to transcription factor activation in the nucleus. Notably, the same transcription factor can be activated by different MAPKs. All the three MAPKs may be involved in the proliferative activity, cell survival or proapoptotic function depending on cell type, MAPK isoform and transcription factor activated

important roles in normal cellular physiology, but the tumorigenesis process "captures" and also uses MAPKs to continuously transmit survival signals to the nucleus [16]. Besides, ERK5 and other atypical MAPKs like ERK3/4, ERK7 have been described. But, ERK1/2, JNKs, and p38 isoforms represent the most studied mammalian MAPKs that is why we focused on these three later MAPKs.

While ERK pathway links preferentially to cell proliferation, differentiation, and death, JNK and p38 MAPK pathways participate in stress signaling thus promoting an inflammatory response as depicted in the Fig. 1. As the association between chronic inflammation and cancer development has been evidenced, an important part for these stress-activated kinases in cancer has emerged. However, besides their involvement in inflammation, the role of JNK and p38 as a regulator of cell proliferation and apoptosis must be considered.

Different parameters govern the MAPK activity. Among them, the duration of MAPK phosphorylation plays a crucial role in the decision of cell fate. For instance, it has been shown that prolonged ERK phosphorylation changes the cell response and leads to cell differentiation instead of cell proliferation [17]. Once phosphorylated MAPK requires a deactivation program to return to basal level. In this context, phosphatases play a key role in the regulation of MAPK pathways activity through dephosphorylation of threonine (Thr) and/or tyrosine (Tyr) residues [18, 19]. Any alteration in the delicate balance between kinase and phosphatase activities may contribute to development and progression of various diseases, including cancer, that explains why phosphatases are under investigation in this area. A slight upregulation or downregulation of the MAPK phosphorylation can alter cell response. Another factor that may determine the MAPK activity is its spatial distribution. MAPKs are essential for the activation of transcription factors necessary for gene expression and regulation of cell cycle [20, 21]. In this context, nuclear translocation of MAPKs appears essential for many of their activities, since the blocking of nuclear activity of ERK, JNK and p38 inhibits many cellular processes like cell proliferation. In this regard, such strategy to reduce tumor cell proliferation has been tested by Plotnikov et al., who used NTS-derived myristoylated phosphomimetic peptide which inhibited the activity of Imp7, a protein involved in the ERK nuclear translocation [22].

ERK Pathway

ERK1 was the first mammalian MAPK to be cloned and characterized [23–26]. It was originally found to be phosphorylated on Tyr and Thr residues in response to growth factors [25, 27, 28]. The ERK signalling pathway is activated by an array of receptor types, including receptor tyrosine kinases (RTKs), G protein-coupled receptors and cytokine receptors [29, 30]. The core of this pathway is involved in activation of the cascade of RAF, MEK, and ERK. Although this cascade is classically shown as linear, its representation should take into account the complexity of the signaling network. Indeed, this is illustrated by the convergence of signaling at MEK1/2 level as presented in the Fig. 1. Besides the RAF proteins (A-RAF, B-RAF and C-RAF) that are the best-studied MEK activators, a number of other MAP kinase kinase kinases (MAP3Ks) like MEKK1or MEKK2 may activate MEK1/2.

The RAF proteins have been intensely studied over the past years, and most of the studies have been focused on C-RAF. Then, with the discovery of B-RAF mutations involved in a large number of tumors, B-RAF has received more attention, specifically in melanomas. However, very little is known about A-RAF. Differences in function and tissue expression among RAF isoforms have been evidenced. For example, B-RAF is frequently overexpressed in cells of neuronal origin [31]. The activation of RAF triggered by various signals like RAS GTPases [21, 32] appears complex and involves phosphorylation/dephosphorylation cycle before reaching the activated state. Importantly, it has been shown that B-RAF requires fewer phosphorylation events than A-RAF and C-RAF for maximal activation [33]. The ability to activate MEK in vitro also differs depending on the isoform: B-RAF is the strongest inducer of MEK activation, followed by C-RAF and A-RAF whose MEK activity is merely detected [34]. Later, it has been reported that heterodimerization was crucial to promote the RAF activity. Indeed, Rushworth et al. have demonstrated that B-RAF and C-RAF heterodimerize in multiple cell lines in response to mitogens [35]. This supports the hypothesis of Matallanas et al. suggesting that C-RAF and A-RAF may act as modulators to enhance the ability of B-RAF to activate the ERK pathway [36]. This pathway is highly regulated as illustrated by the ERK-mediated feedback phosphorylation of B-RAF reducing the lifetime of C-RAF/B-RAF heterodimers [35, 37]. In some other way, ERK may act directly on RAS reducing the efficiency of the RAS/C-RAF association and renders ERK activation transient [38].

Concerning MEK1 and MEK2 kinase isoforms that are directly responsible for the activation of ERK, it has also been assumed that they may have different functions. In fact, the absence of MEK1 provoked an embryonic lethality of the *MEK1*$^{-}$/$^{-}$ mice [39]. By contrast, *MEK2*$^{-}$/$^{-}$ mice are viable and fertile [40]. But, more recently, Aoidi et al. [41] have changed this equation by describing the contribution of both MEK1 and MEK2 in the placenta development and embryo survival. According to this study, a minimal amount of MEK protein, independently of which isoform, was required for embryo survival.

In cell model, by depleting either MEK subtype by siRNA, it was reported that downregulation of MEK1 expression inhibited pancreatic cancer cells and induced G0/G1 arrest [42]. In colon cancer line or pancreatic cancer line, the lack of MEK1 induced an upregulation of MEK2 activity and a sustained strong ERK activity leading to growth arrest. By contrast, when MEK1 activity became predominant as in the absence of MEK2, ERK pathway activation induced cell proliferation [43]. Recently, a differential function for MEK1 and MEK2 has been evidenced in breast cancer cells. The authors have shown that the depletion of MEK2 but not MEK1 reduced the cyclin D1 expression leading to decreased cell survival. Further, the authors have described a link between MEK2 and p38 pathway never described in normal cells [44]. MEK1 and MEK2 are phosphorylated by RAF or MAP3K at Serine (Ser) 218 and Ser 222 and Ser 222 and Ser 226, respectively. Both isoforms have a strategic position in ERK pathway since they are considered the only activators of ERK1/2. MEK1 and MEK2 have been noted to exist as heterodimers. ERK is involved in phosphorylation of MEK1 on Thr292 that impedes the formation of MEK1/MEK2 heterodimers, and promotes dephosphorylation of activating residues Ser 218 and Ser 222 [45, 46]. The direct consequence of the MEK1 phosphorylation is a reduction of MEK1/2 activity and consequently of ERK activation illustrating another negative feedback of ERK on this pathway.

Concerning ERK1 and ERK2 isoforms, different debates are still in progress about functional difference or functional redundancy between them. As inhibitors of B-RAF and MEK1/2 have been approved for the treatment of cancer and they are expected to inhibit their downstream effectors ERK1 and ERK2, it is crucial to understand whether the two isoforms exert specific or redundant functions. Several studies have claimed a redundant role for both isoforms, in which generally, the methodological approach was the reduction of ERK1 and/or ERK2 to clarify their role in cells. Single and combined silencing of ERK1 and ERK2 have shown that their decisive role in growth signaling depend on their expression levels [47]. In other way, Vantaggiato et al. have suggested that ERK1 and ERK2 may assume opposite functions in RAS-mediated signaling since ERK1 negatively regulates the signal induced by ERK2 [48]. Shin et al. have defined that downregulation of ERK2 but not ERK1, abolish oncogenic RAS-induced senescence [49]. In the same way, other groups have demonstrated that ERK2 but not ERK1 depletion significantly reduces global ERK activity that corroborates with the absence of effect on ERK activity after ERK1 knockdown [50, 51]. Importantly, ERK2 is generally more expressed than ERK1 in most mammalian tissues. Such observations address the use of silencing methods to define ERK1 or ERK2 role due to their differential expression in tissues. In addition, this may explain why the impact of ERK2 silencing appears more pronounced in different models; however, the role of ERK1 cannot be neglected as suggested by Frémin et al. [52]. They have demonstrated that the loss of functions due to ERK2 deficiency may be rescued by overexpression of ERK1 and have concluded that ERK1 and ERK2 exert redundant functions in mouse development. The same remains to be demonstrated in cancer or in others diseases. Interestingly, Buscà et al. propose a new concept where total ERK activity and not isoform itself is the critical parameter to achieve ERK functions [53].

The ERK cascade plays a crucial role in multiple cellular processes involved in cell fate [30, 54, 55]. Importantly, the RAS-RAF-MEK-ERK1/2 pathway is one of the most dysregulated signaling pathways in human cancer. For instance, B-RAF mutation frequently occurs in certain types of cancers such as melanoma (50–80% of cases), papillary thyroid carcinoma (~45%), hepatocellular carcinoma (~40%) and colorectal cancer (~10%) [56, 57]. The direct consequence of RAF mutation might be the constitutive activation of ERK1/2. But, constitutive ERK activation is not necessarily linked to mutated component of this pathway. Other factors like epigenetic factors may also play a role in the dysregulation of ERK pathway. The high incidence of human cancers with a constitutively active ERK pathway has encouraged the research of pharmacological inhibitors able to efficiently target different regulators of this cascade.

JNK Pathway

JNK was described, almost 20 years ago, as the protein kinase responsible for activating c-Jun which is a component of the activating protein-1 (AP-1) transcription factor family that may be involved in malignant transformation [58]. Besides, JNK was defined as a stress-activated kinase responding to a large panel of stimuli leading to the production of cytokine, and consequently to the development of chronic inflammation [59]. JNK can be phosphorylated by two distinct MAPKK, MKK4, and MKK7, which cooperate in the JNK activation. In turn, MKK4/7 are phosphorylated by a plethora of MAKKKs, including MEKK1 to −4, MLK1 to −3, Tpl-2, DLK, TAO1/2, TAK1 and ASK1/2 [13, 14]. It has been described, up to now, three JNK isoforms, JNK1/2/3, which have about 85% of homology, but their tissue distribution may vary [60]. While JNK1 and JNK2 are distributed in different organs, JNK3 is mostly expressed in neuronal tissues, testis, and cardiomyocytes, probably predicting functional differences [61]. It has been stated by Gupta et al. that JNK isoforms may act individually on specific transcription factors in vivo. Indeed, JNK2 seems to have a stronger affinity for c-Jun and induces a higher proliferative activity when compared to JNK1 [62].

JNK has been reported to play a significant role in various diseases. In cancer, for instance, JNK seems to have an ambiguous position, acting like a proliferative or death inducer, depending on cell type, tumor stage, and isoform [59]. For example, activation of JNK1 was essential for tumorigenesis in response to RAS activation induced by UV radiation. Furthermore, in childhood sarcoma, JNK1 appeared crucial for cell proliferation, while JNK2 might induce apoptosis [63]. In the same way, another study has suggested that JNK2, in contrast to JNK1, downregulated cellular proliferation in a wide range of cell models [64]. Also, JNK3 was described as an apoptosis inducer in chemoresistant human ovarian cancer cells [65]. In mouse models, the lack of JNK1 or JNK2 favored the development of breast cancer. However, JNK1-deficient mice presented a decrease in gastric carcinogenesis compared to their wild-type counterparts [66]. Mice lacking of JNK1 in the liver were less susceptible than wild-type animals to hepatocellular carcinoma [67]. Considering the different studies cited above it clearly appears that there is no consensus concerning the role of JNK isoforms in tumor cell physiology. These discrepancies must be explained by the use of gene silencing technique which may bias the interpretation of the results. This underlines the necessity to use diverse tools of investigation to better define kinase functions [68] before targeting JNK in cancer. In any case, a selective role of different JNK isoforms depending on tumor types should be further investigated.

p38 Pathway

The p38 MAPK was first identified in 1994 and reportedly triggered by stress stimuli like inflammatory cytokines, UV irradiation, hypoxia, and ischemia. The activation of p38 occurs via its upstream kinase MKK3/MKK6, but MKK4 may also activate p38. MKK3/6 are activated by a plethora of MAPKKKs, including MEKK1 to −3, MLK2/3, ASK1, Tpl2, TAK1, and TAO1/2. The MAPKKK responsible for activating the p38 MAPK pathways appears to be cell type and stimulus-specific [13, 14]. After the identification of p38 (also known as p38α), three other isoforms were also described: p38β/δ/γ, [69]. MKK6 can activate all isoforms of p38, while MKK3 are responsible for phosphorylating preferentially p38α, γ and δ. An important fact is that the expression of these isoforms varies from tissue to tissue: p38α is found in almost all cell types, while p38β is more brain-tissue specific, p38γ is expressed in skeletal muscle and p38δ in endocrine glands [70].

p38 has a key role in the inflammatory response [71, 72]. Once activated, p38 pathway induces the synthesis of pro-inflammatory cytokines by modulating transcriptional factors implicated in cancer development [70]. More precisely, α and β isoforms of p38 are predominant in chronic inflammation [73]. Interestingly, these same isoforms are involved in breast cancer progression, maybe due to their inflammatory properties [74]. Besides, p38 is also involved in cell cycle, controlling its proliferation and survival. In fact, p38 may regulate both the G2/M as well as G1/S cell cycle checkpoint [75–77]. In cancer, the role of p38 is not completely understood [78]. There are several studies describing p38 as a proliferative agent [74, 79]; on the other hand, some studies have defined p38 as an apoptosis inducer [80–82]. Notably, p38 may directly affect tumor growth independently of its role in inflammation. In most of the studies concerning prostate cancers, cancer cells require the activity of p38 to proliferate, indicating that p38 may act as proto-oncogenic protein [83, 84]. Furthermore, overexpression of p38 in its phosphorylated form is also associated with a bad prognosis and with high morbidity rate in colorectal cancer [85]. Besides, analysis of the phenotype of MKK3/6$^{-/-}$ and p38α$^{-/-}$ mice has led to the conclusion that p38 can function as a tumor suppressor. The tumor suppressive effects of p38 may be mediated in different ways since p38 is involved both in the induction of p53-dependent apoptosis and in the negative control of cell cycle progression. A reduction of p38 activity has been shown in hepatocellular carcinomas, where an inverse correlation was established between tumor size and p38 activity. This ambiguous role of p38 pathway may occur due to the existence of four isoforms (p38α/β/δ/γ) acting independently and sometimes leading to opposite effects. The absence of selective p38 isoform inhibitors adds another layer of complexity to intricate crosstalk between proteins of different networks in cancer cells. The heterogeneity of cancer cells and its variable genomic mutations may also contribute to the ambiguous p38 pathway function in cancer cells.

As related above, the properties of ERKs, JNKs, and p38s to provoke cell death or to induce cell proliferation are tumor-dependent indicating that there are no rules concerning their role in cancer.

What Is a "Good" MAPK Inhibitor?

Current efforts to discover kinase inhibitors are concentrated on fundamental hallmarks of cancers like excessive cell proliferation, increased survival or tumor angiogenesis. As reported above, an extensive literature supported a role for MAPKs in these different cellular events and opened new horizons to explore their potential as a therapeutic target in cancer.

Specificity Towards Binding Site

The development of specific MAPK inhibitors themselves has been less successful and only a few compounds have been identified. Interestingly, the idea that MAPK pathways would represent drug targets in cancer therapy emerged in the mid-1990s by the characterization of SB203580 as a selective p38 inhibitor that downregulated TNF-α [71]. The first step towards kinase inhibitor development was selection of ATP cleft as target site. Indeed, binding of ATP to a protein kinase is essential for the kinase's phosphotransferase activity, and thus, the ATP binding pocket was the "target" of most inhibitor screens [86, 87]. The majority of MAPK inhibitors belongs to class of ATP-competitive inhibitors that recognizes the active conformation of the kinase. Accordingly, many compounds have been tested in vitro using enzymatic assays in which kinases were in their active conformation and the strategy to synthesize MAPK inhibitors was to mimic ATP structure. The common problem with kinase inhibitors that compete with ATP binding is their lack of specificity since the ATP-binding pocket is highly conserved among members of the kinase family. This is illustrated by the anthrapyrazole SP600125, one of the earliest and most studied ATP-competitive JNK inhibitor, that has been shown to inhibit 13 other protein kinases [88]. SB203580 represents the other most famous MAPK inhibitor that binds to ATP-binding pocket [71]. But, interestingly, this inhibitor may recognize the active and inactive conformation of the kinase [89]. The binding of a drug to the inactive conformation of the kinase is becoming an attractive approach. The major advantage of this strategy is that the inhibitor will face weaker competition from cellular ATP and even for those classified as ATP-competitive inhibitors. They may act by shifting the equilibrium between inactive and active kinase conformation impeding kinase activation. It has been proposed that SB203580 could stabilize p38α in its inactive conformation that reduces the rate of p38 phosphorylation by MAPKK. This additional mechanism of action of SB203580 may explain its relative specificity towards p38α.

Alternative strategies to inhibit MAP kinase function are currently under investigation. For example, compounds that bind outside the ATP-binding site—at an allosteric site (regulatory site)—and modulate kinase activity in an allosteric manner may represent an attractive alternative. Inhibitors from this category generally exhibit the greatest kinase selectivity because they bind to sites that are specific to a particular kinase. The most well described allosteric kinase inhibitor is CI-1040 (PD184352), previously described by Sebolt-Leopold et al., which decreases MEK1 and MEK2 activity by occupying a pocket adjacent to the ATP binding site [90]. Interestingly, a lot of new MEK1/2 inhibitors belong to this family [91, 92].

Small molecule and peptide-based inhibitors that target the docking site of downstream substrates or the scaffold proteins involved in MAPK cascade are a promising alternative to the traditional ATP-competitive inhibitors with improved efficacy and specificity. For example, JNK-interacting protein-1 (JIP1), a scaffolding protein that promotes JNK activity by facilitating the interaction between JNK and upstream kinases [93, 94] may be a relevant target in cancer. With this focus, a peptide corresponding to the minimal region of JIP1 (pepJIP1) has been developed as an inhibitor of JNK activity by reducing the interaction between JIP1 and JNK [95, 96]. It has been shown that cell-permeable JIP1-based peptides may help to resolve some JNK-dependent diseases. But, several limitations have interfered with the development of peptide-based inhibitors due to physiochemical instability and unsatisfactory pharmacological properties. Other compounds that inhibit the interaction between JIP1 and JNKs have also been characterized that may represent a promising strategy in therapy [97].

Another different way to inhibit protein kinase activity may be targeting of protein substrate binding site to inhibit the activation of downstream kinase or transcription factor phosphorylation. This strategy may have many advantages because this type of inhibitor is specific for selected kinase substrates contrasting with the ATP-competitive inhibitors that would inhibit phosphorylation of all substrate proteins. The same specificity may be expected from the new approaches which include the use of inhibitors of kinase dimerization, as proposed by Herrero et al. In this study, efficiency of a peptide was evaluated which inhibited ERK dimerization and reduced tumor growth in xenografted mice [98]. Besides, as commented above, inhibitor of ERK translocation may represent prototype for the development of new cancer drug.

The challenge of making selective inhibitors with good pharmacological properties remains daunting due to the 518 kinases encoded in the human genome and over 2000 other nucleotide-dependent enzymes, including chaperones, polymerases, reductases, motor proteins and methyltransferases, that may provide potential binding sites [99]. In addition, natural variation in the expression levels of kinases can indirectly alter inhibitor efficiency by changing the total kinase activity in the cell. Kinase inhibitors have been classically tested at the protein level for their potential to inhibit kinase-catalysed phosphotransfer from ATP to a substrate protein or peptide that may sometimes explain their low selectivity. Due to the constraints encountered in cells, the screening of new potential inhibitors may involve not only kinase assays but also critical analysis of downstream effectors and substrates of these kinases in cells where specificity and sensitivity parameters may be evaluated before clinical trials.

Specificity Towards MAPK Isoform

The existence of different isoforms for the same MAPK put into question their redundant or independent activities that may directly influence the MAPK inhibitor efficiency in cancer. This is the case of ERK1 and ERK2 functions, as related above. Such discrepancies may be explained by different cell response evaluated (proliferation, survival, inflammatory response, drug resistance). There are some outstanding questions related to biological outcome associated with the use of ERK isoform selective inhibitors. Up to now, inhibitors targeting ERK1 and ERK2 in an indiscriminate way are yet under investigation in the preclinical stage. The notion that global ERK inhibition would not be recommended in all situation is support by the fact that different studies have reported opposite roles for ERK1 and ERK2 in tumor biology [48, 49, 100, 101]. Interestingly, Aceves-Luquero et al. have involved ERK2 but not ERK1 in resistance to Imatinib Mesylate in a model of chronic myelogenous leukemia sustaining the use of therapeutic approaches based on ERK2 inhibition. ERK inhibitors have been tested in phase I and are ongoing in phase II of clinical trials. So, more related clinical studies should be performed in more advanced stages before the validation of inhibitors of both ERK isoforms as chemotherapeutic agent in cancer treatment.

Existing data clearly suggested that different JNK isoforms may have different or redundant functions in cancer cell [61, 62, 64, 68]. So it appears essential to define

Table 1 p38 pathway inhibitor in clinical trials

Target	Drug	Cancer type	Phase	Interpretation	Sponsor
p38α/β	Ralimetinib	Ovarian	2	Study is ongoing	Lilly Oncology (NCT01663857)
p38α/β	Ralimetinib	Advanced cancer	1	Completed	Eli Lilly and Company (NCT01393990)

when JNK isoforms may cooperate or play opposite role depending on cancer type and cancer stage. This reinforces the necessity to develop inhibitors with more selectivity towards JNK and its isoforms. Recently, it has been shown that JNK3 can be selectively targeted [102]. These results are encouraging and future studies must converge on identification and evaluation of JNK isoform inhibitors with minimum off target effects.

The preservation of the four p38 MAPK isoforms suggests a functional difference between them [69, 88, 103]. The broad body of literature has reported findings related to p38α and p38β. This is due to the fact that generally p38 inhibitors are more selective to α and β isoforms. This is well illustrated by the capacity of SB203580 to inhibit p38α and p38β but not p38γ and p38δ. The differences in chemical inhibitor sensitivity towards isoforms could be attributed to their different substrate specificities and expression patterns [73, 88]. There is only one global inhibitor of p38 described up to now, BIRB 796, that inhibits efficiently α and β isoforms and moderatly γ and δ isoform. But unfortunately, this compound also inhibits JNK2 isoform at the same concentration [88]. The recent interest in the role of p38δ in cancer was based on the fact that p38δ expression and activation were significantly increased in a variety of carcinoma cell lines such as human primary cutaneous squamous carcinoma cells [104], neck and head squamous carcinoma cells and tumors [105], cholangiocarcinoma, and liver cancer cell lines [106]. In the absence of specific inhibitor of p38 isoform, p38δ knocked-down mice were used to confirm the importance of this p38 isoform in the model of chemically induced skin carcinogenesis. These findings paved the way towards development of specific p38 inhibitor [107]. Unfortunately, until now, there are fewer studies related to the use of p38 inhibitors in clinical trials, as depicted in Table 1.

All together, these data show the pertinence to seek new selective inhibitors towards MAPK isoforms in order to clarify their redundant or different functions.

Use of MAPK Inhibitors in Clinical Trials: A Cycle of Hope and Disappointment

The possible use of MAPK pathway inhibitor in cancer has ushered in a new era. Nearly 50% of human malignancies exhibit dysregulated RAS-ERK signaling [32, 108, 109] that justifies the prevalence of clinical trials investigating RAF-ERK pathway inhibitors as shown in Table 2. Targeting of RAS protein was the initial strategy to control signaling pathway involved in tumor progression [110, 111]. However, RAS inhibition did not reach the expected results in clinical trials probably because these inhibitors were unable to target selective proteins. It is well known that mutations in RAS happen quite often in cancer patients. Mutation in RAS induced constitutive activation. In such context, the inhibition of RAS remains challenging.

Completed clinical trials of MEK inhibitors include some disappointments as well as some promising signs of the value of these compounds [92]. The potential for MEK inhibitors as monotherapy and their use in drug combination with RAF inhibitors are currently under clinical investigation and more frequently in melanoma (Table 2). At first, randomized Phase III clinical trial was conducted with the RAF inhibitor sorafenib (Nexavar; Bayer/Onyx Pharmaceuticals) in patients with metastatic melanoma [112, 113], including patients with tumors that carry the B-RAF^{V600E} mutation, but no antitumor activity was observed [114]. This may be because sorafenib, originally developed as a C-RAF and wild-type B-RAF inhibitor, appeared less efficient towards *B-RAF*^{V600E} [115]. Further, B-RAF^{V600E}-selective inhibitors like vemurafenib and dabrafenib entered in clinical trials. But, rapidly paradoxical effects have been noted particularly the activation of RAF instead of its inhibition in cells with wild-type B-RAF, when used at non-saturating concentrations [116].

The MAPK inhibitor saga continued with the use of MEK inhibitors [91]. Indeed, unlike B-RAF, activating mutations in MEK are more rarely encountered in human tumors. Selumetinib (AZD6244; AstraZeneca/Array Biopharma), another allosteric MEK1 and MEK2 inhibitor that is highly selective for MEK1 and MEK2 has been tested using different protocols in patients with biliary and pancreatic cancer [117, 118]. At first, a modest clinical activity of this compound has been reported. In metastatic melanoma, the therapy impact was also moderate but, the trials were not carried out in patients selected for activating mutations in B-RAF [119]. In fact, a correlation has been drawn between sensitivity to MEK inhibitor and the presence of mutations in B-RAF, since MEK inhibitors are more efficient in cells which carry B-RAF mutations [120, 121]. Reconsidering the first results obtained from studies that have been performed without patient selection and after further evaluation, trametinib (Mekinist, GSK1120212; GSK) became the first MEK1/MEK2 inhibitor to be approved by the US Food and Drug Administration (FDA) for the treatment of metastatic melanoma with the B-RAF$^{V600E/K}$ mutation [122]. Going downstream on ERK signaling pathway, there are few ERK inhibitors reported in clinical trials, but tests are just at the beginning and still ongoing. Carlino et al. have reported that inhibition of ERK, rather than MEK, was more efficient at reducing MAPK activity and inhibiting the proliferation of multiple B-RAF inhibitor resistant melanoma cell models but, without inducing cell death [123]. The efficiency of ERK inhibitors has been shown in cell lines in B-RAF/MEK inhibitor resistance model [124, 125]. But, the use of ERK inhibitor in monotherapy may represent a double edge sword. Indeed, the inhibition of ERK may cause the relief of ERK-dependent negative feedback, provoking a sustained activation of ERK cascade and the cell survival. One strategy to inhibit ERK-induced proliferation without affecting negative

Table 2 RAF-ERK pathway inhibitors in clinical trials

Target	Drug	Cancer type	Phase	Interpretation	Sponsor
B-RAF[a]	Vemurafenib	Melanoma	3	Inhibition of B-RAF with vemurafenib improves survival in patients with the most common B-RAF^{V600E} mutation and in patients with the less common B-RAF^{V600K} mutation	Hoffman (NCT01307397)
B-RAF[a] MEK1 and MEK2	Dabrafenib + trametinib vs. vemurafenib	Melanoma	3	Study is ongoing	GlaxoSmith Kline (NCT01597908)
B-RAF[a] MEK1 and MEK2	Dabrafenib in combination with trametinib	Melanoma	3	Modest clinical efficacy in patients with B-RAF inhibitor-resistant melanoma. Increased survival benefit	GlaxoSmith Kline (NCT01072175)
B-RAF[a] MEK1 and MEK2	Dabrafenib in combination with trametinib	Melanoma stage III–IV	2	Study is ongoing. Testing of the superiority of intermittent dosing of dabrafenib and trametinib compared to continuous dosing with these two same agents	National Cancer Institute (NCI) (NCT02196181)
MEK1 and MEK2	Trametinib	Melanoma	3	Increased survival in ongoing trials for B-RAF-mutated melanoma	GlaxoSmith Kline (NCT01245062)
MEK1 and MEK2 immunotherapy	Selumetinib in combination with durvalumab (MEDI4736)	Advanced solid tumors	1	Study is ongoing	AstraZeneca (NCT02586987)
MEK1 and MEK2	Binimetinib	Melanoma	3	Successful trials for mutant-N-RAS melanoma but lack efficacy in ovarian cancer	Array Biopharma (NCT01763164)
ERK1/2	BVD-523	Myelogenous Leukemia or Myelodysplastic Syndromes	1 and 2	Study is ongoing	BioMed Valley Discoveries (NCI201402600) (NCT02296242)

(continued)

Table 2 (continued)

Target	Drug	Cancer type	Phase	Interpretation	Sponsor
MEK1 and MEK2	Selumetinib	Thyroid	2	Well tolerated but the study was negative with regard to the primary outcome. Disappointing results	AstraZeneca (NCI 7918)
MEK1 and MEK2	RO4987655	B-RAF-mutated and non-mutated Melanoma, small cell lung, K-RAS-mutated colorectal	1	Manageable toxicity, a favorable pharmacokinetics/pharmacodynamics profile, and promising preliminary antitumor activity	Hoffmann-La Roche (NCT00817518)
B-RAF RAF and MEK1/2	Vemurafenib Cobimetinib	Melanoma	3	Improvement in progression-free survival among patients with *BRAF* V600–mutated metastatic melanoma, at the cost of some increase in toxicity	Hoffmann-La Roche (NCT01689519)
B-RAF RAF and MEK1/2	Binimetinib Encorafenib	Melanoma	3	Improvement in several clinically relevant endpoints was well tolerated and may offer a new treatment against *N-RAS*-mutant melanoma	Novartis Pharmaceuticals and ArrayBioPharm (NCT01909453)
MEK1 and MEK2	Trametinib	Low-grade ovarian and peritoneal cavity	2 and 3	Study is ongoing	National Cancer Institute (NCT02101788)
MEK1 and MEK2	Refametinib (BAY 86-8766)	Carcinoma hepatolceular	2	This study has been completed. No results published yet	Bayer/Ardea Biosciences (NCT01915589)
MEK1 and MEK2	Pimasertib (AS703026)	Metastatic solid tumors or locally advanced	1	This study has been completed	Merck KGaA (NCT01713036)

Target	Drug	Cancer type	Phase	Interpretation	Sponsor
MEK1 and MEK2	AZD8330	Patients with advanced malignancies with no described treatment	1	This study has been completed. No results published yet.	AstraZeneca (NCT00454090)
ERK	MK-8353/SCH900353	Metastatic melanoma or metastatic corectal cancer	1	This study has been completed. No results published yet	Merck Sharp & Dohme Corp. (NCT01358331)
ERK1/2	RG7842 (GDC0994)	Solid tumors	1	Study is ongoing	Genentech (NCT01875705)
ERK	CC-90003	Metastatic solid tumors or locally advanced	1	This study has been completed. No results published yet	Celgene Corporation (NCT02313012)

[a]Patients with B-RAF^{V600E} mutation-positive have been screened for eligibility

feedback loops, is to avoid ERK1/2 nuclear translocation [22]. This may offer a double advantage in reducing the activation of ERK substrates and at the same time maintaining ERK cytosolic effect like negative feedback loops.

The association of compounds acting at different levels on a same pathway has been tested as shown in the Table 2. The drug association was expected to present a superior efficiency than a single compound but, in long term treatment, resistance emerged either way. So, intermittent therapy has been considered as a strategy to delay the development of resistance mechanisms. Therefore, studies comparing intermittent dosing schedule and continuous treatment with patients treated with B-RAF and MEK inhibitors are ongoing. Other approach to delay resistance includes B-RAF and MEK targeted therapies in association with immunotherapy.

Resistance to MAPK Inhibitor Treatment

Resistance is still an important issue that restrains the long-term responsiveness of the majority of the patients to MAPK inhibitors. Different events may originate drug-resistance phenomenon like target mutation, intratumor heterogeneity, and crosstalk.

As many kinase inhibitors exert their apoptotic properties primarily by inhibiting a specific kinase, there is a strong selective pressure for cells to acquire resistance through mutations in the kinase gene that abolish drug binding. This is illustrated by resistance to the MEK inhibitor AZD6244 reported in melanoma patients that was associated with mutations in MEK1 [126]. MEK1 mutations have been identified to confer resistance to B-RAF inhibitor according to different studies [126, 127]. Recently, MEK2 mutations have also been involved in drug resistance [128–130]. The same occurred concerning ERK1 after long-term treatment with the ERK1/2 inhibitor SCH772984 [131]. Various strategies may be adopted to surmount the problem. One possibility is to develop kinase inhibitor that can tolerate mutation of one or two amino acids in the target. A second possibility is to target the kinase with an association of inhibitors that bind at alternative binding sites. Besides mutation, other change in drug target may occur like its expression that may be increased as exemplified in the study by Wang et al. which described an increase of K-RAS and MEK after long-term treatment with the MEK inhibitor CI-1040 [132] indicating that the inefficiency of a drug may be related to the overexpression of its target.

Resistance may also lead to the upregulation of alternative pathway. In the case of B-RAF inhibitor after long-term treatment, the acquired resistance has been associated with pathway switching, where MAPK signaling is forwarded from B-RAF to C-RAF [133]. In addition to MAPK pathway activation, resistant tumors often show the activation of PI3K/AKT/mTOR pathway [134, 135], this may explain why PI3K inhibitors was classically associated with MAPK inhibitors or other conventional drugs [136].

Surprisingly, some kinase inhibitors have presented paradoxical effects. This is the case of RAF inhibitors that has been reported to increase RAF activities. In the first study describing such paradoxical effect of RAF inhibitor, the authors concluded that RAF kinases suppress their own activation by engaging feedback loops in a MEK-dependent manner [137]. Thereafter, the increased RAF activity in the presence of RAF inhibitor in tumors with wild-type RAF isoforms has been explained by RAF dimerization, membrane localization and increased interaction of RAF with G-RAS [116]. However, it appears that the next generation of RAF inhibitors might evade paradoxical MAPK pathway activation [138]. In the same line, the paradoxical effect of ERK pathway inhibitors observed might be due to the existence of ERK negative feedback loop. The inhibition of ERK may cause the relief of ERK-dependent negative feedback, that may also provoke tumor resistance due to the reactivation of ERK pathway [35, 37].

Crosstalk between Signaling Pathways

Crosstalk between signaling pathways is a common event in cell regulation, which generally depends on cell context and plays a major role in the regulation of biological responses. This may be one of the greatest challenges of using MAPK inhibitors in cancer therapy, once crosstalk between different pathways may implicate an effect that, sometimes, cannot be predicted. A recent study published by Huth et al., described a new connection between MEK2 and p38, suggesting a crosstalk between ERK and p38 pathway [44]. Such phenomenon reveals a greater complexity of the ERK signaling cascade and may explain why ERK inhibition may not be an efficient strategy in all the cases. This illustrates the necessity to develop inhibitors of other MAPK pathways in cancer. In a similar way, Shimo et al. have also described a crosstalk between ERK and p38 pathway, wherein MEK1 inhibition by using PD98059 induced an upregulation of p38 activation [139]. Another interconnection between p38 and JNK pathways is often described due to the fact that both are stress pathways and share upstream activators [140]. Furthermore, crosstalk exists between MAPK and PI3K signaling pathways as cited above [136]. More precisely, MEK downregulation induced by the inhibitor PD0325901 enhances PI3K signaling [141]. Hence, crosstalk could be one of the most common cellular event responsible for drug-resistance phenomenon in cancer therapy. In such context, the association of different MAPK and PI3K inhibitors has been suggested to overcome drug resistance. Indeed, a synergy between both classes of inhibitor has been reported in different studies [142–144]. This kind of association could usefully be extended to the combination of different MAPK pathway inhibitors.

Tumor Heterogeneity

Up to now, research in cancer considers tumors as single entities and underestimates molecular diversity among the various cell types. Indeed, although solid tumors appear from a unique neoplastic cell, consequent mutations occur over time increasing tumor heterogeneity and its resistance to conventional chemotherapeutic drugs [145]. Tumor heterogeneity refers to the existence of subpopulations of cells with

16. Dhillon AS et al (2007) MAP kinase signalling pathways in cancer. Oncogene 26:3279–3290
17. Marshall C (1995) Specificity of receptor tyrosine kinase signaling: transient versus sustained extracellular signal-regulated kinase activation. Cell 80:179–185
18. Farooq A, Zhou MM (2004) Structure and regulation of MAPK phosphatases. Cell Signal 16:769–779
19. Keyse SM (2008) Dual-specificity MAP kinase phosphatases (MKPs) and cancer. Cancer Metastasis Rev 27:253–261
20. Cargnello M, Roux PP (2011) Activation and function of the MAPKs and their substrates, the MAPK-activated protein kinases. Microbiol Mol Biol Rev 75(1):50–83
21. Turjanski AG, Vaqué JP, Gutkind JS (2007) MAP kinases and the control of nuclear events. Oncogene 26:3240–3253
22. Plotnikov A et al (2015) The nuclear translocation of ERK1/2 as an anticancer target. Nat Commun 6:6685
23. Boulton TG et al (1990) An insulin-stimulated protein kinase similar to yeast kinases involved in cell cycle control. Science 249(4964):64–67
24. Cooper JA et al (1982) Similar effects of platelet-derived growth factor and epidermal growth factor on the phosphorylation of tyrosine in cellular proteins. Cell 31:263–273
25. Kazlauskas A, Cooper JA (1988) Protein kinase C mediates platelet-derived growth factor-induced tyrosine phosphorylation of p42. J Cell Biol 106:1395–1402
26. Widmann C et al (1999) Mitogen-activated protein kinase: conservation of a three-kinase module from yeast to human. Physiol Rev 79(1):143–180
27. Dérijard B et al (1995) Independent human MAP-kinase signal transduction pathways defined by MEK and MKK isoforms. Science 267:682–685
28. Ray LB, Sturgill TW (1988) Insulin-stimulated microtubule-associated protein kinase is phosphorylated on tyrosine and threonine in vivo. Proc Natl Acad Sci U S A 85:3753–3757
29. Karnoub AE, Weinberg RA (2008) Ras oncogenes: split personalities. Nat Rev Mol Cell Biol 9:517–531
30. Shaul YD, Seger R (2007) The MEK/ERK cascade: from signaling specificity to diverse functions. Biochim Biophys Acta, Mol Cell Res 1773:1213–1226
31. Storm SM, Cleveland JL, Rapp UR (1990) Expression of raf family proto-oncogenes in normal mouse tissues. Oncogene 5:345–351
32. Roberts P, Der C (2007) Targeting the Raf-MEK-ERK mitogen-activated protein kinase cascade for the treatment of cancer. Oncogene 26:3291–3310
33. Mason CS et al (1999) Serine and tyrosine phosphorylations cooperate in Raf-1, but not B-Raf activation. EMBO J 18:2137–2148
34. Marais R et al (1997) Differential regulation of Raf-1, A-Raf, and B-Raf by oncogenic Ras and tyrosine kinases. J Biol Chem 272(7):4378–4383
35. Rushworth LK et al (2006) Regulation and role of Raf-1/B-Raf heterodimerization. Mol Cell Biol 26:2262–2272
36. Matallanas D et al (2011) Raf family kinases: old dogs have learned new tricks. Genes Cancer 2:232–260
37. Dougherty MK et al (2005) Regulation of Raf-1 by direct feedback phosphorylation. Mol Cell 17:215–224
38. Kiel C, Serrano L (2009) Cell type-specific importance of ras-c-raf complex association rate constants for MAPK signaling. Sci Signal 2:ra38
39. Giroux S et al (1999) Embryonic death of Mek1-deficient mice reveals a role for this kinase in angiogenesis in the labyrinthine region of the placenta. Curr Biol 9:369–372
40. Bélanger L-F et al (2003) Mek2 is dispensable for mouse growth and development. Mol Cell Biol 23(14):4778–4787
41. Aoidi R, Maltais A, Charron J (2016) Functional redundancy of the kinases MEK1 and MEK2: rescue of the Mek1 mutant phenotype by Mek2 knock-in reveals a protein threshold effect. Sci Signal 9:ra9
42. Zhou L et al (2010) MEK1 and MEK2 isoforms regulate distinct functions in pancreatic cancer cells. Oncol Rep 24:251–255

43. Ussar S, Voss T (2004) MEK1 and MEK2, different regulators of the G1/S transition. J Biol Chem 279(42):43861–43869
44. Huth HW et al (2016) MEK2 controls the activation of MKK3/MKK6-p38 axis involved in the MDA-MB-231 breast cancer cell survival: correlation with cyclin D1 expression. Cell Signal. 28(9):1283–1291
45. Catalanotti F et al (2009) A Mek1-Mek2 heterodimer determines the strength and duration of the Erk signal. Nat Struct Mol Biol 16(3):294–303
46. Eblen ST et al (2004) Mitogen-activated protein kinase feedback phosphorylation regulates mek1 complex formation and activation during cellular adhesion. Mol Cell Biol 24:2308–2317
47. Lefloch R, Pouysségur J, Lenormand P (2008) Single and combined silencing of ERK1 and ERK2 reveals their positive contribution to growth signaling depending on their expression levels. Mol Cell Biol 28(1):511–527
48. Vantaggiato C et al (2006) ERK1 and ERK2 mitogen-activated protein kinases affect Ras-dependent cell signaling differentially. J Biol 5:14
49. Shin J et al (2013) Depletion of ERK2 but not ERK1 abrogates oncogenic Ras-induced senescence. Cell Signal 25(12):2540–2547
50. Li F et al (2009) The linker region of Smad2 mediates TGF-beta-dependent ERK2-induced collagen synthesis. Biochem Biophys Res Commun 386:289–293
51. Li J, Johnson SE (2006) ERK2 is required for efficient terminal differentiation of skeletal myoblasts. Biochem Biophys Res Commun 345:1425–1433
52. Frémin C et al (2015) Functional redundancy of ERK1 and ERK2 MAP kinases during development. Cell Rep 12:913–921
53. Buscà R, Pouysségur J, Lenormand P (2016) ERK1 and ERK2 map kinases: specific roles or functional redundancy? Front Cell Developm Biol 4:1–23
54. McCubrey JA et al (2006) Roles of the RAF/MEK/ERK and PI3K/PTEN/AKT pathways in malignant transformation and drug resistance. Adv Enzym Regul 46:249–279
55. Santarpia LL, Lippman S, El-Naggar A (2012) Targeting the mitogen-activated protein kinase RAS-RAF signaling pathway in cancer therapy. Expert Opin Ther Targets 16(1):103–119
56. Holderfield M et al (2014) Targeting RAF kinases for cancer therapy: BRAF-mutated melanoma and beyond. Nat RevCancer 14(7):455–467
57. Huang T et al (2013) MEK and the inhibitors: from bench to bedside. J Hematol Oncol 6:30
58. Bogoyevitch MA, Kobe B (2006) Uses for JNK: the many and varied substrates of the c-Jun N-terminal kinases. Microbiol Mol Biol Rev 70:1061–1095
59. Bubici C, Papa S (2014) JNK signalling in cancer: in need of new, smarter therapeutic targets. Br J Pharmacol 171:24–37
60. Dèrijard B et al (1994) JNK1: a protein kinase stimulated by UV light and Ha-Ras that binds and phosphorylates the c-Jun activation domain. Cell 76:1025–1037
61. Bode AM, Dong Z (2007) The functional contrariety of JNK. Mol Carcinog 46(8):591–598
62. Gupta S et al (1996) Selective interaction of JNK protein kinase isoforms with transcription factors. EMBO J 15(11):2760–2770
63. Chen F (2012) JNK-induced apoptosis, compensatory growth, and cancer stem cells. Cancer Res 72(24):379–386
64. Sabapathy K, Wagner EF (2004) JNK2: a negative regulator of cellular proliferation. Cell Cycle 3(12):1520–1523
65. Yang X et al (2015) Inhibition of JNK3 promotes apoptosis induced by BH3 mimetic S1 in chemoresistant human ovarian cancer cells. Anat Rec 298:386–395
66. Shibata W et al (2008) c-Jun NH2-terminal kinase 1 is a critical regulator for the development of gastric cancer in mice. Cancer Res 68(13):5031–5039
67. Eferl R et al (2003) Liver tumor development: c-Jun antagonizes the proapoptotic activity of p53. Cell 112:181–192
68. Jaeschke A et al (2006) JNK2 is a positive regulator of the cjun transcription factor. Mol Cell 23:899–911

69. Cuenda A, Rousseau S (2007) p38 MAP-kinases pathway regulation, function and role in human diseases. Biochim Biophys Acta 1773:1358–1375
70. Cuadrado A, Nebreda AR (2010) Mechanisms and functions of p38 MAPK signalling. Biochem J 429:403–417
71. Lee JC et al (1994) A protein kinase involved in the regulation of inflammatory cytokine biosynthesis. Nature 372:739–746
72. Schieven GL (2005) The biology of p38 kinase: a central role in inflammation. Curr Top Med Chem 5:921–928
73. Korb A et al (2006) Differential tissue expression and activation of p38 MAPK alpha, beta, gamma, and delta isoforms in rheumatoid arthritis. Arthritis Rheum 54(9):2745–2756
74. Chen L et al (2009) Inhibition of the p38 kinase suppresses the proliferation of human ER-negative breast cancer cells. Cancer Res 69(23):8853–8861
75. Bulavin DV, Amundson SA, Fornace AJ (2002) p38 and Chk1 kinases: different conductors for the G2/M checkpoint symphony. Curr Opin Genet Dev 12:92–97
76. Mikhailov A, Shinohara M, Rieder CL (2004) Topoisomerase II and histone deacetylase inhibitors delay the G2/M transition by triggering the p38 MAPK checkpoint pathway. J Cell Biol 166:517–526
77. Thornton TM, Rincon M (2009) Non-classical p38 map kinase functions: cell cycle checkpoints and survival. Int J Biol Sci 5(1):44–52
78. Koul HK, Pal M, Koul S (2013) Role of p38 MAP kinase signal transduction in solid tumors. Genes Cancer 4:342–359
79. Leelahavanichkul K et al (2014) A role for p38 MAPK in head and neck cancer cell growth and tumor-induced angiogenesis and lymphangiogenesis. Mol Oncol 8(1):105–118
80. Bulavin DV et al (2003) Loss of oncogenic H-ras-induced cell cycle arrest and p38 mitogen-activated protein kinase activation by disruption of Gadd45a. Mol Cell Biol 23(11):3859–3871
81. Kummer JL, Rao PK, Heidenreich A (1997) Apoptosis induced by withdrawal of trophic factors is mediated by p38 apoptosis induced by withdrawal of trophic factors is mediated by p38 mitogen-activated protein kinase *. J Biol Chem 272(33):20490–20494
82. She QB et al (2001) Resveratrol-induced activation of p53 and apoptosis is mediated by extracellular-signal-regulated protein kinases and p38 kinase. Cancer Res 61:1604–1610
83. Che J et al (2013) Expression and clinical significance of the nin one binding protein and p38 MAPK in prostate carcinoma. Int J Clin Exp Pathol 6(11):2300–2311
84. Xu L, Chen S, Bergan RC (2006) MAPKAPK2 and HSP27 are downstream effectors of p38 MAP kinase-mediated matrix metalloproteinase type 2 activation and cell invasion in human prostate cancer. Oncogene 25(2301):2987–2998
85. Fan XJ et al (2014) Phosphorylated p38, a negative prognostic biomarker, complements TNM staging prognostication in colorectal cancer. Tumor Biol 35:10487–10495
86. Liu Y, Gray NS (2006) Rational design of inhibitors that bind to inactive kinase conformations. Nat Chem Biol 2:358–364
87. Pargellis C et al (2002) Inhibition of p38 MAP kinase by utilizing a novel allosteric binding site. Nat Struct Biol 9:268–272
88. Bain J et al (2007) The selectivity of protein kinase inhibitors: a further update. Biochem J 408:297–315
89. Frantz B et al (1998) The activation state of p38 mitogen-activated protein kinase determines the efficiency of ATP competition for pyridinylimidazole inhibitor binding. Biochemistry 37(98):13846–13853
90. Sebolt-Leopold JS et al (1999) Blockade of the MAP kinase pathway suppresses growth of colon tumors in vivo. Nat Med 5:810–816
91. Caunt CJ et al (2015) MEK1 and MEK2 inhibitors and cancer therapy: the long and winding road. Nat Rev Cancer 15:577–592
92. Zhao Y, Adjei AA (2014) The clinical development of MEK inhibitors. Nat Publ Group 11:385–400

93. Whitmarsh AJ (2006) The JIP family of MAPK scaffold proteins. Biochem Soc Trans 34:828–832
94. Yan C et al (2011) Understanding the specificity of a docking interaction between JNK1 and the scaffolding protein JIP1. J Phys Chem B 115:1491–1502
95. Barr RK, Kendrick TS, Bogoyevitch MA (2002) Identification of the critical features of a small peptide inhibitor of JNK activity. J Biol Chem 277:10987–10997
96. Heo Y-S et al (2004) Structural basis for the selective inhibition of JNK1 by the scaffolding protein JIP1 and SP600125. EMBO J 23:2185–2195
97. Stebbins JL et al (2008) Identification of a new JNK inhibitor targeting the JNK-JIP interaction site. Proc Natl Acad Sci U S A 105:16809–16813
98. Herrero A et al (2015) Small molecule inhibition of ERK dimerization prevents tumorigenesis by RAS-ERK pathway oncogenes. Cancer Cell 28:170–182
99. Venter JC et al (2001) The sequence of the human genome. Science 291:1304–1351
100. Aceves-Luquero CI et al (2009) ERK2, but not ERK1, mediates acquired and "De novo" resistance to imatinib mesylate: implication for CML therapy. PLoS One 4(7):1–10
101. Qin J, Xin H, Nickoloff BJ (2012) Specifically targeting ERK1 or ERK2 kills Melanoma cells. J Transl Med 10(1):15
102. Probst GD et al (2011) Highly selective c-Jun N-terminal kinase (JNK) 2 and 3 inhibitors with in vitro CNS-like pharmacokinetic properties prevent neurodegeneration. Bioorg Med Chem Lett 21:315–319
103. Jiang Y et al (1997) Characterization of the structure and function of the fourth member of p38 group mitogen-activated protein kinases, p38delta. J Biol Chem 272(48):30122–30128
104. Haider AS et al (2006) Genomic analysis defines a cancer-specific gene expression signature for human squamous cell carcinoma and distinguishes malignant hyperproliferation from benign hyperplasia. J Invest Dermatol 126:869–881
105. Junttila M et al (2007) P38a and P38D mitogen-activated protein kinase isoforms regulate invasion and growth of head and neck squamous carcinoma cells. Oncogene 26:5267–5279
106. Tan FLS et al (2010) p38delta/MAPK13 as a diagnostic marker for cholangiocarcinoma and its involvement in cell motility and invasion. Int J Cancer 126:2353–2361
107. O'Callaghan C, Fanning LJ, Barry OP (2014) p38delta MAPK: emerging roles of a neglected isoform. Int J Cell Biol 2014:272689
108. Mccubrey JA et al (2007) Roles of the Raf/Mek pathway in cell growth, malignant transformation and drug resistance. Biochim Biophys Acta 1773(8):1263–1284
109. Montagut C, Settleman J (2009) Targeting the RAF-MEK-ERK pathway in cancer therapy. Cancer Lett 283:125–134
110. Cox AD et al (2014) Drugging the undruggable RAS: mission possible? Nat Rev Drug Discov 13:828–851
111. Cox AD, Der CJ (2002) Ras family signaling: therapeutic targeting. Cancer Biol Ther 1:599–606
112. Flaherty KT et al (2013) Phase III trial of carboplatin and paclitaxel with or without sorafenib in metastatic melanoma. J Clin Oncol 31:373–379
113. Hauschild A et al (2009) Results of a phase III, randomized, placebo-controlled study of sorafenib in combination with carboplatin and paclitaxel as second-line treatment in patients with unresectable stage III or stage IV melanoma. J Clin Oncol 27:2823–2830
114. Eggermont AMM, Robert C (2011) New drugs in melanoma: it's a whole new world. Eur J Cancer 47:2150–2157
115. Mangana J et al (2012) Sorafenib in melanoma. Exp Opin Investig Drugs 21:557–568
116. Hatzivassiliou G et al (2010) RAF inhibitors prime wild-type RAF to activate the MAPK pathway and enhance growth. Nature 464:431–435
117. Bekaii-Saab T et al (2011) Multi-institutional phase II study of selumetinib in patients with metastatic biliary cancers. J Clin Oncol 29:2357–2363
118. Bodoky G et al (2012) A phase II open-label randomized study to assess the efficacy and safety of selumetinib (AZD6244 [ARRY-142886]) versus capecitabine in patients with

advanced or metastatic pancreatic cancer who have failed first-line gemcitabine therapy. Investig New Drugs 30:1216–1223
119. Kirkwood JM et al (2012) Phase II, open-label, randomized trial of the MEK1/2 inhibitor selumetinib as monotherapy versus temozolomide in patients with advanced melanoma. Clin Cancer Res 18:555–567
120. Catalanotti F et al (2013) Phase II trial of MEK inhibitor selumetinib (AZD6244, ARRY-142886) in patients with BRAFV600E/K-mutated melanoma. Clin Cancer Res 19:2257–2264
121. Kim DW, Patel SP (2014) Profile of selumetinib and its potential in the treatment of melanoma. OncoTarget Ther 7:1631–1639
122. Samatar AA, Poulikakos PI (2014) Targeting RAS–ERK signalling in cancer: promises and challenges. Nat Rev Drug Discov 13(12):928–942
123. Carlino MS et al (2013) Antiproliferative effects of continued mitogen-activated protein kinase pathway inhibition following acquired resistance to BRAF and/or MEK inhibition in melanoma. Mol Cancer Ther 12:1332–1342
124. Hatzivassiliou G et al (2012) ERK inhibition overcomes acquired resistance to MEK inhibitors. Mol Cancer Therap 11:1143–1154
125. Morris EJ et al (2013) Discovery of a novel ERK inhibitor with activity in models of acquired resistance to BRAF and MEK inhibitors. Cancer Discov 3:742–750
126. Emery CM et al (2009) MEK1 mutations confer resistance to MEK and B-RAF inhibition. Proc Natl Acad Sci U S A 106:20411–20416
127. Wagle N et al (2011) Dissecting therapeutic resistance to RAF inhibition in melanoma by tumor genomic profiling. J Clin Oncol 29:3085–3096
128. Nikolaev SI et al (2011) Exome sequencing identifies recurrent somatic MAP2K1 and MAP2K2 mutations in melanoma. Nat Genet 44:133–139
129. Villanueva J et al (2013) Concurrent MEK2 mutation and BRAF amplification confer resistance to BRAF and MEK inhibitors in melanoma. Cell Rep 4:1090–1099
130. Wagle N et al (2014) MAP kinase pathway alterations in BRAF-mutant melanoma patients with acquired resistance to combined RAF/MEK inhibition. Cancer Discov 4:61–68
131. Jha S et al (2016) Dissecting therapeutic resistance to ERK inhibition. Mol Cancer Ther 15:548–560
132. Wang Y et al (2005) A role for K-ras in conferring resistance to the MEK inhibitor, CI-1040. Neoplasia 7:336–347
133. Montagut C et al (2008) Elevated CRAF as a potential mechanism of acquired resistance to BRAF inhibition in melanoma. Cancer Res 68:4853–4861
134. Mendoza MC, Er EE, Blenis J (2011) The Ras-ERK and PI3K-mTOR pathways: cross-talk and compensation. Trends Biochem Sci 36:320–328
135. Sánchez-Hernández I et al (2012) Dual inhibition of V600EBRAF and the PI3K/AKT/mtor pathway cooperates to induce apoptosis in melanoma cells through a MEK-independent mechanism. Cancer Lett 314:244–255
136. Fruman DA, Rommel C (2014) PI3K and cancer: lessons, challenges and opportunities. Nat Rev Drug Discov 13:140–156
137. Hall-Jackson CA et al (1999) Paradoxical activation of Raf by a novel Raf inhibitor. Chem Biol 6:559–568
138. Zhang C et al (2015) RAF inhibitors that evade paradoxical MAPK pathway activation. Nature 526:583–586
139. Shimo T et al (2007) Specific inhibitor of MEK-mediated cross-talk between ERK and p38 MAPK during differentiation of human osteosarcoma cells. J Cell Commun Signal 1:103–111
140. Wagner EF, Nebreda AR (2009) Signal integration by JNK and p38 MAPK pathways in cancer development. Nat Rev Cancer 9:537–549
141. Zmajkovicova K et al (2013) MEK1 is required for PTEN membrane recruitment, AKT regulation, and the maintenance of peripheral tolerance. Mol Cell 50:43–55

142. Engelman JA et al (2008) Effective use of PI3K and MEK inhibitors to treat mutant Kras G12D and PIK3CA H1047R murine lung cancers. Nat Med 14(12):1351–1356
143. Posch C et al (2013) Combined targeting of MEK and PI3K/mTOR effector pathways is necessary to effectively inhibit NRAS mutant melanoma in vitro and in vivo. Proc Natl Acad Sci U S A 110(10):4015–4020
144. Villanueva J et al (2011) Acquired resistance to BRAF inhibitors mediated by a RAF kinase switch in melanoma can be overcome by co-targeting MEK and IGF-1R/PI3K. Cancer Cell 18(6):683–695
145. Swanton C (2013) Intratumour heterogeneity: evolution through space and time an evolutionary perspective on cancer heterogeneity. Cancer Res 72(19):4875–4882
146. Fisher R, Pusztai L, Swanton C (2013) Cancer heterogeneity: implications for targeted therapeutics. Br J Cancer 108(3):479–485
147. Norum JH, Andersen K, Sørlie T (2014) Lessons learned from the intrinsic subtypes of breast cancer in the quest for precision therapy. Br J Surg 101:925–938
148. Gerlinger M et al (2012) Intratumor heterogeneity and branched evolution revealed by multiregion sequencing. N Engl J Med 366:883–892
149. Navin N et al (2011) Tumour evolution inferred by single-cell sequencing. Nature 472:90–94
150. Seligson DB et al (2009) Global levels of histone modifications predict prognosis in different cancers. Am J Pathol 174:1619–1628
151. Sharma SV et al (2010) A chromatin-mediated reversible drug-tolerant state in cancer cell subpopulations. Cell 141:69–80
152. Almendro V et al (2014) Genetic and phenotypic diversity in breast tumor metastases. Cancer Res 74:1338–1348
153. Talmadge JE, Fidler IJ (2010) AACR centennial series: the biology of cancer metastasis: historical perspective. Cancer Res 70:5649–5669
154. Kreso A et al (2013) Variable clonal repopulation dynamics influence chemotherapy response in colorectal cancer. Science 339:543–548
155. Zahreddine H, Borden KLB (2013) Mechanisms and insights into drug resistance in cancer. Front Pharmacol 4:1–8
156. Nguyen A et al (2016) Highly variable cancer subpopulations that exhibit enhanced transcriptome variability and metastatic fitness. Nat Commun 7:11246
157. Long GV et al (2014) Combined BRAF and MEK inhibition versus BRAF inhibition alone in melanoma. N Engl J Med 371:1877–1888
158. Davies H et al (2002) Mutations of the BRAF gene in human cancer. Nature 417:949–954
159. Majumder B et al (2015) Predicting clinical response to anticancer drugs using an ex vivo platform that captures tumour heterogeneity. Nat Commun 6:6169

Adenosine Signaling Pathways as Potential Therapeutic Targets in Prostate Cancer Disease

Silvia Novío, María Jesús Núñez-Iglesias, and Manuel Freire-Garabal

Abstract Prostate cancer (PCa) is the second main cause of death by cancer in men. Although most PCa are initially responsive to treatment, they are difficult to manage clinically after their progression to a hormone independent state. During the last years different approaches to treating PCa have been assessed based mainly on specific targets such as adenosine receptors (AR), since it is known that their activation can modulate tumour growth. This chapter is intended to: (a) review evidences on expression levels of AR subtypes in PCa cells; (b) highlight the molecular mechanisms underlying the regulation of AR functioning during growth, apoptosis, invasion, migration, and/or metastasis of PCa cells; (c) analyse the potential application of AR ligands in oncologic treatment of PCa. The critical analysis of herein highlighted evidences shows that especially A_3 AR agonists and to a lesser extent A_{2b} AR antagonists, could be useful clinically in controlling the proliferation and metastasis of hormone sensitive and refractory PCa.

Keywords A_{2b} • A_3 • Adenosine • Adenosine receptor(s) • Apoptosis • Cell cycle • Cell proliferation • Invasiveness • Metastatic potential • Prostate cancer

Abbreviations

A_1 AR	Adenosine A_1 receptor
A_{2a} AR	Adenosine A_{2a} receptor
A_{2b} AR	Adenosine A_{2b} receptor
A_3 AR	Adenosine A_3 receptor
AnR	Androgen receptor
AR	Adenosine receptor
cAMP	Cyclic adenosine monophosphate
ERK1/2	Extracellular signal-regulated kinase 1/2
GPCRs	G protein-coupled-receptors

S. Novío (✉) • M.J. Núñez-Iglesias • M. Freire-Garabal
Lennart Levi Stress and Neuroimmunology Laboratory, School of Medicine, University of Santiago de Compostela, C/San Francisco, s/n, Santiago de Compostela 15782, Spain
e-mail: silvia.novio@usc.es; snl@usc.es; mjesus.nunez@usc.es; manuel.freire-garabal@usc.es

A.A. Farooqi, M. Ismail (eds.), *Molecular Oncology: Underlying Mechanisms and Translational Advancements*, DOI 10.1007/978-3-319-53082-6_4

GSK-3ß	Glycogen synthase kinase 3 beta
IKK	IκB kinase
IκB	Inhibitor of κB
MMP	Mitochondrial membrane potential
MTAs	Microtubule-targeting agents
NADPH	Nicotinamide adenine dinucleotide phosphate
NF-κB	Nuclear factor kappa-light-chain-enhancer of activated B cells
PCa	Prostate cancer
PKA	Protein kinase A
PKB/Akt	Protein kinase B
ROS	Reactive oxygen species
SAC	Spindle assembly checkpoint

During the last decades different approaches to treating cancer have been developed. Progress in the field of oncology has been possible because of identification of specific targets such as receptors. When tumour cells over-express these receptors, they become hyper responsive to normal concentrations of ligands; on the contrary, this effect is not observed in normal cells [1]. Knowledge about the functioning of receptors in cancer cells should be taken into account when new anticancer therapeutic strategies are investigated. In this context, adenosine receptors (AR) have aroused great interest emerging as a promising therapeutic strategy. In this chapter we review progress in the knowledge of AR as potential targets to treat prostate cancer (PCa), the most frequent malignant disease in men.

Adenosine

The adenosine is an ubiquitous purine nucleoside expressed in all cells. It is the backbone of ATP and modulates a lot of physiological and pharmacological functions that are mediated by an intracellular effect of adenosine or by extracellular AR [2, 3]. These receptors have been cloned, identified and categorized as A_1, A_{2a}, A_{2b} and A_3 subtypes [4]. They are G protein-coupled-receptors (GPCRs), each AR subclass is encoded by a separate gene and has an unique pharmacological profile and tissue distribution [5, 6]. While the A_{2a} and A_{2b} AR interact with G_S proteins, activating adenylate cyclase and hence increasing the intracellular, A_1 and A_3 AR cause the opposite effect on adenylate cyclase and cAMP concentration since they are coupled with G_i proteins [7, 8]. Likewise, these receptors have different affinity for adenosine [9], it is lower for A_{2b} AR than for A_1 AR, A_{2a} AR and A_3 AR subtypes [2, 5, 10].

The formation of adenosine varies according to microenvironmental conditions. Usually, nanomolar concentrations of adenosine are measured in the extracellular space, which dramatically increase during metabolically unfavourable conditions where hypoxia and/or ischemia are implicated [11]. Thus, it has been corroborated when there is pain [12], inflammation [13], seizures [14], and cancer [15]. However, it must not be forgotten that hypoxia/ischemia-induced increase is a local effect [16].

During the past decade, the modulation of adenosinergic system in the treatment of Parkinson's disease [17], schizophrenia [18], or pain [19] has aroused considerable interest because adenosine plays a major role in the immune system [20], in the central nervous system [21, 22], as an endogenous pain modulator [23], in the mast cell degranulation [24, 25], and in the regulation of cell proliferation and death [11, 16, 26–28] in vitro and in vivo. In relation to the latter function, it has been reported that adenosine and/or its analogs can: (a) induce programmed cell death in endothelial cells [29, 30], astrocytes [31], thymocytes [32]; (b) block apoptosis in granulocytes [33]; (c) stimulate cell proliferation in mesangial and thymocyte cells [28], Swiss mouse 3T3 fibroblasts [28], bone marrow stromal cells [34]. Taking into account the fact that adenosine can influence cell viability; its role in treatment of cancer is highly attractive. Thus, a review of the studies published to date about the participation of adenosinergic system in cancer, and more specifically of its anti-tumoral effects against PCa, is the focus of this chapter.

Prostate Cancer

The human PCa is the most frequent malignant disease and the second main cause of death by cancer in men, playing metastases an important role in the evolution of the disease [35]. The aetiology of PCa is multifactorial. Stacewicz-Sapuntzakis et al. [36] have identified, among other factors, genetic mutations, environmental factors (e.g. diet) and androgens. In relation to the androgens and androgen receptor (AnR) they have been associated with PCa initiation and promotion [37, 38] to such an extent that the growth and progression of PCa is hormone-sensitive in the early stages [39–41].

The first line therapy for PCa is androgen-deprivation therapy together with castration [42]. Although generally human PCa respond well to this treatment, since androgens promote survival of prostate luminal epithelial cells [43], most treated patients relapse with androgen-independent tumours which are unresponsive to further androgen withdrawal [44]. In these cases, chemotherapy with taxanes (docetaxel and paclitaxel) is to date the standard treatment for the hormone-independent stage of PCa [45]. Taxanes are microtubule-targeting agents (MTAs) which bind to tubulin subunits [46, 47], impeding the correct formation of the mitotic spindle and normal chromosome congression and activating the spindle assembly checkpoint (SAC) in a sustained way [48, 49]. These effects lead to prolonged mitosis followed by the induction of apoptosis, that is the ultimate goal of chemotherapy [47, 50]. MTAs have not tumour cell selectivity and also target resting and differentiated cells causing toxicity (e.g. neutropenia and neurotoxicity) that significantly limits their use [46, 51]. Furthermore, another important inconvenience in using MTAs in chemotherapy is their limited efficacy as single agents [52], so they are used in combination with other drugs/agents in order to improve it [53].

The evidence presented above suggests that new treatments for PCa are required. In this sense, efforts are being focused to discover drugs targeting PCa cell proliferation and apoptosis, such as agonists of the G protein-coupled $P2Y_1$ receptor [54]. As it will be commented below in more detail, several studies on the effects of nucleosides in PCa have been conducted.

Adenosine and Prostate Cancer

Expression of Adenosine Receptors in Prostate Cancer Cells

In an effort to find new therapies for PCa, multiple experimental models of PCa have been developed. By far the most useful in vitro model that we have of PCa is cell culture. In spite of the number of cell lines that are available for study is expansive, the triad consisted of PC3, DU 145, and LNCaP cells is the one more frequently used in in vitro studies [55]. The differences among these cells lie in the expression level of tumour suppressor (p53) and pro-apoptotic (Bax) proteins [56, 57] as well as in the androgen sensitivity [57]. Concretely, PC3 are p53 null, Bax positive, androgen-independent cells; DU 145 are p53 mutant, Bax negative, androgen-independent cells; and LNCaP are p53 wild-type, Bax positive, androgen-dependent cells.

The expression level of AR subtypes has been examined in PC3, DU 145, and LNCaP cells, and all of them have been demonstrated in all these cell lines [15, 58–62]. Unfortunately, there are contradictory results among studies which have not been clarified (Table 1).

Table 1 Relative gene expression of adenosine receptors detected by RT-PCR in prostate cancer cells

	Adenosine receptor				
Cell line	A_3 AR	A_{2b} AR	A_{2a} AR	A_1 AR	References
PC3	+++++	++++	++	+	[58, 59]
	+++	++++	++	+	[15]
	+	++++	+++	++	[60]
	+	++++++	+++	++	[62]
DU 145	++++++	++++	++	+	[58, 59]
	++	++++	+++	+	[15]
	+	++++++	++++	++	[62]
	+	++++	++	++	[61]
LNCaP	++++	+++	++	+	[58, 59]
	+++	++++	++	+	[15]
	+	++++++	+++++	++	[62]

"+" Represents the expression level, from + (*the lowest*) to ++++++ (*the highest*)

The expression level of AR is higher in PCa than in normal cells [15]. Mousavi et al. [15] have observed AR expression increases in malignant tumours and PCa cell lines (PC3, DU 145 and LNCaP) compared to normal tissues, although no significant differences are observed between A_1 AR expression in malignant and normal cells. These data confirm the up-regulation of AR demonstrated in cells/tissues of breast carcinoma [63], thyroid carcinoma [64], colon cancers [65, 66], hepatocellular carcinoma [67], leukemia [68], mesothelioma [69] or neuroendocrine tumours [70]. Likewise, these studies suggest that AR, and more specifically A_3 and A_{2b} AR, may contribute to diagnosis and cure of PCa as potential markers for this disease and targets for tumour growth inhibition, respectively. However, further studies are needed to clarify the participation of AR in the process of tumour development, which seemingly may be of crucial importance to health improvement of patients with PCa.

Identification of genes which are activated or repressed by AnR is important in PCa growth [39, 40, 71]. Recently, it has been demonstrated that AnR stimulation can regulate AR expression in androgen-dependent PCa cells. While the expression of AR is increased by the AnR agonist dihydrotestosterone and decreased by the AnR antagonist bicalutamide in LNCaP cells, no change on AR expression is exerted by these compounds in PC3 cells [15]. No hypothesis has been proposed to explain these effects, however this evidence may lay the foundation for the improvement of the hormonal therapy.

Antitumor Properties of Adenosine

The first evidence about the role of the adenosine as antitumor agent against PCa date from the end of the twentieth century and the beginning of the twenty-first century. In this context, different studies demonstrated that nucleotides such as ATP and UTP were cytotoxic to hormone-independent PCa cells [72, 73] by increasing cytosolic calcium [74]. The fact that these nucleotides are metabolized to adenosine [75], suggested that cell death induced by ATP and UTP may be mediated by adenosine. Later, in vivo studies revealed that the activation of AR inhibited the development of PCa in mice [27, 76], supporting the utilization of AR as a target to treat PCa. According to studies published to date, the anti-tumorigenic effect of adenosine includes: (a) suppression of cancer cell viability [3, 16, 27, 58–60, 62, 76–78] by arresting cell-cycle progression [27, 58, 59, 78, 79] and/or induction of apoptosis [27, 58–60, 62, 77, 78]; (b) inhibition of migration and metastatization [16, 27].

Inhibition of Cancer Cell Growth

Several studies have shown that activation of adenosinergic system is implicated in inhibition of PCa growth [27, 58–60, 76, 77] in a permanent manner [77]. Although this anti-proliferative effect has been demonstrated in hormone-sensitive (ALVA, LNCaP) and -insensitive (PC3, PC3-MM, DU 145, AT6.1) PCa cell lines [27, 59, 60, 77], the former are more susceptible to adenosine toxicity [59]. As it has been observed in other tumours including melanoma [80], colon carcinoma [81, 82], breast carcinoma [83–85] and leukemia [86], time-dependent cell growth inhibition is mediated fundamentally by AR [77] either through A_3 AR activation [27, 58, 59] or A_{2b} AR blockade [62], although some research supports the participation of an intracellular pathway [77]. In relation to the former mechanism, it has been shown that the treatment with 1-deoxy-1-[6-[[(3-iodophenyl)methyl]amino]-9*H*–purine-9-yl]-*N*-methyl-beta-D-ribofuranuronamide (IB-MECA), an synthetic selective A_3 AR agonist, reduces in a dose-dependent manner the proliferation of LNCaP [59], ALVA [27], DU 145 [59], PC3 [59, 76], PC3-MM [27] and AT6.1 [27] cells. This same effect is observed in PCa cell lines treated with the selective A_{2b} AR antagonist PSB603 [62]. This evidence suggests that selective A_3 AR agonists and A_{2b} AR antagonists may be potential novel drugs for the treatment of PCa, although no clinical trial has been carried out yet. Mechanisms underlying the growth inhibitory effects of adenosinergic system on PCa are represented in Fig. 1. To date, only molecular mechanisms mediated by A_3 AR have been studied.

As it was commented in section "Prostate Cancer", taxanes led to significantly improved overall survival in patients with androgen-resistant PCa [45], but the administration of these chemotherapeutic agents in combination with other compounds may potentiate their effects, as it has been corroborated by in vitro [78] and in vivo [76] studies. In this sense, Minelli et al. [78] observed that a non-selective AR agonist, 2-chloroadenosine (2-CADO), enhances the cytotoxic effect of chemotherapy against both androgen-dependent and -independent PCa cells. The pretreatment of PC3 or LNCaP cells with 10 mM 2-CADO for 24 h followed by 1 nM docetaxel for 6 days caused a dose-dependent inhibition of cell proliferation, achieving to decrease the effective concentration of docetaxel.

Adenosine and AR ligands (A_3 AR agonists and A_{2b} AR antagonists) can inhibit the PCa cell viability by interfering with the cell cycle control system and/or inducing apoptosis, depending (among other factors) on the concentration used [87]. Thus, Aghaei et al. [59] have shown that the IB-MECA when administered at low concentration (1 μM) is effective in the suppression of PC3, DU 145 and LNCaP cells growth with cytostatic effect, however at 10–100 μM a cytotoxic effect is induced. In any case, both effects are related in the following way: resting cells are more resistant to apoptosis than proliferating cells, although that cells which enter the cell cycle if lack of progression signals eventually suffer apoptosis [88].

Cell Cycle Arrest: Cytostatic Effect of Low-Concentration Adenosine and AR Ligands on Tumour Cell Growth

The cytostatic mechanism of adenosine and AR agonists in PC3, DU 145 and LNCaP cells appears to occur at G1 [58, 59] or S phase [78, 79] of cell cycle. The cell cycle arrest is induced through p53-dependent, Cdk4/cyclin D1-mediated

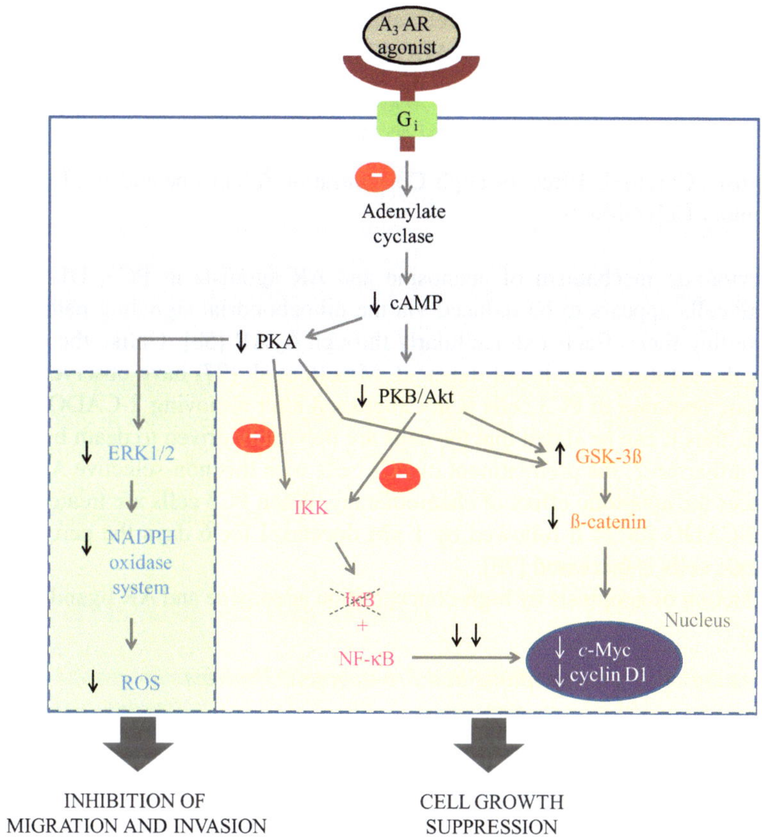

Fig. 1 Molecular mechanisms involved in the inhibition of the growth and metastasis of PCa cells mediated by A_3 AR. Yellow rectangle: pathways involved in the cell growth suppression; green rectangle: pathway involved in the inhibition of cell migration and invasion; gray rectangle: common pathway to both effects. The activation of A_3 AR triggers G_i-protein activation and inhibits adenylate cyclase activity, thereby leading to a decrease in the level of intracellular cAMP. In turn, downstream elements are not activated (level and activity of PKA and PKB/Akt are decreased), so the NF-κB (pink), Wnt (orange) and ERK1/2 mitogen-activated protein kinase (blue) pathways are deregulated. These actions eventually decrease the proliferation and/or migration and invasion of prostate cancer cells [27, 76]. Abbreviations: A_3 AR: adenosine A_3 receptor; cAMP: cyclic adenosine monophosphate; ERK1/2: extracellular signal-regulated kinase 1/2; GSK-3ß: glycogen synthase kinase 3 beta; IκB: inhibitor of κB; IKK: IκB kinase; NADPH: nicotinamide adenine dinucleotide phosphate; NF-κB: nuclear factor kappa-light-chain-enhancer of activated B cells; PKA: protein kinase A; PKB/Akt: protein kinase B; ROS: reactive oxygen species

pathway. Adenosine [58] or IB-MECA [27, 59] notably down regulate the expression of the cyclin D1/Cdk4 complex, responsible for cell cycle progression in early G1 phase, and up regulate the expression of p53 in a concentration-dependent manner in both androgen-independent and -dependent PCa cells. Similar effects have been noted in leukemic [89] and stomach cancer [90] cells. According to studies

References

1. Wang S (2014) Tumor targeted therapies: strategies for killing cancer but not normal cells. Curr Cancer Ther Rev 10:53–61. doi:10.2174/1573394710011408151523322
2. Fredholm BB, Irenius E, Kull B, Schulte G (2001) Comparison of the potency of adenosine as an agonist at human adenosine receptors expressed in Chinese hamster ovary cells. Biochem Pharmacol 61:443–448
3. Jacobson KA, Hoffmann C, Cattabeni F, Abbracchio MP (1999) Adenosine-induced cell death: evidence for receptor-mediated signalling. Apoptosis 4:197–211
4. Jacobson KA, von Lubitz DK, Daly JW, Fredholm BB (1996) Adenosine receptor ligands: differences with acute versus chronic treatment. Trends Pharmacol Sci 17:108–113
5. Fredholm BB, IJzerman AP, Jacobson KA, Linden J, Müller CE (2011) International union of basic and clinical pharmacology. LXXXI. Nomenclature and classification of adenosine receptors—an update. Pharmacol Rev 63:1–34. doi:10.1124/pr.110.003285
6. Gao ZG, Jacobson KA (2011) Emerging adenosine receptor agonists: an update. Expert Opin Emerg Drugs 16:597–602. doi:10.1517/14728214.2011.644786
7. Borea PA, Varani K, Vincenzi F, Baraldi PG, Tabrizi MA, Merighi S et al (2015) The A3 adenosine receptor: history and perspectives. Pharmacol Rev 67:74–102. doi:10.1124/pr.113.008540
8. Poulsen SA, Quinn RJ (1998) Adenosine receptors: new opportunities for future drugs. Bioorg Med Chem 6:619–641
9. Fredholm BB (2014) Adenosine—a physiological or pathophysiological agent? J Mol Med 92:201–206. doi:10.1007/s00109-013-1101-6
10. Ciruela F, Albergaria C, Soriano A, Cuffí L, Carbonell L, Sánchez S et al (2010) Adenosine receptors interacting proteins (ARIPs): behind the biology of adenosine signaling. Biochim Biophys Acta 1798:9–20. doi:10.1016/j.bbamem.2009.10.016
11. Borea PA, Gessi S, Merighi S, Varani K (2016) Adenosine as a multi-signalling guardian angel in human diseases: when, where and how does it exert its protective effects? Trends Pharmacol Sci 37:419–434. doi:10.1016/j.tips.2016.02.006
12. Hu X, Adebiyi MG, Luo J, Sun K, Le TT, Zhang Y et al (2016) Sustained elevated adenosine via ADORA2B promotes chronic pain through neuro-immune interaction. Cell Rep 16:106–119. doi:10.1016/j.celrep.2016.05.080
13. Fredholm BB (2007) Adenosine, an endogenous distress signal, modulates tissue damage and repair. Cell Death Differ 14:1315–1323. doi:10.1038/sj.cdd.4402132
14. Dale N, Frenguelli BG (2009) Release of adenosine and ATP during ischemia and epilepsy. Curr Neuropharmacol 7:160–179. doi:10.2174/157015909789152146
15. Mousavi S, Panjehpour M, Izadpanahi MH, Aghaei M (2015) Expression of adenosine receptor subclasses in malignant and adjacent normal human prostate tissues. Prostate 75:735–747. doi:10.1002/pros.22955
16. Gessi S, Merighi S, Sacchetto V, Simioni C, Borea PA (2011) Adenosine receptors and cancer. Biochim Biophys Acta 1808:1400–1412. doi:10.1016/j.bbamem.2010.09.020
17. Khanfar MA, Al-Qtaishat S, Habash M, Taha MO (2016) Discovery of potent adenosine A2a antagonists as potential anti-Parkinson disease agents. Non-linear QSAR analyses integrated with pharmacophore modeling. Chem Biol Interact 254:93–101. doi:10.1016/j.cbi.2016.05.023
18. Komatsu H (2015) Novel therapeutic GPCRs for psychiatric disorders. Int J Mol Sci 16:14109–14121. doi:10.3390/ijms160614109
19. Ford A, Castonguay A, Cottet M, Little JW, Chen Z, Symons-Liguori AM et al (2015) Engagement of the GABA to KCC2 signaling pathway contributes to the analgesic effects of A3AR agonists in neuropathic pain. J Neurosci 35:6057–6067. doi:10.1523/JNEUROSCI.4495-14.2015
20. Allard B, Beavis PA, Darcy PK, Stagg J (2016) Immunosuppressive activities of adenosine in cancer. Curr Opin Pharmacol 29:7–16. doi:10.1016/j.coph.2016.04.001

21. Burnstock G (2016) An introduction to the roles of purinergic signalling in neurodegeneration, neuroprotection and neuroregeneration. Neuropharmacology 104:4–17. doi:10.1016/j.neuropharm.2015.05.031
22. Mozzicato S, Joshi BV, Jacobson KA, Liang BT (2004) Role of direct RhoA-phospholipase D1 interaction in mediating adenosine-induced protection from cardiac ischemia. FASEB J 18:406–408. doi:10.1096/fj.03-0592fje
23. Burnstock G (2016) Purinergic mechanisms and pain. Adv Pharmacol 75:91–137. doi:10.1016/bs.apha.2015.09.001
24. Iwaki S, Tkaczyk C, Metcalfe DD, Gilfillan AM (2005) Roles of adaptor molecules in mast cell activation. Chem Immunol Allerg 87:43–58. doi:10.1159/000087570
25. Linden J (1994) Cloned adenosine A3 receptors: pharmacological properties, species differences and receptor functions. Trends Pharmacol Sci 15:298–306
26. Burnstock G (2002) Purinergic signaling and vascular cell proliferation and death. Arterioscler Thromb Vasc Biol 22:364–373
27. Jajoo S, Mukherjea D, Watabe K, Ramkumar V (2009) Adenosine A(3) receptor suppresses prostate cancer metastasis by inhibiting NADPH oxidase activity. Neoplasia 11:1132–1145
28. Ohana G, Bar-Yehuda S, Barer F, Fishman P (2001) Differential effect of adenosine on tumor and normal cell growth: focus on the A3 adenosine receptor. J Cell Physiol 186:19–23. doi:10.1002/1097-4652(200101)186:1<19::AID-JCP1011>3.0.CO;2-3
29. Grant MB, Davis MI, Caballero S, Feoktistov I, Biaggioni I, Belardinelli L (2001) Proliferation, migration, and ERK activation in human retinal endothelial cells through A(2B) adenosine receptor stimulation. Invest Ophthalmol Vis Sci 42:2068–2073
30. Meininger CJ, Schelling ME, Granger HJ (1988) Adenosine and hypoxia stimulate proliferation and migration of endothelial cells. Am J Phys 255:H554–H562
31. Ribeiro JA, Sebastiao AM, de Mendonca A (2003) Participation of adenosine receptors in neuroprotection. Drug News Perspect 16:80–86
32. Szondy Z (1994) Adenosine stimulates DNA fragmentation in human thymocytes by Ca(2+)-mediated mechanisms. Biochem J 304:877–885
33. Gao Z, Li BS, Day YJ, Linden J (2001) A3 adenosine receptor activation triggers phosphorylation of protein kinase B and protects rat basophilic leukemia 2H3 mast cells from apoptosis. Mol Pharmacol 59:76–82
34. Costa MA, Barbosa A, Neto E, Sá-e-Sousa A, Freitas R, Neves JM et al (2011) On the role of subtype selective adenosine receptor agonists during proliferation and osteogenic differentiation of human primary bone marrow stromal cells. J Cell Physiol 226:1353–1366. doi:10.1002/jcp.22458
35. Siegel R, Naishadham D, Jemal A (2013) Cancer statistics, 2013. CA Cancer J Clin 63:11–30. doi:10.3322/caac.21166
36. Stacewicz-Sapuntzakis M, Borthakur G, Burns JL, Bowen PE (2008) Correlations of dietary patterns with prostate health. Mol Nutr Food Res 52:114–130. doi:10.1002/mnfr.200600296
37. Koong LY, Watson CS (2014) Direct estradiol and diethylstilbestrol actions on early- versus late-stage prostate cancer cells. Prostate 74:1589–1603. doi:10.1002/pros.22875
38. Tan MH, Li J, Xu HE, Melcher K, Yong EL (2015) Androgen receptor: structure, role in prostate cancer and drug discovery. Acta Pharmacol Sin 36:3–23. doi:10.1038/aps.2014.18
39. Otsuka T, Hamada A, Iguchi K, Usui S, Hirano K (2013) Suppression of metallothionein 3 gene expression by androgen in LNCaP prostate cancer cells. Biomed Rep 1:614–618. doi:10.3892/br.2013.107
40. Xu B, Tang G, Xiao C, Wang L, Yang Q, Sun Y (2014) Androgen deprivation therapy induces androgen receptor-dependent upregulation of Egr1 in prostate cancers. Int J Clin Exp Pathol 7:2883–2893
41. Xu Y, Chen SY, Ross KN, Balk SP (2006) Androgens induce prostate cancer cell proliferation through mammalian target of rapamycin activation and post-transcriptional increases in cyclin D proteins. Cancer Res 66:7783–7792. doi:10.1158/0008-5472.CAN-05-4472
42. Heidenreich A, Bastian PJ, Bellmunt J, Bolla M, Joniau S, van der Kwast T et al (2014) EAU guidelines on prostate cancer. Part 1: screening, diagnosis, and local treatment with curative intent-update 2013. Eur Urol 65:124–137. doi:10.1016/j.eururo.2013.09.046

43. Culig Z, Steiner H, Bartsch G, Hobisch A (2005) Mechanisms of endocrine therapy-responsive and -unresponsive prostate tumours. Endocr Relat Cancer 12:229–244. doi:10.1677/erc.1.00775a
44. Bracarda S, de Cobelli O, Greco C, Prayer-Galetti T, Valdagni R, Gatta G et al (2005) Cancer of the prostate. Crit Rev Oncol Hematol 56:379–396. doi:10.1016/j.critrevonc.2005.03.010
45. Rumohr JA, Chang SS (2006) Current chemotherapeutic approaches for androgen-independent prostate cancer. Curr Opin Investig Drugs 7:529–533
46. Jordan MA, Wilson L (2004) Microtubules as a target for anticancer drugs. Nat Rev Cancer 4:253–265. doi:10.1038/nrc1317
47. Kaestner P, Bastians H (2010) Mitotic drug targets. J Cell Biochem 111:258–265. doi:10.1002/jcb.22721
48. Chan KS, Koh CG, Li HY (2012) Mitosis-targeted anti-cancer therapies: where they stand. Cell Death Dis 3:e411. doi:10.1038/cddis.2012.148
49. Weaver BA, Cleveland DW (2005) Decoding the links between mitosis, cancer, and chemotherapy: the mitotic checkpoint, adaptation, and cell death. Cancer Cell 8:7–12. doi:10.1016/j.ccr.2005.06.011
50. Marzo I, Naval J (2013) Antimitotic drugs in cancer chemotherapy: promises and pitfalls. Biochem Pharmacol 86:703–710. doi:10.1016/j.bcp.2013.07.010
51. Schmidt M, Bastians H (2007) Mitotic drug targets and the development of novel anti-mitotic anticancer drugs. Drug Resist Updat 10:162–181. doi:10.1016/j.drup.2007.06.003
52. Novío S, Freire-Garabal M, Núñez MJ (2014) Target driven preclinical screening for new antimitotic chemotherapy agents. Curr Top Med Chem 14:2263–2271
53. Kattan J, Bachour M, Farhat F, El Rassy E, Assi T, Ghosn M (2016) Phase II trial of weekly docetaxel, zoledronic acid, and celecoxib for castration-resistant prostate cancer. Investig New Drugs 34:474–480. doi:10.1007/s10637-016-0357-4
54. Wei Q, Costanzi S, Liu QZ, Gao ZG, Jacobson KA (2011) Activation of the P2Y1 receptor induces apoptosis and inhibits proliferation of prostate cancer cells. Biochem Pharmacol 82:418–425. doi:10.1016/j.bcp.2011.05.013
55. Cunningham D, You Z (2015) In vitro and in vivo model systems used in prostate cancer research. J Biol Methods 2:e17. doi:10.14440/jbm.2015.63
56. Saha A, Blando J, Silver E, Beltran L, Sessler J, DiGiovanni J (2014) 6-Shogaol from dried ginger inhibits growth of prostate cancer cells both in vitro and in vivo through inhibition of STAT3 and NF-κB signaling. Cancer Prev Res 7:627–638. doi:10.1158/1940-6207.CAPR-13-0420
57. Simone CB 2nd, John-Aryankalayil M, Palayoor ST, Makinde AY, Cerna D, Falduto MT et al (2013) mRNA expression profiles for prostate cancer following fractionated irradiation are influenced by p53 status. Transl Oncologia 6:573–585
58. Aghaei M, Karami-Tehrani F, Panjehpour M, Salami S, Fallahian F (2012) Adenosine induces cell-cycle arrest and apoptosis in androgen-dependent and -independent prostate cancer cell lines, LNcap-FGC-10, DU-145, and PC3. Prostate 72:361–375. doi:10.1002/pros.21438
59. Aghaei M, Panjehpour M, Karami-Tehrani F, Salami S (2011) Molecular mechanisms of A3 adenosine receptor-induced G1 cell cycle arrest and apoptosis in androgen-dependent and independent prostate cancer cell lines: involvement of intrinsic pathway. J Cancer Res Clin Oncol 137:1511–1523. doi:10.1007/s00432-011-1031-z
60. Minelli A, Bellezza I, Tucci A, Rambotti MG, Conte C, Culig Z (2009) Differential involvement of reactive oxygen species and nucleoside transporters in cytotoxicity induced by two adenosine analogues in human prostate cancer cells. Prostate 69:538–547. doi:10.1002/pros.20900
61. Panjehpour M, Movahedian A, Sadeghi H, Eghbali B, Yekdaneh A (2010) Adenosine receptor expression in two different human cancer lines at molecular level. Iranian J Cancer Prevent 3:111–116
62. Wei Q, Costanzi S, Balasubramanian R, Gao ZG, Jacobson KA (2013) A2B adenosine receptor blockade inhibits growth of prostate cancer cells. Purinergic Signal 9:271–280. doi:10.1007/s11302-012-9350-3

63. Mirza A, Basso A, Black S, Malkowski M, Kwee L, Pachter JA et al (2005) RNA interference targeting of A1 receptor-overexpressing breast carcinoma cells leads to diminished rates of cell proliferation and induction of apoptosis. Cancer Biol Ther 4:1355–1360
64. Morello S, Petrella A, Festa M, Popolo A, Monaco M, Vuttariello E et al (2008) Cl-IB-MECA inhibits human thyroid cancer cell proliferation independently of A3 adenosine receptor activation. Cancer Biol Ther 7:278–284
65. Gessi S, Cattabriga E, Avitabile A, Gafa R, Lanza G, Cavazzini L et al (2004) Elevated expression of A3 adenosine receptors in human colorectal cancer is reflected in peripheral blood cells. Clin Cancer Res 10:5895–5901. doi:10.1158/1078-0432.CCR-1134-03
66. Gessi S, Merighi S, Varani K, Cattabriga E, Benini A, Mirandola P et al (2007) Adenosine receptors in colon carcinoma tissues and colon tumoral cell lines: focus on the A(3) adenosine subtype. J Cell Physiol 211:826–836. doi:10.1002/jcp.20994
67. Bar-Yehuda S, Stemmer SM, Madi L, Castel D, Ochaion A, Cohen S et al (2008) The A3 adenosine receptor agonist CF102 induces apoptosis of hepatocellular carcinoma via deregulation of the Wnt and NF-kappaB signal transduction pathways. Int J Oncol 33:287–295
68. Schiedel AC, Lacher SK, Linnemann C, Knolle PA, Müller CE (2013) Antiproliferative effects of selective adenosine receptor agonists and antagonists on human lymphocytes: evidence for receptor-independent mechanisms. Purinergic Signal 9:351–365. doi:10.1007/s11302-013-9354-7
69. Varani K, Maniero S, Vincenzi F, Targa M, Stefanelli A, Maniscalco P et al (2011) A3 receptors are overexpressed in pleura from patients with mesothelioma and reduce cell growth via Akt/nuclear factor-κB pathway. Am J Respir Crit Care Med 183:522–530. doi:10.1164/rccm.201006-0980OC
70. Kalhan A, Gharibi B, Vazquez M, Jasani B, Neal J, Kidd M et al (2012) Adenosine A2A and A2B receptor expression in neuroendocrine tumours: potential targets for therapy. Purinergic Signal 8:265–274. doi:10.1007/s11302-011-9280-5
71. Sun D, Layer R, Mueller AC, Cichewicz MA, Negishi M, Paschal BM et al (2014) Regulation of several androgen-induced genes through the repression of the miR-99a/let-7c/miR-125b-2 miRNA cluster in prostate cancer cells. Oncogene 33:1448–1457. doi:10.1038/onc.2013.77
72. Fang WG, Pirnia F, Bang YJ, Myers CE, Trepel JB (1992) P2-purinergic receptor agonists inhibit the growth of androgen-independent prostate carcinoma cells. J Clin Invest 89:191–196. doi:10.1172/JCI115562
73. Janssens R, Boeynaems JM (2001) Effects of extracellular nucleotides and nucleosides on prostate carcinoma cells. Br J Pharmacol 132:536–546. doi:10.1038/sj.bjp.0703833
74. Olah ME, Stiles GL (1995) Adenosine receptor subtypes: characterization and therapeutic regulation. Annu Rev Pharmacol Toxicol 35:581–606. doi:10.1146/annurev.pa.35.040195.003053
75. Spychala J (2000) Tumor-promoting functions of adenosine. Pharmacol Ther 87:161–173
76. Fishman P, Bar-Yehuda S, Ardon E, Rath-Wolfson L, Barrer F, Ochaion A et al (2003) Targeting the A3 adenosine receptor for cancer therapy: inhibition of prostate carcinoma cell growth by A3AR agonist. Anticancer Res 23:2077–2083
77. Minelli A, Bellezza I, Agostini M, Bracarda S, Culig Z (2006) Mechanism of 2-chloroadenosine toxicity to PC3 cell line. Prostate 66:1425–1436. doi:10.1002/pros.20458
78. Minelli A, Bellezza I, Tucci A, Conte C, Bracarda S, Culig Z (2008) 2-chloroadenosine modulates PAR-1 and IL-23 expression and enhances docetaxel effects on PC3 cells. Prostate 68:360–372. doi:10.1002/pros.20703
79. Bellezza I, Agostini M, Liguori L, Minelli A (2005) Cytostatic effect of the nucleoside analogue 2-chloroadenosine on human prostate cancer cell line. Curr Pharm Anal 1:265–272. doi:10.2174/157341205774597913
80. Madi L, Bar-Yehuda S, Barer F, Ardon E, Ochaion A, Fishman P (2003) A3 adenosine receptor activation in melanoma cells: association between receptor fate and tumor growth inhibition. J Biol Chem 278:42121–42130. doi:10.1074/jbc.M301243200

81. Fishman P, Bar-Yehuda S, Ohana G, Barer F, Ochaion A, Erlanger A et al (2004) An agonist to the A3 adenosine receptor inhibits colon carcinoma growth in mice via modulation of GSK-3 beta and NF-kappa B. Oncogene 23:2465–2471. doi:10.1038/sj.onc.1207355
82. Ma DF, Kondo T, Nakazawa T, Niu DF, Mochizuki K, Kawasaki T et al (2010) Hypoxia-inducible adenosine A2B receptor modulates proliferation of colon carcinoma cells. Hum Pathol 41:1550–1557. doi:10.1016/j.humpath.2010.04.008
83. Lu J, Pierron A, Ravid K (2003) An adenosine analogue, IB-MECA, down-regulates estrogen receptor alpha and suppresses human breast cancer cell proliferation. Cancer Res 63:6413–6423
84. Panjehpour M, Karami-Tehrani F (2004) An adenosine analog (IB-MECA) inhibits anchorage-dependent cell growth of various human breast cancer cell lines. Int J Biochem Cell Biol 36:1502–1509. doi:10.1016/j.biocel.2003.12.001
85. Panjehpour M, Karami-Tehrani F (2007) Adenosine modulates cell growth in the human breast cancer cells via adenosine receptors. Oncol Res 16:575–585
86. Kohno Y, Sei Y, Koshiba M, Kim HO, Jacobson KA (1996) Induction of apoptosis in HL-60 human promyelocytic leukemia cells by adenosine A(3) receptor agonists. Biochem Biophys Res Commun 219:904–910. doi:10.1006/bbrc.1996.0331
87. Fishman P, Bar-Yehuda S, Synowitz M, Powell JD, Klotz KN, Gessi S et al (2009) Adenosine receptors and cancer. Handb Exp Pharmacol 193:399–441. doi:10.1007/978-3-540-89615-9_14
88. Colombel M, Olsson CA, Ng PY, Buttyan R (1992) Hormone-regulated apoptosis results from reentry of differentiated prostate cells onto a defective cell cycle. Cancer Res 52:4313–4319
89. Kim SG, Ravi G, Hoffmann C, Jung YJ, Kim M, Chen A et al (2002) p53-independent induction of Fas and apoptosis in leukemic cells by an adenosine derivative, Cl-IB-MECA. Biochem Pharmacol 63:871–880
90. Kim SY, Kim JE, Lee KW, Lee HJ (2009) Lactococcus lactis ssp. lactis inhibits the proliferation of SNU-1 human stomach cancer cells through induction of G0/G1 cell cycle arrest and apoptosis via p53 and p21 expression. Ann N Y Acad Sci 1171:270–275. doi:10.1111/j.1749-6632.2009.04721.x
91. Portt L, Norman G, Clapp C, Greenwood M, Greenwood MT (2011) Anti-apoptosis and cell survival: a review. Biochim Biophys Acta 1813:238–259. doi:10.1016/j.bbamcr.2010.10.010
92. Raffo AJ, Perlman H, Chen MW, Day ML, Streitman JS, Buttyan R (1995) Overexpression of Bcl-2 protects prostate cancer cells from apoptosis in vitro and confers resistance to androgen depletion in vivo. Cancer Res 55:4438–4445
93. Lin Y, Fukuchi J, Hiipakka RA, Kokontis JM, Xiang J (2007) Up-regulation of Bcl-2 is required for the progression of prostate cancer cells from an androgen-dependent to an androgen-independent growth stage. Cell Res 17:531–536
94. Appel E, Kazimirsky G, Ashkenazi E, Kim SG, Jacobson KA, Brodie C (2001) Roles of BCL-2 and caspase 3 in the adenosine A3 receptor-induced apoptosis. J Mol Neurosci 17:285–292. doi:10.1385/JMN:17:3:285
95. Wu LF, Li GP, Feng JL, Pu ZJ (2006) Molecular mechanisms of adenosine-induced apoptosis in human HepG2 cells. Acta Pharmacol Sin 27:477–484. doi:10.1111/j.1745-7254.2006.00302.x
96. Herr I, Debatin KM (2001) Cellular stress response and apoptosis in cancer therapy. Blood 98:2603–2614
97. Hashemi M, Karami-Tehrani F, Ghavami S, Maddika S, Los M (2005) Adenosine and deoxyadenosine induces apoptosis in oestrogen receptor-positive and -negative human breast cancer cells via the intrinsic pathway. Cell Prolif 38:269–285. doi:10.1111/j.1365-2184.2005.00349.x
98. Shieh DE, Chen YY, Yen MH, Chiang LC, Lin CC (2004) Emodin-induced apoptosis through p53-dependent pathway in human hepatoma cells. Life Sci 74:2279–2290. doi:10.1016/j.lfs.2003.09.060

99. El-Darahali A, Fawcett H, Mader JS, Conrad DM, Hoskin DW (2005) Adenosine-induced apoptosis in EL-4 thymoma cells is caspase-independent and mediated through a non-classical adenosine receptor. Exp Mol Pathol 79:249–258. doi:10.1016/j.yexmp.2005.08.001
100. Sai K, Yang D, Yamamoto H, Fujikawa H, Yamamoto S, Nagata T et al (2006) A(1) adenosine receptor signal and AMPK involving caspase-9/−3 activation are responsible for adenosine-induced RCR-1 astrocytoma cell death. Neurotoxicology 27:458–467. doi:10.1016/j.neuro.2005.12.008
101. Le Bras M, Clément MV, Pervaiz S, Brenner C (2005) Reactive oxygen species and the mitochondrial signaling pathway of cell death. Histol Histopathol 20:205–219
102. Ryter SW, Kim HP, Hoetzel A, Park JW, Nakahira K, Wang X et al (2007) Mechanisms of cell death in oxidative stress. Antioxid Redox Signal 9:49–89. doi:10.1089/ars.2007.9.49
103. Sosa V, Moliné T, Somoza R, Paciucci R, Kondoh H, LLeonart ME (2013) Oxidative stress and cancer: an overview. Ageing Res Rev 12:376–390. doi:10.1016/j.arr.2012.10.004
104. Sies H (1999) Glutathione and its role in cellular functions. Free Radic Biol Med 27:916–921
105. Atmaca M, Fry JR (1996) Adenosine-mediated inhibition of glutathione synthesis in rat isolated hepatocytes. Biochem Pharmacol 52:1423–1428
106. Merighi S, Benini A, Mirandola P, Gessi S, Varani K, Simioni C et al (2007) Caffeine inhibits adenosine-induced accumulation of hypoxia-inducible factor-1alpha, vascular endothelial growth factor, and interleukin-8 expression in hypoxic human colon cancer cells. Mol Pharmacol 72:395–406. doi:10.1124/mol.106.032920
107. Gessi S, Sacchetto V, Fogli E, Merighi S, Varani K, Baraldi PG et al (2010) Modulation of metalloproteinase-9 in U87MG glioblastoma cells by A3 adenosine receptors. Biochem Pharmacol 79:1483–1495. doi:10.1016/j.bcp.2010.01.009

Emerging Role of ncRNAs in Cancer Biology: Techniques for Diagnostic Monitoring and Potential ncRNA-Based Therapies

Palmiro Poltronieri, Oscar F. D'Urso, and Massimo Mallardo

Abstract In the last 10 years, the discovery that the human genome is able to generate a large number of RNAs non coding for proteins (ncRNAs) has changed our way to approach the understanding and studying of biology. In particular, the discovery of several Long ncRNAs (lncRNAs) and microRNAs (miRNAs) with tumor suppressor or oncogenic function, opened new horizons in molecular oncology research, diagnosis and potential therapies.

Cancer types need to be differentiated by cell type of origin, histological features and genes expression. In addition, it has been recently demonstrated the power of lncRNA signatures in diagnosis of many types of cancer and in the prediction of patients survival.

As oncogenic ncRNAs may support survival of the transformed cells, thus leading to therapy resistance, ncRNA silencing therapies could be a valuable approach to be associated with anticancer drugs and chemotherapy treatments.

Blocking of oncomiR may be achieved by introduction of miRNA sponges with multiple complementary sequences, by antisense oligonucleotides, anti-microRNA sequences (with modified oligonucleotides such as locked nucleic acids, phosphorothioate backbone sequences preventing the cleavage, and 2-O-methoxyethyl modified sequences) named antagomirs. On the other hand, detection of deregulated lncRNAs in tumors as diagnostic biomarkers start to be used in the clinical practice.

Keywords Cancer • Disease induced deregulation of genes • Gene isoforms • Differential splicing • Epigenetics • Stability of mRNAs • lncRNA • miRNA

P. Poltronieri (✉) • O.F. D'Urso
CNR-ISPA, Institute of Sciences of Food Productions, National Research Council, Lecce, Italy
e-mail: palmiro.poltronieri@ispa.cnr.it

M. Mallardo
Department of Molecular Medicine and Medical Biotechnology, University of Naples, Naples, Italy

A.A. Farooqi, M. Ismail (eds.), *Molecular Oncology: Underlying Mechanisms and Translational Advancements*, DOI 10.1007/978-3-319-53082-6_5

Acronyms

BANCR	BRAF-activated non-coding RNA
HOTAIR	*Hox* transcript antisense intergenic RNA
HOTTIP	HOMEOBOX A transcript at the distal tip
lincRNA	long interspersed non coding RNA
MALAT1	Metastasis-associated lung adenocarcinoma transcript 1
NGS	Next Generation Sequencing
PAH	Polycyclic aromatic hydrocarbons
PCA3	Prostate cancer 3
SAMMSON	Survival Associated Mitochondrial Melanoma-Specific Oncogenic Noncoding *RNA*

Introduction

Cancer is a complex disease, whose molecular etiology includes both genetic modifications and epigenetic aberrations. At genetic level, carcinogenesis is mediated by DNA damage, oncogene activation and inactivation of tumour suppressor genes, including ncRNAs (see [1], for review). At epigenetic level, lncRNAs are emerging as important mechanisms that contribute to induction of carcinogenicity. The specificity of lncRNA expression is now recognized as an important epigenetic mark acting as a biomarker for cancer assessment following exposure to environmental pollutants [2]. For instance, the lncRNA HOTAIR has been shown to facilitate tumor initiation and progression, is associated with poor prognosis in several cancers, and was found to be altered after exposure to PAHs [3].

Chromosome rearrangements, deletions and point mutations alter the transcriptional, translational and post-transcriptional landscapes. Several methods are available for DNA analysis to identify the insertions, deletions, or single nucleotide variations, in tissues or defined cell types. Molecular genetic information has been used to derive new therapeutic regimens and has accelerated the development and application of "personalised cancer medicine". There are also an increasing appreciation that epigenetic aberrations that are often directly caused by genetic defects resulting in loss- or gain-of-function of epigenetic-regulators also contribute significantly to cancer onset and progression. Molecular lesions after transformation are either DNA-based, including chromosomal amplification, deletion, mutation, and translocation, or epigenetic lesions, such as hypomethylation of DNA sequences at promoter regions or changing the euchromatin opening state through histone marks regulated by Polycomb Repressing Complexes (PRC), and finally there are RNA-based modifications, potentially amenable to RNA intervention for phenotype reprogramming (RNA silencing, RNA decoys, rybozymes, RNA sponges). Finally, circulating extracellular ncRNAs can be detected in the blood and urine samples of patients and they may serve as prognostic, diagnostic and therapy follow up for different diseases including cancer.

Potential Use of ncRNAs as a Disease Biomarkers, Biomarkers for Disease Progression

With the introduction of Laser Capture Microdissection and single cell RNA sequencing, it is now feasible to differentiate the transcriptome throughput of different cell types. Indeed, all cell types possess a unique molecular signature, referred to as biomarkers, which define the principal cellular features such the capabilities of certain genes to be expressed into proteins or ncRNAs and perform their functions among all genes contained into a specific genome. Many cancer types (i.e. breast, colon, lung tumours) are undetectable before the appearance of a solid mass of various millimetres. Thus, RNA has been long studied as biomarker to potentially identify the presence of few cells in the blood stream or in the urine samples revealing the precocious formation of a cancer still undetectable using scanning techniques (TAC, PET, metabolite radioisotopes). For instance, circulating cells originating from thyroid cancers have been investigated by means of Real Time (RT)-PCR using primers specific for few mRNAs expressed only in thyroid cells [4]. Also in the case of brain tumours, there is a necessity to detect as much earlier as possible to presence of cancer cells without surgical intervention [5, 6]. Integration of the knowledge of the cancer genome and epigenome using sophisticated "Omic" technologies (transcriptomics, Deep Super–Serial Analysis of Gene Expression combined with Next-Generation-Sequencing of transcript tags, RNA sequencing and small RNA sequencing) and high throughput functional screening techniques are providing tangible prove of links between genetic/genomic aberrations, epigenetic/epigenomic deregulation and tumorigenesis. Moreover, these information can be translated into clinical use through the finding of genetic and epigenetic biomarkers of cancer development, evolution, heterogeneity and response to therapeutic intervention. Recent studies have evaluated the potential application of tumor-derived circulating ncRNAs as a diagnostic tool for either early detection of systemic cancer, prediction of tumour progression, or as means to monitor the response to therapy. Although ncRNAs do not encode proteins, it is now clear and well documented their role during the steps of tumorigenesis and the development of therapeutic resistance [7–10]. One of the first lncRNA identified as associated to cancer is *MALAT1*. It has also be associated with metastasis and poor prognosis for patients with non-small cell lung cancer (NSCLC) [11]. *MALAT1* resides on chromosome 11q13.1 which has been found to harbor chromosomal translocation breakpoints linked to cancer [12–14]. The *Hox* transcript antisense intergenic RNA *HOTAIR* represents a good example of how lncRNAs can be involved in aetiology of cancer, chromatin remodeling and, in turn, it represents a cancer biomarker. Moreover, high expression of *HOTAIR* correlates with worse survival in many cancer types [15]. Both *HOTAIR and MALAT1* lncRNAs can be detected in urine and blood samples of patients. For example, they are considered, together with *TUG1* and *GASS*, sensitive biomarkers of PHAs exposure and PAHs-induced DNA damage [2]. HOTAIR was recently proposed as diagnostic biomarker of colorectal cancer (CRC) and liver metastases correlating with a poor prognosis [16]. *HOTAIR, H19* and *MEG3* have been found to be associated with miRNAs in gastric cancer (GC), generating regulatory crosstalk across the transcriptome [17, 18]. Finally, the lncRNA *Prostate Cancer 3* (*PCA3*), can be easily detected in urine samples by RT-PCR. It is considered as a prostate cancer marker and it is now used on routine basis in the clinical practice. Also microRNAs represent an useful source of cancer biomarkers. Recently, the expression pattern of seven miRNAs (*miR-10b, miR-21, miR-125b, miR-145, miR-155 miR*-191 and *miR-382*) showed specific characteristics in serum of breast cancer patients compared to healthy controls and those miRNA were proposed as breast cancer biomarkers [19]. Another work showed that 38 microRNAs in whole blood were significantly de-regulated in patients with pancreatic cancer compared with controls [20]. Meta-analysis permitted the identification of circulating microRNAs as novel potential biomarkers for gastric cancer detection [21]. All together these reports demonstrate that miRNAs are effective diagnostic biomarkers for cancer but, differently to lncRNAs, a single molecule is not enough for the diagnosis but rather a specific signature.

Non-coding RNAs and microRNAs: RNAs as Active Components of Cellular Processes and Signalling Pathways, Relationship with Pathological States and Cancer

RNAs are now recognised to be active components of many cellular processes and signalling pathways, and represent the major output of DNA. A large number of non-protein coding transcripts has been discovered in recent years, with most of them appearing to be functional, with a specific phenotype linked to down-regulation or overexpression [22]. Transcripts may be processed into mature, shorter sequences, and constitute several functional classes: dual mRNAs with ribo-regulation role and producing small peptides, long, interspersed non-coding RNAs (lincRNA), antisense RNAs and small RNAs (sRNA) of various lengths. Non-coding RNAs (ncRNAs) regulate key biological processes during development or in pathological contexts by mechanisms distinct from protein-mediated interactions. The ncRNAome is considered the entirety of all ncRNAs in a specific organ or cell type. Thus, RNAs are a hidden layer of regulation of the active genetic information that is translated in the cell specific output and phenotype. RNAs are part of and assemble chromatin remodelling complexes, ribonucleoproteins; RNA splicing complexes, mRNA maturation complexes, RNA-binding proteins involved in transport to long distances and compartmentalisation; RNA riboswitches; RNA decoys; circular RNAs (closed mRNA); natural antagomiRs and miRNA sponges.

Small non-coding RNAs deregulation has been linked to several types of cancers, such as breast [23] and endometrial cancers [24]. To evaluate differential expression of small RNAs, NGS platforms and sequencing of small RNAs has been combined with bioinformatics and ad-hoc pipelines [25].

Among sncRNAs, microRNAs (miRNAs) constitute one of the best investigated classes. Lacking or de-regulated expression of certain miRNAs is, amongst others, associated with oncogenesis and cardiovascular, endocrine or neurological disorders. The link between certain microRNAs and their overexpression in cancer types has been shown: for instance, overexpression of *miR-17-92* cluster has been observed in several diseases [26, 27], such as human lung cancer, where it enhances cell proliferation [28]. For instance, miRNA expression and biogenesis has been shown induced by estrogen receptor beta in hormone-responsive breast cancer [29].

This finding brought to the definition of cancer-overexpressed miRNAs as oncomiRs. Detection of overexpressed oncomiRs has been one of the emerging fields of cancer diagnostics [30], with several platforms shown to be suitable for this aim, most recently also digital PCR [31]. On the contrary, the finding of microRNAs within deleted regions of chromosomes and the functional characterization of their involvement in cancers has led to the definition of suppressor microRNAs.

The localization of human *miR-15a/miR-16* cluster at the 13q14 chromosomal breakpoint or deletion sites has suggested their involvement in the aetiology of the chronic lymphocytic leukemia (CLL) and multiple myeloma [32].

Since their discovery, miRNAs were associated with different functions in major signaling pathways, cellular processes and tissue morphogenesis. MicroRNAs exert their function in cooperation with Argonaute proteins by post-transcriptional gene silencing (RNA silencing) of messenger RNAs (mRNAs). Binding of a miRNA to a target mRNA either results in translational repression or miRNA-mediated degradation subsequent to cleavage of the target mRNA by the Argonaute endonuclease. The binding sites for miRNAs are often present in the 3′ untranslated region (3′ UTR) of mRNAs, especially in mammals. Additionally, miRNA-binding sites may be present in the coding sequence of mRNAs: these binding sites are linked to translational repression. Even though miRNA binding site predictions are often exclusively focused on these 3′ UTRs, identification of truly used binding sites is pursued using several approaches, such as cell transformation with plasmids carrying a reporter gene tailed with a target 3′UTR sequence specific for each microRNA.

Furthermore, the widespread alternative polyadenylation in eukaryotes generates mRNAs with alternative (non-canonical) 3′ ends. Recently, multiple polyadenylation sites were identified in more than 50% of all human genes, and as a consequence these genes encode mRNAs that harbour different miRNA binding sites in their 3′ UTRs.

Alternative polyadenylation (APA) as well as single-nucleotide polymorphisms (SNPs) affect miRNA targeting of transcripts from different individuals and tissues [33, 34]. Especially, APA is known to contribute to variations in miRNA-mRNA interplay in animals [35]. SNPs in miRNA sequences have been associated with better or poorer response to treatment, tumor susceptibility [36], and prognosis [37], or in healthy bone tissue [38] and in ageing processes.

The total number of mRNAs subject to miRNA-mediated decay can be determined by high-throughput techniques combined with NGS analysis. In view of these complex regulatory mechanisms, analyses of complementing miRNA and mRNA datasets may provide a more complete understanding of cellular states.

RNA complexes involved in splicing and in mRNA polyadenylation are often in competition with binding sites on mRNAs and with structural RNAs involved in the assembling of spliceosomes and other protein complexes. Alternative splicing has been shown in various types of cancers, such as estrogen-dependent breast cancer [39]. Thus, small RNAs and long RNAs shape the evolution of protein-coding genes in eukaryotes.

Circulating, secretory miRNAs are often abundant and very stable in blood [40] and urine samples, protected from ribonucleases by proteins and lipid membranes within exosome particles, an important prerequisite for clinical biomarker tests [41, 42]. Furthermore, these miRNAs remain stable at harsh conditions including boiling, low/high pH, extended storage, freeze-thaw cycles. Circulating miRNAs in the blood of cancer patients could play the same important roles as miRNAs in tissues. Exosomes have been shown to have an active role intercellular signaling [43]. Even for circulating miRNAs, there are findings showing the use of some circulating miRNA species as biomarker of certain cancer types [44–47].

RT-PCR methodology has been introduced and applied extensively in several technology settings. For instance, as a method to confirm the data obtained by DNA microarrays, after appropriate selection of candidate genes. Often the hybridisation signals and the value of expression found using RT-PCR are quite different, showing potential biases between the fluorescence-based method or caused by inappropriate primers or oligonucleotide sequence. A second method of choice is following the analysis of SuperSAGE (serial analysis of gene expression) data, to confirm the over-expression values of specific isoforms of genes using Taqman validated primers.

Deregulated ncRNAs and Their Potential Effects on Cancer Therapies

As above explained, from a clinical point of view, non-coding RNAs aberrations show high diagnostic and prognostic values. Among lincRNAs, several types have been linked to better or poorer prognosis and malignant phenotypes. Among them, *SAMMSON*, was deregulated in melanoma [48, 49], *BANCR* in melanoma [50] in hepatocellular carcinoma (HCC) [51] in small cell lung cancer (SCLC) [52] gastric cancer [53] and in osteosarcoma [54]. *HOTTIP* was found up-regulated and associated with poor prognosis in osteosarcoma [55] and in gastric cancer [56]. CCAT2 was found correlated to poor prognosis in gastric cancers [57].

Lnc2Cancer is a manually curated database of experimentally supported lncRNAs associated with various human cancers [58]. In ovarian (OV) cancer, two protective lncRNAs, *RP11-284N8.3.1* and *AC104699.1.1*, were differentially expressed throughout the progression of malignant OV and also independently predictive of the survival of patients [17, 18].

In Fig. 1 are shown several ncRNAs with their roles in cellular processes, individuated as potential targets for therapeutic intervention in different types of cancers.

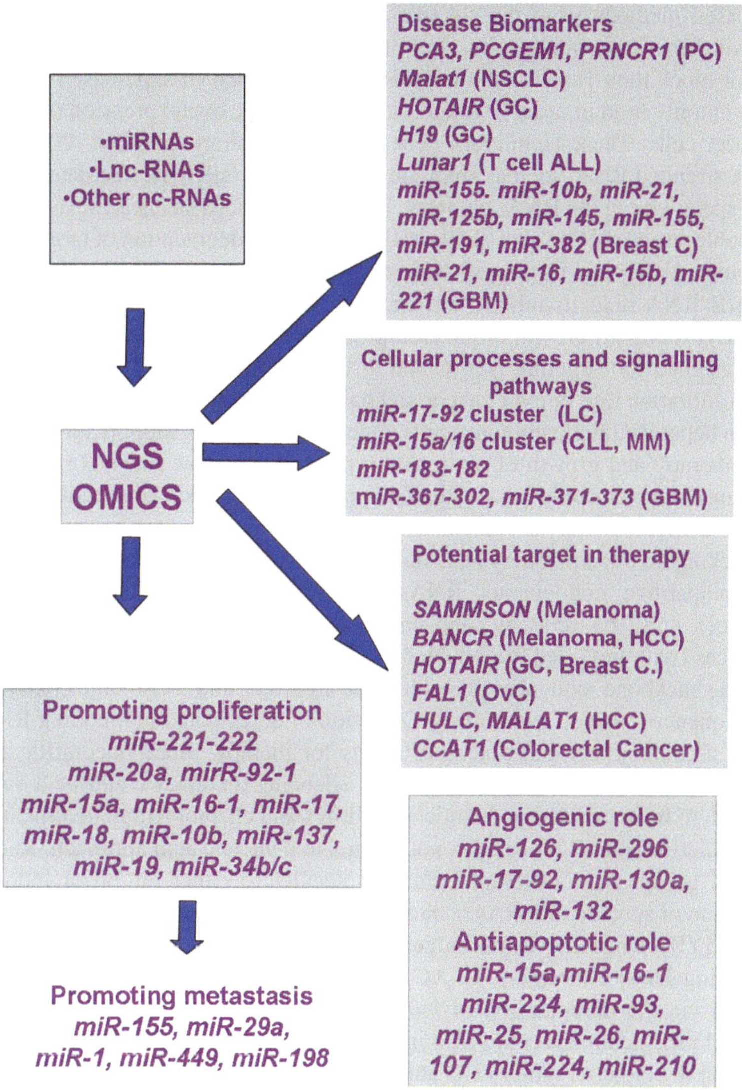

Fig. 1 A selection of lncRNAs and miRNAs with a role in cellular processes related to development of various types of cancers, such as cell proliferation,angiogenesis, antiapoptotic activity

It is clear that the improvement of the knowledge on the nature and roles of non-coding RNAs will enhance our capability to develop therapeutic treatment against cancer via the modulation of these RNA molecules. Moreover, the progress in nucleic acid drug design linked to advanced computational simulation will prompt the development of agents to intervene the malignant effects of non-coding RNAs.

Most of the attempts for therapeutic strategies targeting lncRNAs were performed depleting the oncogenic lncRNAs in cancer cells [59]. So far, the nucleic acid-based methods were the elective approaches to target RNA molecules, and they were able to normalize the level of deregulated lncRNAs, modify their structures or block their functional motifs. RNA interference (RNAi)-based techniques are commonly used in order to inhibit or even block the overexpression of lncRNAs in cancer cells. These techniques generally employ short stretched (20–30 nt) of double-stranded RNA, such as small interfering RNA (siRNA), that determines the target specificity in the RNAi pathway. Inhibition of lncRNAs is achieved thanks to the double stranded RNA that elicits a RISC-mediated degradation of target lncRNA molecules. Using this technique, were designed siRNAs able to specifically target *HOTAIR* RNA able to inhibit cell invasion ability of breast cancer cells [16]. Similarly, xenograft growth of pancreatic cancer cells [60] was also inhibited. siRNAs designed for targeting *HULC* and *MALAT1* showed the ability to inhibit the cell proliferation rate in liver cancer and halted cell cycle progression (reviewed in [61]) in hepatocellular carcinoma cells. Oncogenic ncRNAs support survival during chemotherapy and growth of malignant types linked to low survival rate: ncRNA silencing therapies could be a valuable approach to be associated with anticancer drugs and chemotherapy treatments.

Blocking an oncomiR may be achieved by introduction of miRNA sponges [62] and competitive endogenous RNAs (ceRNA) with multiple complementary sequences [18, 63–65], by antisense oligonucleotides [66], anti-microRNA sequences (with modified oligonucleotides such as locked nucleic acids, phosphorothioate backbone sequences preventing the cleavage, and 2-O-methoxyethyl modified sequences) named antagomirs. Detection of deregulated non-coding RNAs in tumors as biomarkers and potential targets for therapy. Since oncomiRs support survival during chemotherapy, microRNA silencing therapies could be a valuable approach to be associated with anticancer drugs and chemotherapy treatments.

Modulation of miRNA level is not limited to a nucleic acid approach. Recently, different groups have developed small molecules to either inhibit or induce the expression of specific miRNAs in cancer cells. Small molecule inhibitor of *miR-21* AC1MMYR2 could block the biogenesis of mature *miR-21* from *pre-miR-21* by attenuating Dicer cleavage [67]. AC1MMYR2 could suppress tumor growth and invasion via the upregulation of *miR-21* functional targets such as PTEN [68]. AC1MMYR2 treatment could also induce the reversal of epithelial-mesenchymal transition in epithelial tumor cells and orthotopic nude mouse model [67]. In addition to *miR-21*, the level of *miR-122* can also be modified by small molecules. Both inhibitors and activators were generated that are capable of inducing the down-regulation or upregulation of *miR-122* transcriptionally [69]. Study showed that inhibitors of *miR-122* could inhibit HCV replication in liver cells, as *miR-122* is a cellular component required by the hepatitis C virus (HCV) for viral replication. Moreover, activation of *miR-122* could elicit a proapoptotic effect in cancer cells. Thus small molecules could up-regulate *miR-122* in the hepatocellular carcinoma cells, and subsequently increase caspase expression, leading to cell apoptosis and reduced cell viability.

Several miRNA activators have been studied and applied to up-regulate the expression of the tumor suppressor *miR-34a* [70, 71]. A natural product, Rubone, was screened out that was capable of transcriptionally upregulating *miR-34a* level in hepatocellular carcinoma cells [72]. The study showed that Rubone could increase *miR-34a* promoter activities and p53 occupancy on miR-34a promoter in both wild-type and mutant p53 cells. Rubone inhibited hepatocellular carcinoma growth without showing hepatocyte toxicity [69].

Biogenesis of mature miRNA provides another mechanism for modulating miRNA level. Inhibition of miRNAs can be achieved by interfering with the maturation of the precursor molecules of miRNA. Aptamers, short DNA or RNA oligonucleotides or peptides that have a stable 3-dimensional structure in vivo, are compounds blocking pre-miRNA maturation. The binding relies on the fitting of the aptamer with the 3-dimensional shape of the targets [73]. Studies showed that aptamer could reduce the level of miRNAs through targeting the apical loop domain of pri-microRNA molecules, and block the biogenesis of mature microRNA. An aptamer was screened, selectively interacting with the target *pri-miR-18a*, and inhibit the binding of hnRNP A1 to the apical loop of pri-microRNA which was able to interrupt *miR-18a* maturation [74]. *miR-17-92* cluster gives rise to a set of oncogenic microRNAs which target SOCS1, PTEN and BIM, among others. An aptamer was developed that could abrogate the biogenesis of miRNAs at the entire *miR-17-92* cluster. The introduction of miR-*17-92* aptamer could block the maturation of *miR-17*, *miR-18a* and *miR-19b* in retinoblastoma cell lines, leading to the induction of cell cycle arrest and apoptosis [75]. In addition to being the drug targets, miRNAs can be regarded as the drug used in cancer treatment. Ectopically introducing miRNAs that repress the level of oncogenic protein coding mRNAs is another potential therapeutic strategy against cancers. Like siRNAs, mimics of miRNA can be employed as therapeutic agents to target specific oncogene or oncogenic network based on its endogenous gene silencing ability of miRNAs [76]. In this way, instead of reversing the loss of miRNAs, the aim of the miRNAs introduction is to induce gain of functions in cancer cells that elicits tumor suppressing effects. Such idea has been verified by the study in which the level of oncogene BCR/ABL was suppressed by synthetic miRNAs [77]. miRNA-based anticancer therapy has great potential as reports showed there is apparent lack of adverse effects in normal tissues when administrated with miRNA-based agent.

Among anti-microRNA oligonucleotides, there are those containing modified oligonucleotides (locked nucleic acids, phosphorothioate backbone sequences that prevent their cleavage, the 2-O-methoxyethyl modified sequences). Among antagomirs, there are RNA sponges [78] and circular RNAs with multiple miR binding sites [66], miRNA inhibitors conjugated to gold and lipid nanoparticles [79, 80] or transferrin-coated nanoparticles [81]. Thus, antagomir therapeutics targeting microvesicles in the brain could take the lead in the near future in the treatment of brain cancers in substitution of invasive surgical intervention.

Taken together, treatment with siRNA or ectopic miRNA agonists and antagonists seem to be all promising therapeutic advancement.

Real Time PCR in Quantification of Non-coding RNAs

To date, no reliable circulating biomarkers for the detection and risk stratification of gliomas have been identified, while few intracellular miRNAs (*miR-155, miR-21*) have been detected at high levels in glioblastoma tumours [6, 82, 83].

In one study on circulating miRNAs, 48 plasma samples of patients with glial tumors, 48 control patients with various neurological disorders, 36 patients with B-cell lymphoma of the CNS (BCNSL) and 16 patients with brain metastases or leptomeningeal secondary involvement originated from various carcinomas were analyzed [5]. The study was based on samples sent routinely to the laboratory. RNA was extracted from whole blood and serum samples that were obtained at the time of surgical treatment. Circulating RNA was extracted from serum prepared by centrifugation starting from 10 mL of whole blood that were obtained at the time of surgical treatment. In their study, a four-miRNA signature was identified as a predictor for overall survival in glioma at various staging and in other malignancies. A higher expression of miR-15b and remarkably decreased expression of *miR-21* were found in plasma samples from patients with glioma. *MiR-15b* was the most abundant miRNA in blood samples showing an eight-fold higher expression levels in blood samples from patients with glioma. *MiR-21*, which also has been found overexpressed in CSF samples from patients with glioma [84], is one of the most consistently expressed microRNA in cancer.

In a wide array of studies on microRNAs, various amplification platforms have been developed and applied, either in the form of Rolling Cycle Amplification (RCA) of adaptors added to the 5′ and 3′ ends, combining a miR-sequence specific primer and a tag-based reverse primer.

The Kreatech microRNA labelling kit was initially developed to label miRNAs hybridised onto miRNA arrays, making use of KREAPURE clean up column that separate the RNA fractions. Nowadays several products are available and in need to be tested before optimisation of assay conditions.

Two methods have been developed to detect specific miRNAs by qPCR. The first makes use of miRNA-specific reverse transcription (stem–loop) primers while the second technique uses universal reverse transcription primers. A number of fluorescent-based technologies exist for qPCR, but both SYBR Green and TaqMan have been successfully used for miRNA detection.

Using SYBR Green based qPCR assay, the efficiency of the PCR assay needs to be determined by running a ten-fold serial dilution (standard curve) for the miRNA. Every 3.32 cycle threshold should represent a ten-fold amplification, which is equal to 100% efficiency. In addition to running a standard curve, it is also important to perform a ‘melt’ or ‘dissociation’ curve. This is essential for SYBR Green based qPCR as the dye is incorporated into any double stranded DNA formed during qPCR (including primer dimers). A single peak (i.e. one PCR product) should be present in the melt curve.

Several methods are available combined with Taqman probes. One method initially uses stem–loop miRNA specific primers that bind to the 3′-portion of miRNA molecules that are individually reversed transcribed. Then, the product (cDNA) is quantified using conventional assays such as TaqMan miRNA assays that include a miRNA-specific forward primer, reverse primer and a dye-labelled probe. Each assay is similar in terms of amplicon length, primers are pre-designed and pre-validated. In conclusion, separate reverse transcription reactions for each miRNA of interest and reference genes must be performed.

Another method adds a common sequence poly(A)tail to the 3′-end of all miRNAs and then reverse transcribes all miRNAs in a certain sample by using a universal primer. qPCR is then performed with a SYBR Green fluorescent dye using a linear miRNA specific primer, designed by the user and universal qPCR primer.

Protocol for Set Up of Real Time PCR Reactions

Total RNA is extracted using a TRIZOL (Invitrogen). miRNA fraction can be isolated using a PureLink™ miRNA Isolation Kit (Invitrogen) following manufacturer's instructions. The RNA concentration is determined by measuring a 2 μL aliquot on a NanoDrop ND-3300 spectrophotometer. A check of RNA integrity is performed using the Agilent Bioanalyser. TaqMan miRNA assays (Applied Biosystems) were set up. In brief, 10 μL of total RNA solution was used for the reverse transcription reaction using a Superscript Reverse Transcriptase followed by in-tube amplification with Taq Gold polymerase. Real-time PCR was performed using a 7500 Real-Time PCR System according to the manufacturer's protocol (Applied Biosystems). Cycling conditions were as follows: 95 °C for 10 min and 40 cycles of 15 s at 95 °C and 60 s at 60 °C. Fluorescent data are converted into cycle threshold (Ct) measurements using the 7500 SDS system software (version 1.2.3; Applied Biosystems). Each sample is run in duplicate. Mean Ct values and standard deviations are calculated for all miRNAs. Several house-keeping genes can be used, but generally the actin expression values have been used, to obtain the relative quantification of each gene monitored in different cell types.

For microRNA quantification in bodily fluids (plasma, serum, cerebrospinal fluid), an immediate need for a small housekeeping miRNA exists because other classes of small RNAs, such as the snoRNA *RNU6B*, cannot not be used for normalization due to instability in presence of RNases. In published work [5], *miR-24* was proposed for normalisation and showed to be applicable to the analysis of miRNAs in various types of tumors. The amount of target miRNA was normalized relative to the amount of *miR-24* (ΔCt = ΔCt *miRx* − ΔCt *miR-24*). Relative expression levels (RELs) were reported as 2 − ΔCt.

The comparison of miRNA data in plasma collected from patients with gliomablastoma (WHO IV) and the other glioma grades (WHO II and II), revealed significantly decreased expression of *miR-16* in plasma samples from patients with glioblastoma (WHO IV). This was an initial study on few miRNAs as serum biomarkers in glioblastoma [5]. Further studies may reveal additional deregulated miRNAs based on the databases of human microRNAs that nowadays contain several thousand sequences: miRNA biomarkers could predict disease recurrence after surgery to provide an early detection method for the progression of disease after surgery.

Detection of lncRNAs and miRNAs in Urine Samples

Circulating extracellular ncRNAs from other tissues within the body can be delivered to renal epithelial cells and released into the urine bound to RNA-binding proteins (soluble fraction) or packaged into microvesicles such as exosomes. Thus the ncRNAs must be extracted from the urine after differential ultracentrifugation on both supernatant (soluble fraction) by standard protocol such as Trizol and on the pellets (exosomal fraction) as described [85]. The total RNAs extracted (each sample is a pool of soluble plus exosomal fractions), need to be retro-transcribed and can be further analyzed by microarray choosing miRNA or lncRNA microarray platform. Following, comparing samples deriving from cancer patients and normal ones will the ncRNAs, potentially biomarkers of a specific cancer, can be identified through random variance model (RVM). RVM, F-test will have been used for analysis. After the significance and false discovery rate (FDR) analysis, will select differentially expressed genes according to the statistical significance of t-test after adjustment with the Benjamini and Hochberg correction for multiple comparisons. The cut-off for t-test P-values will be <0.001. Validation of microarray data can be performed by quantitative real-time PCR (qRT-PCR).

As *PCA3*, a prostate cancer biomarker, represents the best example of ncRNA currently used in the clinical practice we want to point out that it can be easily detected from urine samples using the Real Time PCR technique. Thus, once a ncRNA is identified as biomarker, it offers the possibility to perform, on a routine basis, a rapid, efficient, sensitive and non invasive disease assessment.

Comparing Methods and Complementation with Further Analyses: DNA Array Expression

In a different experimental setting, we monitored the differential expression of non-coding RNA candidates and other less representative transcripts often not present in commercial DNA microarrays by comparing several cell lines representative of various different tumours and the NB4 and HL-60 cell lines induced to differentiate by ATRA (All-trans retinoic acid) and histone deacetylase inhibitors (HDACI) such as niacin and butyrate [86].

The following cancer cell lines were used. Breast cancer: MCF-7, SKBR3, HS-578T, MDA-MD-231. Brain cancer: CCF-STTG1, Be(2)C, DAOY, CHP-212. Testis cancer: 833KE, NT2, Tera-1, 2102EP. Colon cancer: SW1116, LS174-T, Caco-2, WiDr. Lung cancer: GLC-4, GLC-34, H226, SW1573. Total RNA was provided by Prof. Wiemer, Erasmus Medical Centre, Rotterdam. Rhabdomyosarcoma: Embryonal RMS (T174, TE441, Ruch2) and Alveolar RMS (TE617, TE381, RD, Hs729, RH4, RH30) cell lines were provided by M. Kool, Amsterdam Medical Centre. TE381 and RD are ARMS cell lines with identical progenitor cells.

After a preliminary screening through hybridization on an in-house made Ribochip array containing more than 400 ncRNA candidate genes, 10% of the transcripts were found differentially expressed showing in several cases cell type specificity. The aim of this work initially was to screen 491 candidate transcripts using the DNA array to focus on those expressed at detectable levels, and then to make an estimate of quantitative differences in expression using the RT-PCR method on a selection of randomly chosen transcripts.

AK055935, found highly expressed also in brain and testis cancer cell lines, is a patented probe for use in neuroblastoma cancers. Few genes were found expressed in almost all the cancer cell lines, such as *AK092435, AK130351, AK131003* and *BC035189*. Possibly, the mechanisms controlling the regulation of their expression in cancer cells was lost, through alteration of transcriptional factors or epigenetic control. Other genes, whose expression levels fell in most cases under the arbitrary threshold of 1 fluorescence unit, were found at detectable levels in a limited number of cancer cell lines.

Undifferentiated and differentiated NB4 cells were also analyzed for the expression of ncRNAs using the DNA microarrays. Only a small number of transcripts were found differentially expressed in NB4 cells during the treatments. *AK025078 (SLC26A2), AK027179, AK055935, AK125234* and *BC030949* were less expressed in differentiated NB4 cells than in proliferating NB4 cells. *BC030949 (BC025181)* contains a 50 amino acid-long ORF potentially coding for an isoform of a PTPN11-like non-receptor tyrosine phosphatase, and was linked to juvenile leukaemia.

The cluster of genes found downregulated in differentiated NB4 cells could be referred to ontogeny groups required either for proliferation, cell cycling or cell survival [86].

On the other side, few genes detected in some of the cancer cell lines, as *AK023690, AK097380, AK098425, AK128567, BC035189* and *AL110204*, were found expressed at higher levels in differentiated NB4 cells in respect to proliferating NB4 cells [86]. The genes clustering together in cancer cells and in differentiated NB4 cells may be grouped in an ontogeny class of cellular homeostasis, being regulated at transcriptional level and inducible by transcription factors.

Sixteen genes, among those found deregulated on DNA microarrays, were validated by real-time PCR. RT-PCR was performed on 16 cancer cell lines, those whose RNA was available and of good quality. These transcripts showed significant changes between cancer cell lines, and in respect to the controls, brain RNA or testis reference RNA.

The RT-PCR of 11 transcripts was performed using undifferentiated and differentiated NB4 cells. The results showed that *H19* was downregulated after NB4 differentiation, whereas *AK021516* and *AK092435* were overexpressed in differentiated NB4 cells. Meningioma samples were also analyzed for the expression of ncRNAs using semi-quantitative RT-PCR, compared to the expression obtained from normal brain RNA. Four genes were confirmed varying their expression levels. *AK092435* and *H19* were found overexpressed, whereas *AK022994* and *AK027352* were downregulated in meningioma [82].

The intensity of signals detected in the Ribochip arrays did not perfectly matched the real-time PCR data. In some case, as *AK097934* in DAOY cell line, both the Ribochip and the RT-PCR revealed an expression higher that in the remaining cell lines. The differences in intensity of fluorescence may vary depending on many factors, i.e. the design of the oligonucleotide probes, the presence of secondary structures, the set up of hybridization conditions and the lack of automated washing station to perform the experiments uniformly. Many authors suggested to extend the hybridization time over the 24 h, since prolonged times approach more reliably a situation of equilibrium.

In the case of *AK098425*, RT-PCR results were similar in all the cell lines, but the Ribochip results showed higher differences in intensity values in different cell lines. In CACO-2 cells, AL122122 RT-PCR showed lower expression levels that in other cell lines, but the Ribochip signal was high. We thus assumed the Ribochip data as qualitative data without a high confidence on quantitative estimates. Due to the bias introduced using the Ribochip data, we compared the results on the cell lines on the basis of RT-PCR data (unpublished results).

In addition, few experiments using the Northern blot method were performed, to show the size of the expressed transcripts. Using the *AK128567* PCR product as probe, the obtained signals showed the presence of a 3400 base long mRNA and a smaller transcript of about 2800 bases. The GenBank reported length of *AK128567* is 3384 bases. The coding sequence of *AK128567* overlaps with several ESTs reported in other databases, each with one exon falling within the *AK128567* sequence (*BG503445* isolated from embryonal carcinoma, *DB471951* from hippocampus, and *BG255077* from adenocarcinoma). It may be possible that *AK128567* is further processed or that the probe used in this work recognizes the transcripts containing these reported ESTs.

The data on differential expression of selected genes using ARMS cell lines were coherent. TE381 and RD are cell lines with identical progenitor cells. In these lines the expression results were reproducible, reflecting the similar phenotype.

A prototype of dual transcripts potentially peptide-coding and functioning as riboregulators is provided by *H19*. This extensively studied npcRNA was found expressed in many cancer cell lines [22]. In SKBR3 breast cancer cells, over-expressing the ERB-B2 kinase, *H19* was found expressed at levels higher than in the well studied MCF-7 hormone-sensitive cell line. The process of differentiation in NB4 cells corresponded to a decrease in *H19* expression [86]. This finding supports the general opinion that non-coding RNAs exhibit dynamical alteration in their level of expression in response to a specific physiological stimulus in patterns that parallel the behaviour of mRNAs, and suggests that their transcription is functional and that their expression is controlled by tight mechanisms.

H19 has a predictive value for tumour recurrence in bladder cancer. While *H19* expression is downregulated after birth [87], the endometrium and ovary are two of the very few tissues that retain the ability to express the *H19* gene in adult life. *H19* expression increases in the carotid artery after injury, suggesting its role during wound healing. While *H19* RNA does not provide any growth advantage for the cells when cultured in 10% FCS, it enabled cells to overcome the stress caused by serum starvation, with no significant difference in apoptotic rate. This finding showed the importance of *H19* gene expression in tumours under stress conditions when growth factor availability is limited. It is interesting to note that several genes that are upregulated in the presence of *H19* also are induced by hypoxic stress. Hypoxia is considered a tumour gateway, with progression along the angiogenic pathway. *H19* gene is responsible for positively regulating the thioredoxin gene at the post-transcriptional level, thioredoxin being a key protein of the oxidative stress response and accumulates in many cancerous tissues, such as breast carcinomas in which an overexpression of the *H19* gene was shown [22]. Hypoxia and serum starvation both the consequence of a poorly vascularised tumour, considered a normal stage of tumour development, may be thus two factors causing the overexpression of the mRNAs shown in this work. *AK027352*, a gene regulated by hypoxia, was found over-expressed in various cell lines. However, in the analysis of NB4 cells using the RT-PCR method, the transcript showed unchanged expression levels in undifferentiated and differentiating cells. *AK001558* is a gene found over-expressed in microglial cells after 1 h induced by oestrogens, upregulated at the sixth hour through the oxygen radical response. *AK001558* was found over-expressed in many cancer cells lines, and showed similar high expression levels also in non-differentiated NB4 cells (relative expression values, obtained as ratio of *AK001558/actin* as control) [86]. It is possible that this transcript remains expressed at detectable levels in differentiated NB4 cells in response to ROS or other environmental factors.

The function of some npcRNA as tumour suppressor and of others as oncogenes is not yet well understood. The genes falling into the ontogeny group "proliferation" may include either genes activated as direct, causative agents, or in a response to proliferation signals associated with tumour cell growth. In many cases the resistance to apoptosis or the proliferation ability may have consequences on tumour development. The association of some of the studied genes in cancer cells, or their involvement in diseases, through gene expression studies using a more comprehensive human transcript set, may provide more clues on their ontology class, and consequently on their function.

Recently it was shown that many human transcripts, as also *H19*, codify for small RNA species [88]. It is possible that some of the human hypothetical transcripts considered in this study may also generate small RNAs.

In conclusion, this study was brought on a large set of human npc-RNAs and hypothetical unknown transcripts, with the attempt to relate their function through the differential expression in proliferating and non-proliferating cells.

Conclusions

There is a general confidence that further advancements in knowledge of miRNAs and other RNA transcripts will provide new ways for personalized medicine as well as diagnosis, prognostic support, therapy and treatment of human cancers.

References

1. Chakravarthi BV, Nepal S, Varambally S (2016) Genomic and epigenomic alterations in cancer. Am J Pathol 186(7):1724–1735. doi:10.1016/j.ajpath.2016.02.023. Review
2. Gao C, He Z, Li J, Li X, Bai Q, Zhang Z, Zhang X, Wang S, Xiao X, Wang F, Yan Y, Li D, Chen L, Zeng X, Xiao Y, Dong G, Zheng Y, Wang Q, Chen W (2016) Specific long non-coding RNAs response to occupational PAHs exposure in coke oven workers. Toxicol Rep 3:160–166
3. Bollati V, Baccarelli A, Hou L, Bonzini M, Fustinoni S, Cavallo D, Byun HM, Jiang J, Marinelli B, Pesatori AC, Bertazzi PA, Yang AS (2007) Changes in DNA methylation patterns in subjects exposed to low-dose benzene. Cancer Res 67(3):876–880
4. Ishikawa T, Miwa M, Uchida K (2006) Quantitation of thyroid peroxidase mRNA in peripheral blood for early detection of thyroid papillary carcinoma. Thyroid 16:435–442
5. D'Urso IP, D'Urso OF, Gianfreda DC, Mezzolla V, Storelli C, Marsigliante S (2015) miR-15b and miR-21 as circulating biomarkers for diagnosis of glioma. Curr Genomics 16(5):304–311. doi:10.2174/1389202916666150707155610
6. Poltronieri P, D'Urso PI, Mezzolla V, D'Urso OF (2013) Potential of anti-cancer therapy based on anti-miR-155 oligonucleotides in glioma and brain tumours. Chem Biol Drug Des 81:79–84
7. Esquela-Kerscher A, Slack FJ (2006) OncomiRs-microRNAs with a role in cancer. Nat Rev Cancer 6:259–269
8. Gibb EA, Vucic EA, Enfield KSS, Stewart GL, Lonergan KM, Kennett JY, Becker-Santos DD, MacAulay CE, Lam S, Brown CJ, Lam WL (2011) Human cancer long non-coding RNA transcriptomes. PLoS One 6(10):e25915
9. Hung T, Wang Y, Lin MF, Koegel AK, Kotake Y, Grant GD, Horlings HM, Shah N, Umbricht C, Wang P, Wang Y, Kong B, Langerød A, Børresen-Dale AL, Kim SK, van de Vijver M, Sukumar S, Whitfield ML, Kellis M, Xiong Y, Wong DJ, Chang HY (2011) Extensive and coordinated transcription of noncoding RNAs within cell-cycle promoters. Nat Genet 43(7):621–629
10. Yang Y, Li H, Hu B, Liu J, Wang J (2013) The noncoding RNA expression profile and the effect of lncRNA AK126698 on cisplatin resistance in non-small-cell lung cancer cell. PLoS One 8(5):65309
11. Ji P, Diederichs S, Wang W, Böing S, Metzger R, Schneider PM, Tidow N, Brandt B, Buerger H, Bulk E, Thomas M, Berdel WE, Serve H, Müller-Tidow C (2003) MALAT-1, a novel noncoding RNA, and thymosin bold italic beta4 predict metastasis and survival in early-stage non-small cell lung cancer. Oncogene 22:8031–8041. doi:10.1038/sj.onc.1206928
12. Ren S, Wang F, Shen J, Sun Y, Xu W, Lu J, Wei M, Xu C, Wu C, Zhang Z, Gao X, Liu Z, Hou J, Huang J, Sun Y (2013) Long non-coding RNA metastasis associated in lung adenocarcinoma transcript 1 derived miniRNA as a novel plasma-based biomarker for diagnosing prostate cancer. Eur J Cancer 49:2949–2959
13. Ren S, Liu Y, Xu W, Sun Y, Lu J, Wang F, Wei M, Shen J, Hou J, Gao X, Xu C, Huang J, Zhao Y, Sun Y (2013) Long noncoding RNA MALAT-1 is a new potential therapeutic target for castration resistant prostate cancer. J Urol 190(6):2278–2287
14. Ma KX, Wang HJ, Li XR, Li T, Su G, Yang P, Wu JW (2015) Long noncoding RNA MALAT1 associates with the malignant status and poor prognosis in glioma. Tumour Biol 36(5):3355–3359
15. Malek E, Jagannathan S, Driscoll JJ (2014) Correlation of long non-coding RNA expression with metastasis, drug resistance and clinical outcome in cancer. Oncotarget 5(18):8027–8038
16. Gupta RA, Shah N, Wang KC, Kim J, Horlings HM, Wong DJ, Tsai MC, Hung T, Argani P, Rinn JL, Wang Y, Brzoska P, Kong B, Li R, West RB, van de Vijver MJ, Sukumar S, Chang HY (2010) Long non-coding RNA HOTAIR reprograms chromatin state to promote cancer metastasis. Nature 464(7291):1071–1076. doi:10.1038/nature08975

17. Guo Q, Cheng Y, Liang T, He Y, Ren C, Sun L, Zhang G (2015) Comprehensive analysis of lncRNA-mRNA co-expression patterns identifies immune-associated lncRNA biomarkers in ovarian cancer malignant progression. Sci Rep 5:17683
18. Guo LL, Song CH, Wang P, Dai LP, Zhang JY, Wang KJ (2015) Competing endogenous RNA networks and gastric cancer. World J Gastroenterol 21(41):11680–11687
19. Mar-Aguilar F, Mendoza-Ramirez JA, Malagoòn-Santiago I, Espino-Silva PK, Santuario-Facio SK, Ruiz-Flores P, Rodriguez-Padilla C, Resendez-Perez D (2013) Serum circulating microRNA profiling for identification of potential breast cancer biomarkers. Dis Markers 34:163–169
20. Schultz NA, Dehlendorff C, Jensen BV, Bjerregaard JK, Nielsen KR, Bojesen SE, Calatayud D, Nielsen SE, Yilmaz M, Holländer NH, Andersen KK, Johansen JS (2014) MicroRNA biomarkers in whole blood for detection of pancreatic cancer. JAMA 311(4):392–404. doi:10.1001/jama.2013.284664
21. Zhu X, Lv M, Wang H, Guan W (2014) Identification of circulating microRNAs as novel potential biomarkers for gastric cancer detection: a systematic review and meta-analysis. Dig Dis Sci 59(5):911–919. doi:10.1007/s10620-013-2970-9. Review
22. Mallardo M, Poltronieri P, D'Urso OF (2008) Non-protein coding RNA biomarkers and differential expression in cancers. A review. J Exp Clin Cancer Res 27:19
23. Hashim A, Rizzo F, Marchese G, Ravo M, Tarallo R, Nassa G, Giurato G, Santamaria G, Cordella A, Cantarella C, Weisz A (2014) RNA sequencing identifies specific PIWI-interacting small non-coding RNA expression patterns in breast cancer. Oncotarget 5(20):9901–9910
24. Ravo M, Cordella A, Rinaldi A, Bruno G, Alexandrova E, Saggese P, Nassa G, Giurato G, Tarallo R, Marchese G, Rizzo F, Stellato C, Biancardi R, Troisi J, Di Spiezio Sardo A, Zullo F, Weisz A, Guida M (2015) Small non-coding RNA deregulation in endometrial carcinogenesis. Oncotarget 6(7):4677–4691
25. Giurato G, De Filippo MR, Rinaldi A, Hashim A, Nassa G, Ravo M, Rizzo F, Tarallo R, Weisz A (2013) iMir: an integrated pipeline for high-throughput analysis of small non-coding RNA data obtained by smallRNA-Seq. BMC Bioinformatics 14:362. doi:10.1186/1471-2105-14-362
26. Concepcion CP, Bonetti C, Ventura A (2012) The miR-17-92 family of microRNA clusters in development and disease. Cancer J 18(3):262–267
27. Mendell JT (2008) miRiad Roles for the miR-17-92 cluster in development and disease. Cell 133:217–222. Review
28. Hayashita Y, Osada H, Tatematsu Y, Yamada H, Yanagisawa K, Tomida S, Yatabe Y, Kawahara K, Sekido Y, Takahashi T (2005) A polycistronic microRNA cluster, miR-17-92, is overexpressed in human lung cancers and enhances cell proliferation. Cancer Res 65:9628–9632
29. Paris O, Ferraro L, Grober OM, Ravo M, De Filippo MR, Giurato G, Nassa G, Tarallo R, Cantarella C, Rizzo F, Di Benedetto A, Mottolese M, Benes V, Ambrosino C, Nola E, Weisz A (2012) Direct regulation of microRNA biogenesis and expression by estrogen receptor beta in hormone-responsive breast cancer. Oncogene 31(38):4196–4206
30. Ferracin M, Negrini M (2015) Micromarkers 2.0: an update on the role of microRNAs in cancer diagnosis and prognosis. Expert Rev Mol Diagn 15(10):1369–1381
31. Mangolini A, Ferracin M, Zanzi MV, Saccenti E, Ebnaof SO, Poma VV, Sanz JM, Passaro A, Pedriali M, Frassoldati A, Querzoli P, Sabbioni S, Carcoforo P, Hollingsworth A, Negrini M (2015) Diagnostic and prognostic microRNAs in the serum of breast cancer patients measured by droplet digital PCR. Biomark Res 3:12. doi:10.1186/s40364-015-0037-0
32. Pekarsky Y, Croce CM (2015) Role of miR-15/16 in CLL. Cell Death Differ 22:6–11
33. Müller S, Rycak L, Afonso-Grunz F, Winter P, Zawada AM, Damrath E, Scheider J, Schmäh J, Koch I, Kahl G, Rotter B (2014) APADB: a database for alternative polyadenylation and microRNA regulation events. Database (Oxford). pii: bau076
34. Müller S, Raulefs S, Bruns P, Afonso-Grunz F, Plötner A, Thermann R, Jäger C, Schlitter AM, Kong B, Regel I, Roth WK, Rotter B, Hoffmeier K, Kahl G, Koch I, Theis FJ, Kleeff J, Winter P, Michalski CW (2015) Next-generation sequencing reveals novel differentially regulated mRNAs, lncRNAs, miRNAs, sdRNAs and a piRNA in pancreatic cancer. Mol Cancer 14:94

35. Afonso-Grunz F, Müller S (2015) Principles of miRNA-mRNA interactions: beyond sequence complementarity. Cell Mol Life Sci 72(16):3127–3141
36. Nicoloso MS, Sun H, Spizzo R, Kim H, Wickramasinghe P, Shimizu M, Wojcik SE, Ferdin J, Kunej T, Xiao L, Manoukian S, Secreto G, Ravagnani F, Wang X, Radice P, Croce CM, Davuluri RV, Calin GA (2010) Single-nucleotide polymorphisms inside microRNA target sites influence tumor susceptibility. Cancer Res 70(7):2789–2798
37. Yoon KA, Yoon H, Park S, Jang HJ, Zo JI, Lee HS, Lee JS (2012) The prognostic impact of microRNA sequence polymorphisms on the recurrence of patients with completely resected non-small cell lung cancer. J Thorac Cardiovasc Surg 144(4):794–807
38. Dole NS, Delany AM (2016) MicroRNA variants as genetic determinants of bone mass. Bone 84:57–68
39. Dago DN, Scafoglio C, Rinaldi A, Memoli D, Giurato G, Nassa G, Ravo M, Rizzo F, Tarallo R, Weisz A (2015) Estrogen receptor beta impacts hormone-induced alternative mRNA splicing in breast cancer cells. BMC Genomics 16:367. doi:10.1186/s12864-015-1541-1
40. Hunter MP, Ismail N, Zhang X, Aguda BD, Lee EJ, Yu L, Xiao T, Schafer J, Lee ML, Schmittgen TD, Nana-Sinkam SP, Jarjoura D, Marsh CB (2008) Detection of microRNA expression in human peripheral blood microvesicles. PLoS One 3:e3694
41. Ma R, Jiang T, Kang X (2012) Circulating microRNAs in cancer: origin, function and application. J Exp Clin Cancer Res 31:38
42. Tsang JC, Lo YM (2007) Circulating nucleic acids in plasma/serum. Pathology 39:197–207
43. Valadi H, Ekstrom K, Bossios A, Sjostrand M, Lee JJ, Lotvall JO (2007) Exosome-mediated transfer of mRNAs and microRNAs is a novel mechanism of genetic exchange between cells. Nat Cell Biol 9:654–659
44. Godfrey AC, Xu Z, Weinberg CR, Getts RC, Wade PA, DeRoo LA, Sandler DP, Taylor JA (2013) Serum microRNA expression as an early marker for breast cancer risk in prospectively collected samples from the Sister Study cohort. Breast Cancer Res 15:R42
45. Heneghan HM, Miller N, Lowery AJ, Sweeney KJ, Newell J, Kerin MJ (2010) Circulating microRNAs as novel minimally invasive biomarkers for breast cancer. Ann Surg 251:499–505
46. Mitchell PS, Parkin RK, Kroh EM, Fritz BR, Wyman SK, Pogosova-Agadjanyan EL, Peterson A, Noteboom J, O'Briant KC, Allen A, Lin DW, Urban N, Drescher CW, Knudsen BS, Stirewalt DL, Gentleman R, Vessella RL, Nelson PS, Martin DB, Tewari M (2008) Circulating microRNAs as stable blood-based markers for cancer detection. Proc Natl Acad Sci U S A 105:10513–10518
47. Tsujiura M, Ichikawa D, Komatsu S, Shiozaki A, Takeshita H, Kosuga T, Konishi H, Morimura R, Deguchi K, Fujiwara H, Okamoto K, Otsuji E (2010) Circulating microRNAs in plasma of patients with gastric cancers. Br J Cancer 102:1174–1179
48. Goding CR (2016) Targeting the lncRNA SAMMSON reveals metabolic vulnerability in melanoma. Cancer Cell 29(5):619–621
49. Leucci E, Vendramin R, Spinazzi M, Laurette P, Fiers M, Wouters J, Radaelli E, Eyckerman S, Leonelli C, Vanderheyden K, Rogiers A, Hermans E, Baatsen P, Aerts S, Amant F, Van Aelst S, van den Oord J, de Strooper B, Davidson I, Lafontaine DL, Gevaert K, Vandesompele J, Mestdagh P, Marine JC (2016) Melanoma addiction to the long non-coding RNA SAMMSON. Nature 531(7595):518–522
50. Li R, Zhang L, Jia L, Duan Y, Li Y, Bao L, Sha N (2014) Long non-coding RNA BANCR promotes proliferation in malignant melanoma by regulating MAPK pathway activation. PLoS One 9(6):e100893
51. Zhou T, Gao Y (2016) Increased expression of LncRNA BANCR and its prognostic significance in human hepatocellular carcinoma. World J Surg Oncol 14(1):8. doi:10.1186/s12957-015-0757-5
52. Sun M, Liu XH, Wang KM, Nie FQ, Kong R, Yang JS, Xia R, Xu TP, Jin FY, Liu ZJ, Chen JF, Zhang EB, De W, Wang ZX (2014) Downregulation of BRAF activated non-coding RNA is associated with poor prognosis for non-small cell lung cancer and promotes metastasis by affecting epithelial-mesenchymal transition. Mol Cancer 13:68. doi:10.1186/1476-4598-13-68

53. Li L, Zhang L, Zhang Y, Zhou F (2015) Increased expression of LncRNA BANCR is associated with clinical progression and poor prognosis in gastric cancer. Biomed Pharmacother 72:109–112
54. Peng ZQ, Lu RB, Xiao DM, Xiao ZM (2016) Increased expression of the lncRNA BANCR and its prognostic significance in human osteosarcoma. Genet Mol Res 15(1). doi: 10.4238/gmr.15017480
55. Li F, Cao L, Hang D, Wang F, Wang Q (2015) Long non-coding RNA HOTTIP is up-regulated and associated with poor prognosis in patients with osteosarcoma. Int J Clin Exp Pathol 8(9):11414–11420
56. Ye H, Liu K, Qian K (2016) Overexpression of long noncoding RNA HOTTIP promotes tumor invasion and predicts poor prognosis in gastric cancer. Onco Targets Ther 9:2081–2088
57. Wang CY, Hua L, Yao KH, Chen JT, Zhang JJ, Hu JH (2015) Long non-coding RNA CCAT2 is up-regulated in gastric cancer and associated with poor prognosis. Int J Clin Exp Pathol 8(1):779–785
58. Ning S, Zhang J, Wang P, Zhi H, Wang J, Liu Y, Gao Y, Guo M, Yue M, Wang L, Li X (2016) Lnc2Cancer: a manually curated database of experimentally supported lncRNAs associated with various human cancers. Nucleic Acids Res 44(D1):D980–D985. doi:10.1093/nar/gkv1094
59. Li CH, Chen Y (2013) Targeting long non-coding RNAs in cancers: progress and prospects. Int J Biochem Cell Biol 45(8):1895–1910. doi:10.1016/j.biocel.2013.05.030. Review
60. Kim K, Jutooru I, Chadalapaka G, Johnson G, Frank J, Burghardt R, Kim S, Safe S (2013) HOTAIR is a negative prognostic factor and exhibits pro-oncogenic activity in pancreatic cancer. Oncogene 32(13):1616–1625. doi:10.1038/ onc.2012.193
61. Gutschner T, Diederichs S (2012) The hallmarks of cancer: a long non-coding RNA point of view. RNA Biol 9(6):703–719. doi:10.4161/rna.20481. Epub **2012** Jun 1. Review
62. Moshiri F, Callegari E, D'Abundo L, Corrà F, Lupini L, Sabbioni S, Negrini M (2014) Inhibiting the oncogenic mir-221 by microRNA sponge: toward microRNA-based therapeutics for HCC. Gastroenterol Hepatol Bed Bench 7(1):43–54
63. Dai Q, Li J, Zhou K, Liang T (2015) Competing endogenous RNA: a novel posttranscriptional regulatory dimension associated with the progression of cancer. Oncol Lett 10(5):2683–2690
64. Wang P, Zhi H, Zhang Y, Liu Y, Zhang J, Gao Y, Guo M, Ning S, Li X (2015) miRSponge: a manually curated database for experimentally supported miRNA sponges and ceRNAs. Database (Oxford). pii: bav098
65. Zhang J, Fan D, Jian Z, Chen GG, Lai PB (2015) Cancer specific long noncoding RNAs show differential expression patterns and competing endogenous RNA potential in hepatocellular carcinoma. PLoS One 10(10):e0141042
66. Stenvang J, Petri A, Lindow M, Obad S, Kauppinen S (2012) Inhibition of microRNA function by antimiR oligonucleotides. Silence 3:1
67. Bidros DS, Liu JK, Vogelbaum MA (2010) Future of convection enhanced delivery in the treatment of brain tumors. Future Oncol 6:117–125
68. Gabriely G, Yi M, Narayan RS, Niers JM, Wurdinger T, Imitola J, Ligon KL, Kesari S, Esau C, Stephens RM, Tannous BA, Krichevsky AM (2011) Human glioma growth is controlled by microRNA-10b. Cancer Res 71:3563–3572
69. Young DD, Connelly CM, Grohmann C, Deiters A (2010) Small molecule modifiers of microRNA miR-122 function for the treatment of hepatitis C virus infection and hepatocellular carcinoma. J Am Chem Soc 132:7976–7981
70. Daige CL, Wiggins JF, Priddy L, Nelligan-Davis T, Zhao J, Brown D (2014) Systemic delivery of a miR34a mimic as a potential therapeutic for liver cancer. Mol Cancer Ther 13(10):2352–2360. doi:10.1158/1535-7163.MCT-14-0209
71. Farooqi AA, Fayyaz S, Shatynska-Mytsyk I, Javed Z, Jabeen S, Yaylim I, Gasparri ML, Panici PB (2016) Is miR-34a a well-equipped swordsman to conquer temple of molecular oncology? Chem Biol Drug Des 87(3):321–334. doi:10.1111/cbdd.12634
72. Xiao Z, Li CH, Chan SL, Xu F, Feng L, Wang Y, Jiang JD, Sung JJ, Cheng CH, Chen Y (2014) A small-molecule modulator of the tumor-suppressor miR34a inhibits the growth of hepatocellular carcinoma. Cancer Res 74:6236–6247

73. Mayer G, Raddatz MS, Grunwald JD, Famulok M (2007) RNA ligands that distinguish metabolite-induced conformations in the TPP riboswitch. Angew Chem Int Ed Engl 46:557–560
74. Lünse CE, Michlewski G, Hopp CS, Rentmeister A, Cáceres JF, Famulok M, Mayer G (2010) An aptamer targeting the apical-loop domain modulates pri-miRNA processing. Angew Chem Int Ed Engl 49:4674–4677
75. Subramanian N, Kanwar JR, Kanwar RK, Krishnakumar S (2015) Blocking the maturation of oncomiRNAs using pri-miRNA-17~92 aptamer in retinoblastoma. Nucleic Acid Ther 5:47–52
76. Bouchie A (2013) First microRNA mimic enters clinic. Nat Biotechnol 31(7):77
77. Li CH, Chen Y (2015) Small and long non-coding RNAs: novel targets in perspective cancer therapy. Curr Genomics 16:319–326
78. Lee JB, Hong J, Bonner DK, Poon Z, Hammond PT (2012) Self-assembled RNA interference microsponges for efficient siRNA delivery. Nat Mater 11:316–322
79. Di Martino MT, Leone E, Amodio N, Foresta U, Lionetti M, Pitari MR, Cantafio ME, Gullà A, Conforti F, Morelli E, Tomaino V, Rossi M, Negrini M, Ferrarini M, Caraglia M, Shammas MA, Munshi NC, Anderson KC, Neri A, Tagliaferri P, Tassone P (2012) Synthetic miR-34a mimics as a novel therapeutic agent for multiple myeloma: in vitro and in vivo evidence. Clin Cancer Res 18:6260–6270
80. Kim JH, Yeom JH, Ko JJ, Han MS, Lee K, Na SY, Bae J (2011) Effective delivery of anti-miRNA DNA oligonucleotides by functionalized gold nanoparticles. J Biotechnol 1553:287–292
81. Huang X, Schwind S, Yu B, Santhanam R, Wang H, Hoellerbauer P, Mims A, Klisovic R, Walker AR, Chan KK, Blum W, Perrotti D, Byrd JC, Bloomfield CD, Caligiuri MA, Lee RJ, Garzon R, Muthusamy N, Lee LJ, Marcucci G (2013) Targeted delivery of microRNA-29b by transferrin-conjugated anionic lipopolyplex nanoparticles: a novel therapeutic strategy in acute myeloid leukemia. Clin Cancer Res 19:2355–2367
82. D'Urso PI, D'Urso OF, Storelli C, Mallardo M, Gianfreda CD, Montinaro A, Cimmino A, Pietro C, Marsigliante S (2012) miR-155 is up-regulated in primary and secondary glioblastoma and promotes tumour growth by inhibiting GABA receptors. Int J Oncol 41:228–234
83. Skog J, Wurdinger T, van Rijn S, Meijer DH, Gainche L, Sena-Esteves M, Curry WT, Carter BS Jr, Krichevsky AM, Breakefield XO (2008) Glioblastoma microvesicles transport RNA and proteins that promote tumour growth and provide diagnostic biomarkers. Nat Cell Biol 10:1470–1476
84. Baraniskin A, Kuhnhenn J, Schlegel U, Maghnouj A, Zollner H, Schmiegel W, Hahn S, Schroers R (2012) Identification of microRNAs in the cerebrospinal fluid as biomarker for the diagnosis of glioma. Neuro Oncol 14:29–33
85. Chang TY, Huang TS, Wang HW, Chang SJ, Lo HH, Chiu YL, Wang YL, Hsiao CD, Tsai CH, Chan CH, You RI, Wu CH, Tsai TN, Cheng SM, Cheng CC (2014) miRNome traits analysis on endothelial lineage cells discloses biomarker potential circulating microRNAs which affect progenitor activities. BMC Genomics 15:802. doi:10.1186/1471-2164-15-802
86. Rossi A, D'Urso OF, Gatto G, Poltronieri P, Ferracin M, Remondelli P, Negrini M, Caporaso MG, Bonatti S, Mallardo M (2010) Non-coding RNAs change their expression profiles after retinoid induced differentiation of the promyelocytic cell line NB4. BMC Res Notes 3:24
87. Manoharan H, Babcock K, Willi J, Pitot HC (2003) Biallelic expression of the H19 gene during spontaneous hepatocarcinogenesis in the albumin SV40 T antigen transgenic rat. Mol Carcinog 38:40–47
88. Cai X, Cullen BR (2007) The imprinted H19 noncoding RNA is a primary microRNA precursor. RNA 13:1–4

Exosomes: New Biomarkers for Targeted Cancer Therapy

Chiara Martinelli

Abstract Exosomes have emerged as novel and important mediators of intercellular communication. They contain bioactive molecules including proteins, DNA, mRNA and miRNA, which are transferred from donor to target cells, leading to exchanges of genetic information and reprogramming of the recipients. Recently, it has been suggested that tumor cells release increased amounts of exosomes which are involved in tumor initiation, growth, progression, metastasis, and multidrug resistance. Exosomal shuttling between cells contributes to transfer material from tumor to immune and stromal cells, favoring the escape from immune surveillance and the formation of a conditioned tumor niche. The critical involvement of exosomes in cancer has evidenced important roles both for diagnostic and therapeutic purposes. Exosomes can be exploited as biomarkers for diagnosis and as targets for therapy. They can be considered potential therapeutic agents. Due to their high loading efficiency and biocompatibility they can be used as vehicles for delivering targeted anti-cancer drugs with low immunogenicity and toxicity.

Keywords Exosomes • Cancer • Tumorigenesis • Metastasis • Diagnosis • Therapy Drug delivery

Abbreviations

AEX	Ascites derived exosomes
AFM	Atomic force microscopy
APC	Antigen presenting cells
ASC	Adipose-derived stem cells
BM-MSC	Bone marrow mesenchymal stromal cells
CD	Cytosine deaminase
CML	Chronic myelogenous leukemia
CTX	Cyclophosphamide
DMA	Dimethyl amiloride

C. Martinelli (✉)
Department of Biosciences, University of Milan, Milan, Italy
e-mail: chiara.martinelli@protonmail.com

A.A. Farooqi, M. Ismail (eds.), *Molecular Oncology: Underlying Mechanisms and Translational Advancements*, DOI 10.1007/978-3-319-53082-6_6

ECM	Extracellular matrix
EBV	Epstein Barr virus
EGFR	Epidermal growth factor receptor
ELISA	Enzyme-linked immunosorbent assay
ESCRT	Endosomal sorting complex required for transport
EV	Extracellular vesicle
FACS	Fluorescence activated cell sorting
GM-CSF	Granulocyte-macrophage colony-stimulating factor
HSPG	Heparan sulfate proteoglycans
IAP	Inhibitors of apoptosis
IGF1R	Insulin-like growth factor receptor 1
ISEV	International society for extracellular vesicles
lncRNA	long non coding RNA
MDR	Multidrug resistance
MDSC	Myeloid derived suppressor cells
MHC	Major histocompatibility complex
mRNA	messenger RNA
MIF	Macrophage migration inhibitory factor
miRNA	micro RNA
MM	Multiple myeloma
MRI	Magnetic resonance
MSC	Mesenchymal stem cells
MVB	Multivesicular Bodies
NFkB	Nuclear factor kappa-light-chain-enhancer
NK	Natural killer
NPC	Nasopharyngeal carcinoma
NSCLC	Non-small cell lung cancer
PDAC	Pancreatic ductal adenocarcinoma
piRNA	piwi-interacting RNA
pre-miRNA	precursor micro RNA
RGD	Arg-Gly-Asp
RISC	RNA induced silencing complex
RTC	Reticulocytes
RT-PCR	Real time polymerase chain reaction
RVG	Rabies viral glycoprotein
scaRNA	small Cajal body-specific RNA
shRNA	short hairpin RNA
siRNA	small interfering RNA
SMCNCs	Superparamagnetic magnetite colloidal nanocrystal clusters
SNARE	Soluble NSF attachment protein receptor
snoRNA	small nucleolar RNA
SPION	Superparamagnetic iron oxide nanoparticles
TEM	Transmission electron microscopy
TGF-ß	Transforming growth factor ß
TLR	Toll-like receptor

TRAIL	Tumor necrosis factor-related apoptosis-inducing ligand
tRNA	transfer RNA
TSAP	Tumor suppressor-activated pathway
UPRT	Uracil phosphoribosyltransferase

Introduction

Exosomes are defined as a family of nanovesicles with a diameter size ranging from 30 to 150 nm, secreted by the vast majority of our body's cells, both in physiological and pathological conditions [1–4]. They display a cup-like shape and they are constituted by a bilayer-lipid membrane that presents peculiar proteins on its surface (i.e., tetraspanins) [5]. Exosomes can be physiologically found in almost any extracellular fluid in our body (i.e., urine, blood, amniotic fluid, saliva and cerebrospinal fluid) [6, 7]. They were originally described by Trams et al., as "exfoliations" from normal and neoplastic cell lines, and later proved to be involved in a pathway responsible for the elimination of unnecessary materials from reticulocytes [8–11]. These studies suggested their major role in secreting biomolecules from the cells, when lysosomal pathways were lacking. Nowadays, exosomes are defined as vesicles formed in endosomal compartments [12], able to carry biological material and to shuttle between cells, therefore participating in intercellular communication [5]. The content of exosomes is essential for their classification and for their function, as they carry messenger and micro RNA (mRNA, miRNA) [13], proteins, peptides, lipids [14, 15], and occasionally DNA [16, 17].

An updated collection of the content and composition of exosomes is reported in ExoCarta and to date, 9769 proteins, 3408 mRNAs, and 2838 miRNAs have been recognized as exosome contents [18, 19].

The essential feature of exosomes is that they are able to shuttle between cells carrying a plethora of molecules that maintain their function after reaching recipient cells and transmit signals. Exosomes can participate both in physiological processes (immune defence, antigen presentation, waste removal, stem cell maintenance etc.) [20, 21] and in many pathological conditions (viruses' pathogenesis, degenerative and prion diseases and inflammation) [22]. Importantly, exosomes have been shown to be implicated in the survival and proliferation of cancer cells and metastasis [23–25], but at the same time they can be potentially exploited as new tools for the treatment, detection and prognosis of cancer [26, 27]. The population of exosomes that can be obtained from a sample is very heterogeneous, thus making very challenging the determination of their specificity and the correlation to a precise phenotype. Nowadays, exosomes can be isolated from cells under normal and stressed conditions. Usually, exosomes are purified by ultracentrifugation combined with sucrose gradient and immuno-purification on conjugated beads. After isolation, exosomes can be characterized by western immuno-blot and fluorescence activated cell sorting (FACS) (size, shape, membrane markers) and visualized by transmission electron microscopy (TEM). The specific contents of exosomes are currently identified by quantitative real time polymerase chain reaction (RT-PCR), nucleic acid sequencing, western immuno-blot and enzyme linked immunosorbent assay (ELISA).

The International Society for Extracellular Vesicles (ISEV) has recently defined the minimal criteria to identify extracellular vesicles. One of the first rules used to define extracellular vesicles is their protein composition: several analyses have shown that many of the most commonly found proteins in exosome preparations are only "enriched" and not "specific". Therefore, they can be defined as common markers of different kinds of extracellular vesicles. In particular, by performing an analytic identification of the protein composition, it is possible to describe four different classes of proteins that can be found in extracellular vesicles: (1) transmembrane or lipid-bound extracellular proteins; (2) cytosolic proteins; (3) intracellular proteins independent from cellular/endosomal membranes; (4) extracellular proteins that can be isolated together with extracellular vesicles [28].

Importantly, the characterization of single vesicles within a mixture needs TEM or atomic force microscopy (AFM) image acquisition in order to precisely identify isolated vesicles. Size distribution of extracellular vesicles is needed to grant diameter measurement. There is a continuous need to match data obtained by all these different characterization techniques. Studies in vitro of the functional activity need to be supported by adequate controls in order to give a precise quantification of the real functionality of the isolated extracellular vesicles [28].

In this chapter, we will describe the novel emerging roles of exosomes in intercellular communication and cancer. Their involvement in tumorigenesis, growth, progression and metastasis will be analyzed, highlighting their ability to transfer material from tumor cells to the surrounding environment. Finally, we will report recent findings demonstrating their crucial roles as biomarkers for diagnosis, targets for therapy and drug delivery carriers.

Exosomes: Biogenesis, Content and Fate

Exosomes clearly differ from shedding microvesicles, that directly form by membrane budding [1, 10]. They originate by invagination of early endosomal membranes into the lumen of the compartment in a process that creates multivesicular bodies (MVBs) (Fig. 1). Their most important feature, as compared to endosomes, is that the extracellular leaflet of the plasma membrane is fully preserved in its orientation as an extracellular part of their membrane and it presents typical endosomal components. The most commonly identified proteins bound on the lipid bilayer cover a broad spectrum of immune-modulating and cell recognizing ubiquitous molecules (i.e., cytoskeletal proteins, transporters, integrins and heat shock family proteins). Moreover, the exosomal membrane presents many proteins related to MVBs (i.e., flotillins, annexins, GTPases, Rab, and SNAREs) and involved in their biogenesis (i.e., Alix, Tsg101), transducers (i.e., β-catenin) and membrane-associated proteins (i.e., tetraspanins) [29–31], essential for intercellular communication and targeting to recipient cells [32]. Some exosomal membranes can expose on their surface Major Histocompatibility Complex (MHC) molecules. All these

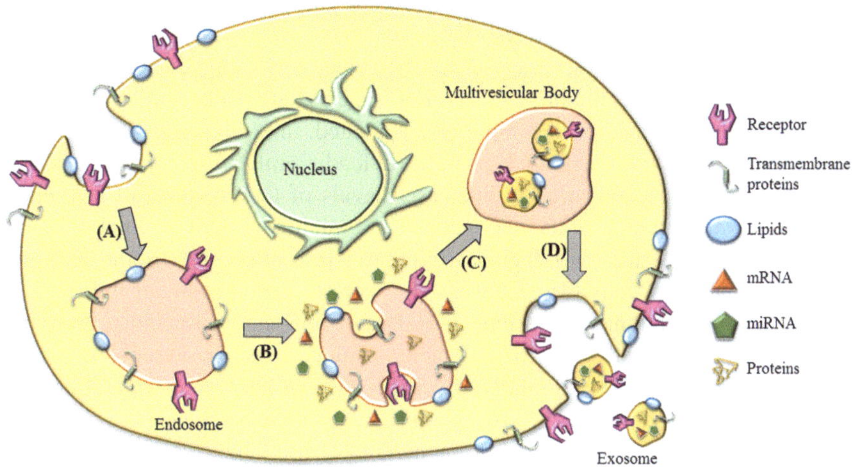

Fig. 1 Biogenesis of exosomes. (**a**) The plasma membrane invaginates and creates an endosome that engulfs macromolecules and other contents within the extracellular environment. Proteins located on the plasma membrane are found on the endosomal membrane. (**b**) Invagination of the endosomal membrane creates (**c**) a multivesicular body (MVB). Intracellular proteins and RNAs are packaged into the microvesicles contained in the MVB. (**d**) MVB fuses with the plasma membrane and releases exosomes into the extracellular environment

specific markers are considered essential for the identification of exosomes and are particularly attractive as putative novel targets for diagnosis and therapy [33].

Two main pathways are involved in the biogenesis and sorting of exosomes: the Endosomal Sorting Complex Required for Transport (ESCRT)-dependent pathway and the ESCRT-independent pathway. The first one is essential for endosomal sorting and secretion of ubiquitinylated membrane proteins [34], it requires Alix, and it includes: ESCRT-0, responsible for loading ubiquinated proteins on the endosomal surface; ESCRT-I and ESCRT-II, responsible for membrane budding; ESCRT-III, responsible for membrane separation. The ESCRT-independent pathway exploits lipids, such as sphingosine-1-phosphate and ceramide, microdomains enriched with tetraspanins, and the enzyme sphingomyelinase [35]. Recently, it has been reported that exosomes can be produced by a pathway that involves syndecan heparan sulfate proteoglycans and syntenin [36], together with the accessory proteins Alix, GTPase ADP Ribosylation Factor 6 (ARF6), proteolipid protein D2, and endoglycosidase heparinase [37].

Different cellular components are involved in exosome biogenesis: cytoskeletal proteins, molecular motors, molecular switches like GTPases, fusion and tethering proteins such as SNAREs [4]. During secretion, MVBs containing exosomes are directed to the target cell membrane and later they fuse by the assistance of mediating proteins Rab GTPases, like Rab27a/b (they affect size and localization of MVBs), Rab3 (it coordinates MVBs binding to the recipient cells), Rab11 and Rab35 [38–40]. Mesenchymal stem cells (MSCs) release increased amounts of exosomes respect to slowly proliferating cells and recently, it has been demonstrated that their ability can be experimentally forced by transfecting the MYC gene [41, 42]. Exosomes that are not secreted, normally undergo lysosomal degradation. In particular, MVBs with membranes poor in cholesterol and that present peculiar compositions are directed to the lysosomes [43].

Exosomes contain a wide variety of cargos, selectively sorted during the process of biogenesis. Only specific proteins and RNA species are packed and the underlying mechanisms have not been completely elucidated. Interestingly, it has been suggested a putative role for ESCRT-II complex in loading mRNA into exosomes [44]. Exosome secretion is favoured by increased levels of Ca^{2+} in the cell cytoplasm [45]. Moreover, variation in the endogenous and microenvironmental pH has been demonstrated to interfere with their secretion: low pH enhances exosome secretion and uptake by target cells [46]. Cancer cells secrete exosomes under influence of both oncogenes and tumor suppressors [47]. It has been demonstrated that the tumor suppressor-activated pathway (TSAP) is able to induce exosome secretion under the regulation of p53 [48, 49]. Similarly, overexpression of heparanase in cancer cells enhances exosome secretion [50]. Intriguingly, an opposite mechanism of inhibition of secretion has been described in normal mammary epithelial cells underlining the action of finely tuned regulation systems [51]. Small non-coding RNAs and particularly miRNAs are the most abundant molecules present in exosomes [42], together with piwi-interacting RNA (piRNA), small nucleolar RNA (snoRNA), Small Cajal body-specific RNA (scaRNA), silencing RNA (siRNA), transfer RNA (tRNA) fragments, and vault RNA [52]. It is important to consider that endogenous exosomes are made from fragments of the plasma membrane and preserve its original orientation therefore inheriting the glycome, the glycocalyx from the originating cells with its innate immune tolerance.

Exosomes communicate with target cells through different mechanisms (1) interaction with cell membrane receptors; (2) fusion with cell membrane; (3) phagocytosis. Several proteins are involved in the process of uptake, such as Tim1/4 for B cells [53] and ICAM-1 for APCs [54]. For example, melanoma cells uptake exosomes by fusion, facilitated by low pH [55]. Phagocytosis is specifically exploited by phagocytic cells [56]. Generally, the process of uptake is energy dependent [57]. It has been demonstrated that cancer cell derived exosomes use heparan sulfate proteoglycans (HSPGs) present on the cell membranes for internalization and their depletion and/or inhibition of their synthesis greatly reduces exosome uptake [58].

Exosomes and Cancer

By a biological point of view, cancer is a complex and intricate network of interconnected players. Communication between cancer cells and their microenvironment is crucial in regulating tumor progression and spreading. Recent evidences indicate that exosomes have a key role in cancer, contributing to its development, progression and to the creation of metastases. Cancer exosomes are able to manipulate immune cells by carrying material from tumor cells, suppress specific T-cell immunity favoring the escape from immune surveillance, and can participate in drug resistance to anti-cancer therapies.

Tumorigenesis, Angiogenesis, Metastasis

Exosomes can be uptaken by recipient cells and modulate their activities in a persistent and efficient way. They are responsible for the intercellular communication between tumor cells and the surrounding tissues, they carry oncogenic proteins and nucleic acids and they promote cancer development and progression, metastasis, and drug resistance (Fig. 2). Exosomes can act as pro-tumoral agents, as deduced from their increased levels in the plasma of cancer patients correlating with tumor progression [59, 60]. Many studies in the last years have demonstrated and corroborated the complex roles of exosomes in cancer, even though the exact underlying mechanisms have not been fully elucidated.

The material carried by exosomes plays a preeminent role in mediating their intercellular functions. In the last years, in vitro and in vivo researches have underlined the essential function of miRNAs in regulating many cellular processes and their involvement as tumor suppressors or cancer promoters. In particular, many efforts have been made in order to unravel the multiple roles of miR-421, miR-155 and miR-650 [61]. Studies focused on prostate cancer progression have demonstrated that miRNAs interact with many different cellular components creating a network implied in the regulation of genome integrity [62]. Moreover, it has been

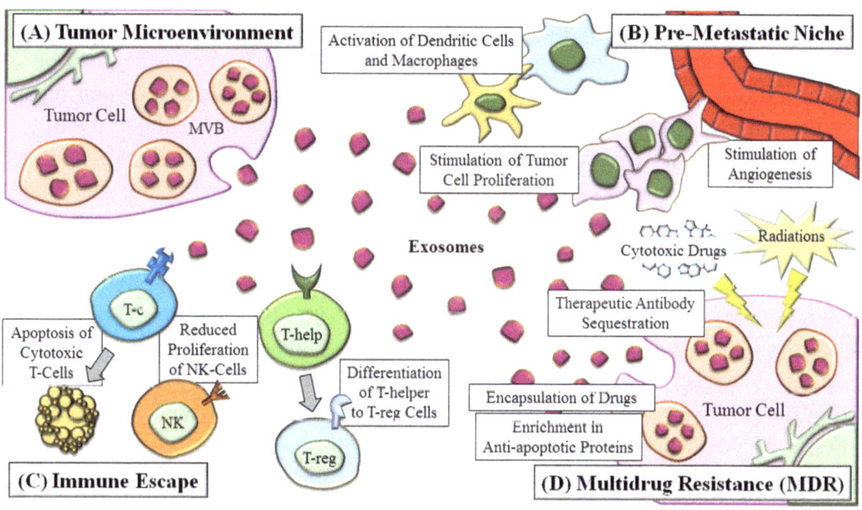

Fig. 2 Exosomes are involved in many different pathological processes. (**a**) Exosomes (*purple dots*) secreted by cancer cells modify local tumor microenvironment and promote tumor cell proliferation. (**b**) Exosomes are able to reach distant sites and promote the creation of a pre-metastatic niche. Stimulation of angiogenesis induces endothelial and stromal cell differentiation. (**c**) Exosomes interfere with normal immune response and prevent the recognition of tumor cells (immune escape). Cytotoxic T-cells are forced to apoptosis, natural killer cells undergo reduced proliferation and T-helper cells differentiate into a T-regulatory phenotype. (**d**) Exosomes are involved in multidrug resistance. They can sequester therapeutic antibodies, encapsulate drugs administered to tumor cells and engulf anti-apoptotic proteins

shown that miRNAs can regulate tumor necrosis factor-related apoptosis-inducing ligand (TRAIL)-mediated signaling, a pathway that is disrupted in prostate cancer cells [63]. Intriguingly, miRNAs are also involved into post-transcriptional regulation of tumor suppressors and oncogenes: in leukemia cells positive for BCR-ABL1, it has been reported that miRNAs can positively and negatively regulate BCR-ABL1-mediated signaling pathways [64]. In a therapeutic perspective, further understanding of miRNA roles will be necessary in order to restore the activity of the tumor suppressors while targeting the oncogenic ones.

Exosomes from cancer cells have been shown to be able to induce normal cell transformation (Fig. 2, panel A). As an example, prostate cancer cell-derived exosomes are involved in the transformation of adipose-derived stem cells (ASCs) [65], with consequent delivery of oncogenic proteins (Ras superfamily of GTPases), mRNAs, and miRNAs (miR-125b, miR-130b, and miR-155). Similarly, exosomes isolated from breast cancer cells can efficiently silence mRNAs in normal epithelial cells by transferring precursor microRNAs (pre-miRNAs) together with RNA-induced silencing complex (RISC)-loading complex proteins, ultimately contributing to tumorigenesis [66]. These observations are further supported by in vivo experiments demonstrating that exosomes isolated from serum of breast cancer patients coinjected with normal epithelial cells can induce neoplasia in mice [66].

Recent studies have reported that exosomes can also interfere with cancer cell proliferation, promoting tumor growth. Tumors can be defined as a network of different kinds of cells strictly interconnected and constitutively essential in determining the physiology, behavior and spreading of cancer [67]. The accumulation of mutations, neoangiogenesis, increased proliferation and invasion of distant organs are the common traits of tumor progression. Increasing evidences support the role of tumor exosomes in delivering information able to modify stroma and malignant cell functions [68]. Exosomes can contribute to oncogenic transfer [69–71] and angiogenesis [72], induce drug resistance and immune suppression (Fig. 2, panel B). Valadi et al. were the first to demonstrate that exosomes from mouse mast cells are able to transfer RNAs to human mast cells [13] and that carried mRNA transcripts can originate functional proteins in recipient mast cells. Similar observations came from lung derived exosomes that transport lung-specific and functional mRNAs to bone marrow cells [73]. Interestingly, exosome transfer in glioma cells is able to stimulate proliferation through delivery of a mutant epidermal growth factor receptor (EGFRvIII) that causes increased expression of anti-apoptotic genes [69]. Similarly, exosome mediated transfer of mutant KRAS from colon cancer cells can enhance the 3D growth of wild-type colon cells [74]. Exosomes isolated from a highly metastatic melanoma cell line can induce the conversion of bone marrow progenitor cells to a pro-vasculogenic and pre-metastatic phenotype via the MET receptor [75].

The cross-talk between tumor stromal cells and tumor cells is essential for tumorigenesis. In chronic myelogenous leukemia (CML), secreted exosomes are able to induce release of IL-8 by bone marrow stromal cells promoting leukemia onset [76]. Similarly, exosomes released from bone marrow mesenchymal stromal cells (BM-MSCs) of multiple myeloma (MM) patients are involved in increased growth of MM cells due high levels of carried oncogenic proteins, inflammatory agents, and adhesion molecules [77].

Finally, uptake of exosomes containing protein survivin in cancer cells is able to make them resistant to apoptosis induced by genotoxic agents [78].

Another important aspect in the process of tumorigenesis is the creation of new blood vessels, essential to deliver nutrients and to overcome hypoxia in the growing tumor cells (Fig. 2, panel B) [79]. Exosomes have been demonstrated to be involved in proangiogenic pathways activated by hypoxia conditions in vascular cells [80–82]. Notably, glioblastoma cells grown in hypoxic conditions can release exosomes containing peculiar proteins able to induce creation of ex vivo microvasculature and neovascularization of tumor tissues in xenografted animals [72]. Multiple myeloma cells grown under hypoxic condition have been reported to generate exosomes loaded with a specific miRNA, miR-135b, which is able to inhibit the activity of proteins that normally block tube formation in endothelial cells [83]. Moreover, exosomes secreted by squamous carcinoma cells grown under hypoxic conditions can increase their metastatic potential and decrease vessel branching and tissue intercellular adhesion [81]. Exosome carrying pro-angiogenic factors to endothelial cells can induce the upregulation of specific genes involved in angiogenesis and cause abnormal proliferation, migration, and diffusion [84]. The role of miRNAs in exosome mediated angiogenesis has been frequently highlighted in many recent studies. Exosomes secreted by metastatic breast cancer cells contain and transfer miR-105 that disrupts cellular adhesion favoring vascular permeability [85]. Likewise, leukemia cells release miR-92a enriched exosomes responsible for increased endothelial cell migration and neovascularization [86]. Hypoxic K562 cells produce miR-210 enriched exosomes causing a pro-angiogenic phenotype [87]. Finally, glioblastoma cells secrete exosomes containing an oncogenic epidermal growth factor receptor (EGFR) that, once transferred, leads to a cascade of events leading to transformation, uncontrolled proliferation and neovascularization [69].

Involvement of exosomes in creating systemic changes can be an explanation of metastatic dissemination, the major cause of cancer patients' deaths [75]. Unfortunately, very few therapies are available for treating patients with diffused metastases [88]. Metastasis comprehends a series of steps starting with dissemination from the primary tumor, survival and immune-escape, intravasation into the blood vessels, extravasation at targeting secondary sites with growth of metastatic neoformations [89]. This concept was exposed for the first time by the "seed and soil" hypothesis which explained the non randomness of the seeding at secondary organs [89]. The essential step necessary for the successful colonization of distant organs relies on the accumulation of modifications in the target tissues and in their surrounding microenvironment (defined as pre-metastatic niche formation, Fig. 2, panel B) primed by factors released in primary tumor sites [90–92]. Exosomes contribute to the metastatic process by increasing tumor cell migration and subsequent invasion of distant sites for metastases onset. Exosomes secreted by EBV-positive nasopharyngeal carcinoma (NPC) cells enhance migration and invasiveness of EBV-negative NPC cells [93]. Evaluating the presence of miRNAs and analyzing their increased levels when released by tumor cells is indicative of the presence of highly metastatic cells [94]. Exosomes coming from gastrointestinal stromal tumor cells can transform progenitor smooth muscle cells to a pre-metastatic phenotype [95]. By in vitro and in vivo imaging it has been demonstrated that highly metastatic breast cancer cells can transfer exosomes both to tumoral and normal lung cells, educating stromal cells [24]. Recent studies have shown that exosomes released by stromal cells and targeted to breast cancer cells are successively modified in their content, increasing their detrimental effects on tumor growth and metastasis [96]. Exosome secretion from cancer cells is a prerequisite for their continuous migration to secondary organs: the process induces autocrine signaling caused by transported fibronectin [97]. Interestingly, inhibition of exosome biogenesis blocked cell movements, thus allowing to conclude that cancer exosomes are essential for the delivery of extracellular matrix (ECM) molecules and regulation of integrins and cellular adhesion. Notably, exosomes secreted by pancreatic ductal adenocarcinomas (PDAC) expressing high levels of macrophage migration inhibitory factor (MIF) have been demonstrated to cause TGF-β production in liver Kupffer cells. As a result, hepatic stellate cells produce higher amounts of fibronectin (FN) and bone marrow derived cells are recruited favouring the formation of a pre-metastatic niche. Patients affected by PDAC secrete exosomes carrying high quantities of MIF, correlating with the development of liver metastases [98]. Exosomes released from activated CD8+ T-cells promote cancer cell diffusion and lung metastasis mediated by the Fas/FasL pathway [99]. The metastatic potential of exosomes can be also boosted by delivery of oncogenic miRNAs to target cells. Exosomes isolated from macrophages activated by IL-4 and carrying miR-223 enhance the metastatic potential of targeted breast cancer cells [100]. It has been demonstrated that delivery of miR-221/222 from MSCs to gastric cancer cells significantly increases cell migration [101]. Metastasis can be promoted by miRNAs present in tumor secreted exosomes that can bind toll-like receptor (TLR) exposed on immune cells [102]. Recently, it has been shown that some tumor cell lines secrete exosomes containing inhibitors of apoptosis (IAPs) that are then circulated as a defence mechanism from tumor proliferating cells [103]. Intriguingly, an in vivo imaging technique has been set up in order to follow the shuttling of extracellular vesicles (EVs) between cancer cells [104]. Recently, microvesicles have been related to the possibility of modifying the phenotype of stromal cells by stimulating angiogenesis and formation of lung premetastatic niche [105]. Interestingly, it has been shown that not only cancer cells release exosomes but also normal stromal cells can secrete vesicles able to increase the spreading of several cancer cell types [96]. Mesenchymal stem cells release exosomes that stimulate mobility and invasiveness of MCF7 breast cancer cells mediated by upregulation of Wnt signaling [23]. Finally, exosomes originated from T-cells can promote invasion and migration of murine B16 melanoma cells to the lungs [99].

Tumor Immune Escape and Multidrug Resistance

Exosomes can interfere with the normal immune system functions acting as immunosuppressive agents that uphold tumorigenesis. As an example, activation of the death receptor pathway can induce apoptosis of CD8+ T-cells [106]. Further T-cell dysregulation can be induced by the proliferation of regulatory T-cells and the inhibition of effector T-cells growth [107]. Exosomes can also inhibit the cytotoxic functions proper of natural killer (NK) cells [108]. In the last years, it has been shown that cancer exosomes can suppress specific T-cell immunity and push the transformation of innate immune cells towards a pro-tumor phenotype (Fig. 2, panel C) [75, 109]. Exosomes derived from human colorectal cancer and melanoma cells block the differentiation of peripheral blood monocytes to functional dendritic cells and direct them towards myeloid-derived suppressor cells (MDSCs) [110], immature cells with multiple immunosuppressive functions [111]. Exosomes secreted from breast cancer cells promote accumulation of MDSCs by a prostaglandin E2 and TGF-beta mediated pathway [109]. This effect has been confirmed in cancer patients and correlated with poor prognosis and overall survival [111]. Some cancer derived exosomes have been demonstrated able of inducing apoptosis in activated T-cells due to the presence of death ligands FasL and TRAIL [112, 113]. This effect was verified in ovarian cancer patients that release exosomes enriched in FasL able to induce T-cell apoptosis [113]. Pre-treatment of mice with exosomes derived from mammary cancer showed enhanced tumor cell proliferation due to suppression of activation of natural killer cells necessary to remove cancer cells [114]. Human NPC cell-derived exosomes impair T-cell activity, which is connected with upregulation of miRNAs in exosomes [115, 116]. The presence of ligands for NKG2D on the membrane of exosomes originated by human prostate cancer cells has been demonstrated to be responsible for the downregulation of NKG2D expression on NK and CD8+ T-cells, determining the impairment of their cytotoxic functions [117].

Exosomes participate in the development of drug resistance to anti-cancer therapies in tumor cells through a plethora of mechanisms (Fig. 2, panel D). Recent work has proven the role of exosomes derived from tumor cells in delivering proteins and miRNAs conferring multidrug resistance (MDR) to target cells in vivo. It has been demonstrated that targeted therapies, like radiation and chemotherapy, stimulate secretion of exosomes enriched with anti-apoptotic proteins [118]. In response to radiation, HeLa cells secrete exosomes containing survivin, a protein involved in the suppression of apoptosis and regulation of mitosis [119]. Exosomes participate in the development of drug resistance also by encapsulating administered therapeutic molecules and exporting them from tumor cells [120, 121]. This phenomenon is very similar to the sequestration of cytotoxic drugs by melanosomes during therapy of aggressive melanomas [122]. Recent findings show that cisplatin-resistant cancer cells produce exosomes containing larger amounts of cisplatin as compared to the cytoplasm of parental cells [123]. Targeted antibodies dispensed during therapy can be sequestered by exosomes. Lymphoma exosomes display CD20, a receptor able to bind therapeutic antibodies and making useless this kind of therapeutic treatment [124]. Stromal cells secrete particular exosomes that may contribute to drug resistance. For example, it has been observed that the activation of multiple survival pathways by exosomes released from BM-MSC causes resistance to bortezomib in myeloma cells [124]. Exosomes can also subtract other molecules, like cisplatin and trastuzumab, to tumor cells [106]. Recent works demonstrate that miRNAs can be packaged in exosomes secreted by specific chemoresistant cancer cells [125]. These observations support the hypothesis of drug resistance acquisition mediated by exosome during intercellular communication [15]. MSC derived exosomes are involved in promoting chemotherapeutic drug resistance in gastric cancer cells by activating the calcium/calmodulin-dependent protein kinase (CaM-Ks) and Raf/MEK/ERK kinase cascade [126].

Exosomes in Cancer Diagnosis and Therapy

Nowadays, exosomes are recognized as ideal biomarkers for diagnosis and therapy (Fig. 3). Improvements in the isolation from body fluids and in the characterization of their internal cargo, that reflects the pathological condition of the parental cells, have helped in the discovery and validation of new markers in human cancers that can be used as potential diagnostic and prognostic factors. Moreover, the increased ability in loading exosomes with small molecules and drugs for cancer therapy and the enhanced efficiency in targeting specific tissues are promoting their use as physiological carriers in clinical therapy.

Biomarkers for Diagnosis

It has been demonstrated that the levels of exosomes increase in the plasma of ovarian cancer patients, correlating to the tumor stage [127]. The high abundance of miRNAs in exosomes and the proven specific miRNA profile of tumors [128] have suggested them to be diagnostic and prognostic indicators for many different

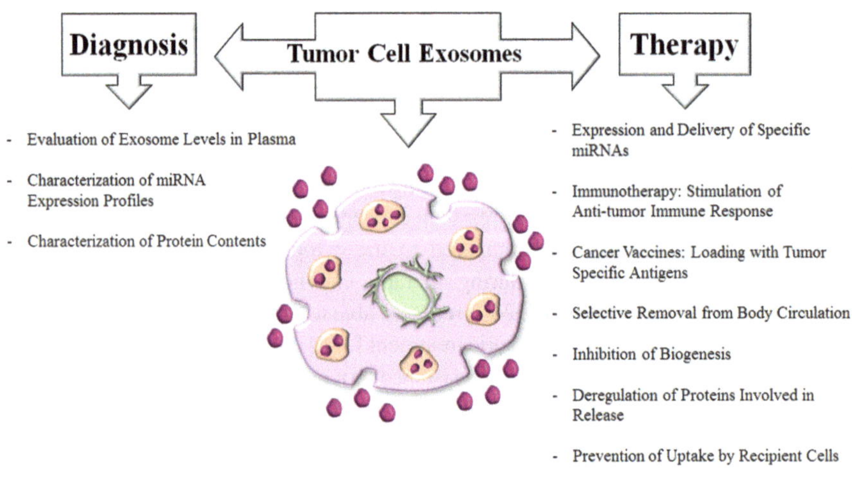

Fig. 3 Tumor cell exosomes can be exploited both as biomarkers for cancer diagnosis (on the *left*) and for tumor targeted therapy (on the *right*)

cancers (i.e., glioblastoma, lung, pancreatic, prostate, breast cancer and esophageal squamous cell carcinoma) [129–135]. Exosomes can be isolated and characterized in their content (miRNA, proteins) in patients affected by colorectal carcinoma and pancreatic cancer and used as useful diagnostic tools [136–138]. A lot of different cancer exosomes can be actually characterized and adopted as biomarkers: analysis of the protein content of melanoma exosomes [139, 140], analysis of the miRNAs content of esophageal adenocarcinoma [141] and gastric cancer [142], profiling of the protein content of cholangiocarcinoma [143], non-small cell lung cancer [144], and glioma [145].

Very recently, research on exosomes as biomarkers has opened a new way to a more focused approach towards specific cancer diagnosis. In particular, the presence of cell surface proteoglycan, glypican-1, on cancer exosomes has contributed to the discrimination between healthy individuals and early/late stage patients affected by pancreatic cancer, strikingly with absolute specificity and sensitivity [146]. Evaluation of the presence of long non-coding RNAs (lncRNAs) has been defined as novel exosomal biomarker [147, 148], especially if present in serum of gastric cancer patients [149].

Tools for Targeted Therapy

Exosomes containing miR-150 have been demonstrated to be able to reduce endothelial cell migration and to inhibit the functions of effector T-cells. When 293T cells were transduced with miRNAs and cell culture medium was collected and used to culture un-conditioned 293T cells, higher expression of the specific miRNAs was observed due to the uptake of released exosomes [150, 151]. Many studies clearly support the concept of combining miRNA- and exosome-based therapies as innovative tools for cancer therapy. Interesting works have demonstrated the applicability of MSC-derived exosomes. Exosomes collected from these cells and carrying the tumor suppressor miR-146b were intratumorally injected in a xenograft model of glioblastoma, inhibiting tumor growth [152, 153]. In vitro experiments in glioblastoma cells demonstrated the efficacy of delivered anti-miRs in knockdown of oncogenic miRNA and consequent increased cell sensitivity to specific chemotherapy [154, 155].

Exosomes have also been exploited for immunotherapy and many examples can be reported. In particular, tumor peptide-pulsed exosomes isolated from dendritic cells can suppress tumor cell proliferation in a T-cell dependent way [156]. On the other side, exosomes secreted by tumor cells carry and present tumor antigens to dendritic cells inducing a specific CD8+ T-cell-dependent immune response against tumors [157]. Intriguingly, dendritic cell-derived exosomes have entered clinical trials for colorectal cancer, metastatic melanoma, and non-small cell lung cancer (NSCLC) [158]. These modified vesicles were able of inducing specific T-cell immune responses and tumor regression [159–161]. A novel immunotherapeutic strategy can be envisaged by creating vaccines based on tumor derived exosomes containing molecules necessary to target cancer cells. [162]. The principle is to stimulate an anti-tumor immune response against tumors by using exosomes containing tumor specific antigens. Exosomes derived from antigen-presenting dendritic cells have been shown very efficient for this purpose [163] and in 2010 the first exosome based cancer vaccine has been approved for the treatment of metastatic prostate cancer [158].

Recently, exosomes have been proved to be valuable cancer vaccines. Tumor growth can be decreased by administering exosomes carrying α-galactosylceramide and tumor-specific antigens able to stimulate cancer-specific adaptive immune responses [164]. For example, in primary and metastatic melanoma models cancer exosomes loaded with tumor antigens have been shown to efficiently induce anti-tumor immune responses [165].

An interesting option that can be considered when treating cancer involves removal of exosomes from the body's circulation, keeping in mind that, despite their prominent role in cancer progression, exosomes retain also important physiological functions essential for normal intercellular communication. Therefore, removing the totality of exosomes from the body could be detrimental and selective removal of exosomes could become feasible only after univocal identification of the molecules present on the pathogenic exosomes. Depletion of exosomes is an innovative approach to treat patients presenting advanced tumors [166]. Dimethyl amiloride (DMA), a drug used to treat hypertension, inhibits exosome formation and mediates immunosuppressive function of mouse and human myeloid derived suppressor cells in colorectal cancer patients [167]. However, these kinds of treatment in prostate cancer patients did not give similar results, indicating cell-type specific responses [168]. Exosome depletion and inhibition of MDSC functions by DMA in mice restored the anti-tumor efficacy of cyclophosphamide (CTX). A company has recently developed an adjunct therapeutic treatment "HER2osome", able to reduce tumor-secreted HER2 positive exosomes and selectively inhibit HER2-positive breast cancer proliferation (Aethlon Medical, Inc.). The clinical efficacy of this approach is currently under evaluation.

Innovative strategies to remove tumor exosomes from the circulation have been recently proposed. Some extracorporeal hemofiltration devices have been produced [166], with the aim of reducing the risk of drug toxicity due to classical chemotherapy. By applying these strategies, patient's blood is selectively depleted of cancer derived exosomes. It has to be noted that, eventhough these approaches can reveal extremely valuable for their efficiency, they are not selective towards malignant exosomes and the effects of aspecifically depleting also healthy exosomes needs to be carefully evaluated.

Inhibition of exosome biogenesis can be obtained by using sphingomyelinase inhibitors (e.g. GW4869), which prevent their budding into MVBs through reduction of ceramide [169]. This approach has been proved to be effective in vivo: when the inhibitor was administered to Lewis Lung carcinoma bearing mice a significant reduction in lung metastases was clearly appreciable [169]. Finally, besides interfering with the process of exosome formation and release by inhibiting the endosomal pathway, another possibility could be targeting members of the ESCRT machinery, like syndecan proteoglycan and adaptor syntenin.

Interestingly, the adoption of RNAi to inhibit specific genes is becoming more and more frequent both in basic research and in clinical application [170]. RNAi and small molecule mediated inhibition of proteins involved in exosome biogenesis can effectively reduce their production and release from diseased cells, avoiding the diffusion of pathological phenotypes. In particular, by using short hairpin RNAs (shRNAs), the translation of exosome-producing systems like ESCRT proteins and/or GTPases can be prevented [171]. These systems allow for long term silencing in target tissues following exosome delivery. RNAi of Rab27a in melanoma cells clearly blocked exosome production and bone marrow education, and reduced their metastatic potential [75]. Targeting GTPases involved in the fusion of MVBs to the cell membrane can be useful for inhibiting secretion of cancer exosomes. As an example, secretion of malignant exosomes and consequent cell migration capacity were reduced after knockdown of Rab27a and Syt7 [97].

Another possible strategy for inhibiting the tumorigenic effects of tumor exosomes is to avoid recipient cell uptake. This idea was tested by means of blocking phosphatidylserine with diannexin [172]. However, it is important to consider that blocking exosome functions can inadvertently cause problems in normal physiological pathways.

Exosomes as Drug Delivery Carriers

The peculiar properties of exosomes, particularly their excellent biodistribution, biocompatibility and stability in circulation make them invaluable tools for nucleic acid or drug delivery [173]. The great potential of exosomes for targeted therapy is based on the fact that they are natural carriers in the body and therefore they will exert less toxicity and elicit lower immune responses once injected into the patients' circulation. Loading of a specific cargo can be accomplished by (1) endogenous overexpression of RNA species and molecules of interest in producer cells, that will physiologically package them into exosomes, or by (2) exogenous loading (co-incubation or electroporation) [174]. A third possibility would be to exploit viral packaging systems to load exosomes with specific cargos [175].

The mechanisms of exosome uptake in target cells have not yet fully understood. It has been hypothesized that exosomes can be uptaken and compartimentalized in MVBs of primary and secondary target cells [176]. In particular, exosome membrane constitution is crucial for their ability to target cells [177]. Interestingly, lipidic vesicles mimicking exosome membranes are unable to fuse with cells, suggesting that also the protein component is equivalently essential for their activity. Notably, exosomes do not accumulate in the liver, in fact Rabies viral glycoprotein (RVG)-exosomes were shown to almost completely bypass liver accumulation and only minimal amounts of curcumin via exosomes were appreciable following intranasal administration [178].

Exosome delivery of small interfering RNA (siRNA) has been tested because of their relevant potential in gene-based therapies [179–181] and due to the fact that it has to be overcome the common issue of low stability when injected in systemic circulation [182, 183]. In vitro experiments have shown that delivery of Rad51- and Rad52-siRNA mediated by exosomes resulted in specific gene knockdown and reduced cell viability and proliferation in fibrosarcoma [180]. Exosome-delivered siRNA revealed effective also in post-transcriptional gene silencing and caused apoptosis in target cancer cells [180, 181].

A new strategy adopted in order to obtain a better cell/tissue targeting is to modify exosomes by fusing specific ligands to proteins exposed on their lipidic bilayer. As an example, exosomes isolated from immature dendritic mouse cells were engineered to express Arg-Gly-Asp (RGD)-Lamp2b peptide fused to a tumor-targeting integrin. Intravenous injection of these vesicles, loaded with doxorubicin, was shown to efficiently target integrin-positive breast cancer cells and to inhibit tumor growth [180].

Exosomes can be produced also by ad hoc cell lines that must be immune-tolerated (i.e., immature dendritic cells [184]) and must insert on the exosome membrane the right surface proteins necessary to obtain the binding to the correct final target. Human MSC cells can be considered ideal candidates as producers of exosomes with excellent immunosuppressive activity and loaded with molecules for targeted therapy [41]. Exosomes isolated from MSCs have been tested as carriers for active drugs such as paclitaxel. When targeted to mouse breast cancer cells, they were able to deliver molecules causing down-regulation of VEGF with subsequent decrease in tumor growth and suppression of angiogenesis [185].

One interesting possibility is to exploit exosomes as carriers for loaded chemotherapeutics. In vivo experiments demonstrated that doxorubicin loaded exosomes inhibited the growth of breast and colon adenocarcinoma xenografts [186, 187]. Moreover, enhanced efficacy of doxorubicin was appreciable when immature dendritic cells derived exosomes were targeted to the tumor tissue. Concomitantly, there were significantly less adverse effects on major organs [186, 188]. Encapsulation in exosomes of cucurbitacin I, a potent anti-inflammatory molecule, and administration to a murine model of glioblastoma showed enhanced activity and reduction in the tumor mass volume [189, 190]. Creation of engineered exosomes carrying cytosine deaminase (CD) and uracil phosphoribosyltransferase (UPRT) have been obtained by transfecting HEK 293T cells. An orthotopic model of schwannoma was treated with these isolated exosomes in combination with the chemotherapeutic prodrug 5-fluorocytosine. Interestingly, the prodrug was efficiently converted to the active 5-fluorouracil and 5-fluoro-deoxyuridine monophosphate and significant tumor cell apoptosis and regression were obtained [191, 192]. These kinds of studies clearly display the potential and the increasing applicability of exosomes as cancer therapy treatments.

Recent studies have focused on the isolation of reticulocyte derived exosomes (RTC), potential drug carriers due to their inability to elicit immune responses and cancer-prone reactions in recipient cells [193, 194]. Qi et al. combined these features to the properties of superparamagnetic magnetite colloidal nanocrystal clusters (SMCNCs) (i.e., self-assembly and growth in solution, significant increase in nanocrystal magnetization, while retaining their superparamagnetic behaviour)

[195, 196] in order to separate exosomes from blood and to provide them with a strong targeting capacity. They anchored multiple superparamagnetic nanoparticles to obtain a cluster on the RTC exosomes for in vivo studies: drug-loaded exosome-based vehicle delivery enhanced cancer targeting under an external magnetic field and suppressed tumor growth.

Exosomes Based Therapies in Clinical Development

Several clinical trials based on the application of exosomes for cancer targeted therapy are actually in progress or just completed. In a phase I study, exosomes were isolated from dendritic cells, loaded with antigenic peptides and used as cancer vaccines in stage III/IV melanomas. Outstandingly, no significant toxicity was observed while a considerable increase in NK cell number and reactivity were detected [162]. The same kind of approach was successfully applied to NSCLC patients [160]. Second generation dendritic cell derived exosomes combined with chemotherapy were employed in the treatment of unresectable NSCLC. Patients were treated both with chronic low doses of chemotherapeutics and with exosomes, obtaining immunostimulatory effects on T-cells and tumor growth arrest [197]. Similarly, autologous ascites-derived exosomes (Aex) used in combination with GM-CSF in the treatment of colorectal cancer showed enhanced efficacy due to activated cytotoxic T-cell response [198].

In a recent phase I clinical trial on aggressive glioma, cancer cells were isolated and treated with an antisense molecule to inhibit the expression of insulin-like growth factor receptor 1 (IGF1R). When these cells, confined in small biodiffusion chambers, were re-implanted into the abdomen of the patients, they underwent apoptosis and secreted exosomes eliciting a potent immune response mediated by T-cells [199].

Significantly, two clinical trials are evaluating the potential of plant derived exosomes for cancer therapy: (1) grape-derived exosome-like nanoparticles are being evaluated in the treatment of oral mucositis and potential reduction of side effects after radio- and chemotherapy in head and neck cancers [200], (2) exosomes loaded with curcumin are being tested for the treatment of colorectal cancer [201]. The fact that exosomes are efficiently performing in clinical trials further corroborates the importance of developing new drug delivery systems based on these innovative nanocarriers.

Conclusions and Future Perspectives

The emerging roles of exosomes as nanovesicles with several physiological and pathological functions increasingly underline the importance of their study both for basic research and clinical applications. Exosomes can act as carriers for proteins and nucleic acids and are responsible for intercellular communication. Furthermore, they display a great potential as non-invasive diagnostic biomarkers and as carriers for targeted drug delivery.

In the last years, researches have unraveled their involvement in cancer, indicating a plethora of pathways in which they participate, from tumorigenesis, to tumor microenvironment modulation, to phenomena like tumor immune escape and multidrug resistance. Eventhough in vitro and in vivo data have proven their multiple roles, the mechanisms through which exosomes act in cancer patients have not been fully elucidated. Many technical challenges need to be addressed and overcome in order to completely exploit their potential: usually, low concentrations of vesicles are obtained after isolation and time consuming and expensive procedures are currently needed in order to get ultra-pure preparations.

Some questions remain open: which are the exact relations between healthy and oncogenic exosome-mediated signaling? How are cancer exosomes able to corrupt healthy exosomes? Exosomal signaling is complex and their ability to act simultaneously by means of different cellular contents makes very difficult a univocal understanding of their tasks. Further investigations are required in order to correlate their contribution and involvement in signaling pathways to the observed phenotypes.

The possibility to modify their intricate communication networks is the main aim of research efforts. There is increasing interest in the introduction of personalized cancer therapy: ad hoc treatments based on each individual's features and biology can be set and exosomes could be used for this purpose. They are perfectly biocompatible, they have reduced toxicity and immunogenicity, they display great stability in body fluids and they can be loaded with specific molecules to target a specific tissue. Ideally, it would become feasible to isolate exosomes from patients, load them with desired drugs and then inject back in order to obtain the required personalized response.

Ongoing clinical trials will help in clarifying the complex roles of exosomes in cancer and they will give necessary indications on the proper modifications that would be needed for the creation of the ideal translational drug based on these nanovesicles.

References

1. Vlassov AV, Magdaleno S, Setterquist R, Conrad R (2012) Exosomes: current knowledge of their composition, biological functions, and diagnostic and therapeutic potentials. Biochim Biophys Acta 1820:940–948
2. Théry C, Ostrowski M, Segura E (2009) Membrane vesicles as conveyors of immune responses. Nat Rev Immunol 9:581–593
3. Thery C (2015) Cancer: diagnosis by extracellular vesicles. Nature 523:161–162
4. Colombo M, Raposo G, Thery C (2014) Biogenesis, secretion, and intercellular interactions of exosomes and other extracellular vesicles. Annu Rev Cell Dev Biol 30:255–289
5. Mathivanan S, Ji H, Simpson RJ (2010) Exosomes: extracellular organelles important in intercellular communication. J Proteomics 73:1907–1920

6. Witwer KW, Buzás EI, Bemis LT, Bora A, Lässer C, Lötvall J, Nolte-'t Hoen EN, Piper MG, Sivaraman S, Skog J, Théry C, Wauben MH, Hochberg F (2013) Standardization of sample collection, isolation and analysis methods in extracellular vesicle research. J Extracell Vesicles 2:10.3402
7. Jia S, Zocco D, Samuels ML, Chou MF, Chammas R, Skog J, Zarovni N, Momen-Heravi F, Kuo WP (2014) Emerging technologies in extracellular vesicle-based molecular diagnostics. Expert Rev Mol Diagn 3:307–321
8. Trams EG, Lauter CJ, Salem N, Heine U (1981) Exfoliation of membrane ecto-enzymes in the form of micro-vesicles. Biochim Biophys Acta 645:63–70
9. Pan BT, Johnstone RM (1983) Fate of the transferrin receptor during maturation of sheep reticulocytes in vitro: selective externalization of the receptor. Cell 33:967–978
10. Johnstone RM, Adam M, Hammond JR, Orr L, Turbide C (1987) Vesicle formation during reticulocyte maturation. Association of plasma membrane activities with released vesicles (exosomes). J Biol Chem 262:9412–9420
11. Johnstone RM, Mathew A, Mason AB, Teng K (1991) Exosome formation during maturation of mammalian and avian reticulocytes: evidence that exosome release is a major route for externalization of obsolete membrane proteins. J Cell Physiol 147:27–36
12. Raposo G, Nijman HW, Stoorvogel W, Liejendekker R, Harding CV, Melief CJ, Geuze HJ (1996) B lymphocytes secrete antigen-presenting vesicles. J Exp Med 183:1161–1172
13. Valadi H, Ekström K, Bossios A, Sjöstrand M, Lee JJ, Lötvall JO (2007) Exosome mediated transfer of mRNAs and microRNAs is a novel mechanism of genetic exchange between cells. Nat Cell Biol 9:654–659
14. Simpson RJ, Lim JW, Moritz RL, Mathivanan S (2009) Exosomes: proteomic insights and diagnostic potential. Expert Rev Proteomics 6:267–283
15. Zhao L, Liu W, Xiao J, Cao B (2014) The role of exosomes and "exosomal shuttle microRNA" in tumorigenesis and drug resistance. Cancer Lett 356:339–346
16. Kahlert C, Melo SA, Protopopov A, Tang J, Seth S, Koch M, Zhang J, Weitz J, Chin L, Futreal A, Kalluri R (2014) Identification of double-stranded genomic DNA spanning all chromosomes with mutated KRAS and p53 DNA in the serum exosomes of patients with pancreatic cancer. J Biol Chem 289:3869–3875
17. Thakur BK, Zhang H, Becker A, Matei I, Huang Y, Costa-Silva B, Zheng Y, Hoshino A, Brazier H, Xiang J, Williams C, Rodriguez-Barrueco R, Silva JM, Zhang W, Hearn S, Elemento O, Paknejad N, Manova-Todorova K, Welte K, Bromberg J, Peinado H, Lyden D (2014) Double-stranded DNA in exosomes: a novel biomarker in cancer detection. Cell Res 24:766–769
18. Mathivanan S, Simpson RJ (2009) ExoCarta: a compendium of exosomal proteins and RNA. Proteomics 9:4997–5000
19. ExoCarta. http://www.exocarta.org/. Accessed 17 July 2016
20. Lo Cicero A, Stahl PD, Raposo G (2015) Extracellular vesicles shuffling intercellular messages: for good or for bad. Curr Opin Cell Biol 35:69–77
21. Lee Y, El Andaloussi S, Wood MJ (2012) Exosomes and microvesicles: extracellular vesicles for genetic information transfer and gene therapy. Hum Mol Genet 21(R1):R125–R134
22. El Andaloussi S, Mäger I, Breakefield XO, Wood MJA (2013) Extracellular vesicles: biology and emerging therapeutic opportunities. Nat Rev Drug Discov 12:347–357
23. Luga V, Wrana JL (2013) Tumor-stroma interaction: revealing fibroblast-secreted exosomes as potent regulators of Wnt-planar cell polarity signaling in cancer metastasis. Cancer Res 73:6843–6847
24. Suetsugu A, Honma K, Saji S, Moriwaki H, Ochiya T, Hoffman RM (2013) Imaging exosome transfer from breast cancer cells to stroma at metastatic sites in orthotopic nude-mouse models. Adv Drug Deliv Rev 65:383–390
25. Kumar B, Garcia M, Murakami JL, Chen CC (2016) Exosome mediated microenvironment dysregulation in leukemia. Biochim Biophys Acta 1863:464–470
26. Katsuda T, Kosaka N, Ochiya T (2014) The roles of extracellular vesicles in cancer biology: toward the development of novel cancer biomarkers. Proteomics 14:412–425

27. Raimondo S, Corrado C, Raimondi L, De Leo G, Alessandro R (2015) Role of extracellular vesicles in hematological malignancies. Biomed Res Int 2015:821613
28. Lötvall J, Hill AF, Hochberg F, Buzás EI, Di Vizio D, Gardiner C, Gho YS, Kurochkin IV, Mathivanan S, Quesenberry P, Sahoo S, Tahara H, Wauben MH, Witwer KW, Théry C (2014) Minimal experimental requirements for definition of extracellular vesicles and their functions: a position statement from the International Society for Extracellular Vesicles. J Extracell Vesicles 3:26913
29. Raposo G, Stoorvogel W (2013) Extracellular vesicles: exosomes, microvesicles, and friends. J Cell Biol 200:373–383
30. Riteau B, Faure F, Menier C, Viel S, Carosella ED, Amigorena S, Rouas-Freiss N (2003) Exosomes bearing HLA-G are released by melanoma cells. Hum Immunol 64:1064–1072
31. Caby MP, Lankar D, Vincendeau-Scherrer C, Raposo G, Bonnerot C (2005) Exosomal like vesicles are present in human blood plasma. Int Immunol 17:879–887
32. Anand PK (2010) Exosomal membrane molecules are potent immune response modulators. Commun Int Biol 3:405–408
33. Kreimer S, Belov AM, Ghiran I, Murthy SK, Frank DA, Ivanov AR (2015) Mass-spectrometry-based molecular characterization of extracellular vesicles: lipidomics and proteomics. J Proteome Res 14:2367–2384
34. Raiborg C, Stenmark H (2009) The ESCRT machinery in endosomal sorting of ubiquitylated membrane proteins. Nature 458:445–452
35. Colombo M, Moita C, van Niel G, Kowal J, Vigneron J, Benaroch P, Manel N, Moita LF, Thery C, Raposo G (2013) Analysis of ESCRT functions in exosome biogenesis, composition and secretion highlights the heterogeneity of extracellular vesicles. J Cell Sci 126:5553–5565
36. Baietti MF, Zhang Z, Mortier E, Melchior A, Degeest G, Geeraerts A, Ivarsson Y, Depoortere F, Coomans C, Vermeiren E, Zimmermann P, David G (2012) Syndecan-syntenin-ALIX regulates the biogenesis of exosomes. Nat Cell Biol 14(7):677–685
37. Friand V, David G, Zimmermann P (2015) Syntenin and syndecan in the biogenesis of exosomes. Biol Cell 107:331–341
38. Bobrie A, Krumeich S, Reyal F, Recchi C, Moita LF, Seabra MC, Ostrowski M, Thery C (2012) Rab27a supports exosome-dependent and -independent mechanisms that modify the tumor microenvironment and can promote tumor progression. Cancer Res 72:4920–4930
39. Ostrowski M, Carmo NB, Krumeich S, Fanget I, Raposo G, Savina A, Moita CF, Schauer K, Hume AN, Freitas RP, Goud B, Benaroch P, Hacohen N, Fukuda M, Desnos C, Seabra MC, Darchen F, Amigorena S, Moita LF, Thery C (2010) Rab27a and Rab27b control different steps of the exosome secretion pathway. Nat Cell Biol 12:1–13 (sup)
40. Hsu C, Morohashi Y, Yoshimura S, Manrique-Hoyos N, Jung S, Lauterbach MA, Bakhti M, Grønborg M, Möbius W, Rhee J, Barr FA, Simons M (2010) Regulation of exosome secretion by Rab35 and its GTPase activating proteins TBC1D10A-C. J Cell Biol 189(2):223–232
41. Yeo RW, Lai RC, Zhang B, Tan SS, Yin Y, Teh BJ, Lim SK (2013) Mesenchymal stem cell: an efficient mass producer of exosomes for drug delivery. Adv Drug Deliv Rev 65:336–341
42. Chen K, Rajewsky N (2007) The evolution of gene regulation by transcription factors and microRNAs. Nat Rev Genet 8:93–103
43. Wubbolts R, Leckie RS, Veenhuizen PT, Schwarzmann G, Mobius W, Hoernschemeyer J, Slot JW, Geuze HJ, Stoorvogel W (2003) Proteomic and biochemical analyses of human B cell-derived exosomes. Potential implications for their function and multivesicular body formation. J Biol Chem 278:10963–10972
44. Irion U, St. Johnston D (2007) bicoid RNA localization requires specific binding of an endosomal sorting complex. Nature 445:554–558
45. Savina A, Furlan M, Vidal M, Colombo MI (2003) Exosome release is regulated by a calcium-dependent mechanism in K562 cells. J Biol Chem 278(22):20083–20090
46. Parolini I, Federici C, Raggi C, Lugini L, Palleschi S, De Milito A, Coscia C, Iessi E, Logozzi M, Molinari A, Colone M, Tatti M, Sargiacomo M, Fais S (2009) Microenvironmental pH is a key factor for exosome traffic in tumor cells. J Biol Chem 284(49):34211–34222

47. Yu JL, May L, Lhotak V, Shahrzad S, Shirasawa S, Weitz JI, Coomber BL, Mackman N, Rak JW (2005) Oncogenic events regulate tissue factor expression in colorectal cancer cells: implications for tumor progression and angiogenesis. Blood 105(4):1734–1741
48. Yu X, Harris SL, Levine AJ (2006) The regulation of exosome secretion: a novel function of the p53 protein. Cancer Res 66(9):4795–4801
49. Lespagnol A, Duflaut D, Beekman C, Blanc L, Fiucci G, Marine JC, Vidal M, Amson R, Telerman A (2008) Exosome secretion, including the DNA damage-induced p53-dependent secretory pathway, is severely compromised in TSAP6/Steap3-null mice. Cell Death Differ 15(11):1723–1733
50. Thompson CA, Purushothaman A, Ramani VC, Vlodavsky I, Sanderson RD (2013) Heparanase regulates secretion, composition, and function of tumor cell-derived exosomes. J Biol Chem 288(14):10093–10099
51. Riches A, Campbell E, Borger E, Powis S (2014) Regulation of exosome release from mammary epithelial and breast cancer cells—a new regulatory pathway. Eur J Cancer 50(5):1025–1034
52. Janas T, Janas MM, Sapon K, Janas T (2015) Mechanisms of RNA loading into exosomes. FEBS Lett 589:1391–1398
53. Miyanishi M, Tada K, Koike M, Uchiyama Y, Kitamura T, Nagata S (2007) Identification of Tim4 as a phosphatidylserine receptor. Nature 450(7168):435–439
54. Segura E, Nicco C, Lombard B, Véron P, Raposo G, Batteux F, Amigorena S, Théry C (2005) ICAM-1 on exosomes from mature dendritic cells is critical for efficient naive T-cell priming. Blood 106(1):216–223
55. Tian T, Wang Y, Wang H, Zhu Z, Xiao Z (2010) Visualizing of the cellular uptake and intracellular trafficking of exosomes by live-cell microscopy. J Cell Biochem 111(2):488–496
56. Feng D, Zhao WL, Ye YY, Bai XC, Liu RQ, Chang LF, Zhou Q, Sui SF (2010) Cellular internalization of exosomes occurs through phagocytosis. Traffic 11(5):675–687
57. Escrevente C, Keller S, Altevogt P, Costa J (2011) Interaction and uptake of exosomes by ovarian cancer cells. BMC Cancer 11:108
58. Christianson HC, Svensson KJ, van Kuppevelt TH, Li JP, Belting M (2013) Cancer cell exosomes depend on cell-surface heparan sulfate proteoglycans for their internalization and functional activity. Proc Natl Acad Sci U S A 110(43):17380–17385
59. Szajnik M, Derbis M, Lach M, Patalas P, Michalak M, Drzewiecka H, Szpurek D, Nowakowski A, Spaczynski M, Baranowski W, Whiteside TL (2013) Exosomes in plasma of patients with ovarian carcinoma: potential biomarkers of tumor progression and response to therapy. Gynecol Obstet (Sunnyvale) Suppl 4:003
60. Logozzi M, De Milito A, Lugini L, Borghi M, Calabrò L, Spada M, Perdicchio M, Marino ML, Federici C, Iessi E, Brambilla D, Venturi G, Lozupone F, Santinami M, Huber V, Maio M, Rivoltini L, Fais S (2009) High levels of exosomes expressing CD63 and caveolin-1 in plasma of melanoma patients. PLoS One 4:e5219
61. Farooqi AA, Qureshi MZ, Coskunpinar E, Naqvi SK, Yaylim I, Ismail M (2014) miR-421, miR-155 and miR-650: emerging trends of regulation of cancer and apoptosis. Asian Pac J Cancer Prev 15:1909–1912
62. Farooqi AA, Naqi A, Qureshi MZ, Rana A, Khan A, Riaz AM, Afzal SM, Rasheed N, Bhatti S (2012) Prostate cancer is known by the companionship with ATM and miRNA it keeps: craftsmen of translation have dual behaviour with tailors of life thread. Cell Biochem Funct 30(7):611–617
63. Farooqi AA, De Rosa G (2013) TRAIL and microRNAs in the treatment of prostate cancer: therapeutic potential and role of nanotechnology. Appl Microbiol Biotechnol 97:8849–8857
64. Farooqi AA, Nawaz A, Javed Z, Shahzad Bhatti S, Ismail M (2013) While at Rome miRNA and TRAIL do whatever BCR-ABL commands to do. Arch Immunol Ther Exp (Warsz) 61:59–74
65. Abd Elmageed ZY, Yang Y, Thomas R, Ranjan M, Mondal D, Moroz K, Fang Z, Rezk BM, Moparty K, Sikka SC, Sartor O, Abdel-Mageed AB (2014) Neoplastic reprogramming of patient-derived adipose stem cells by prostate cancer cell-associated exosomes. Stem Cells 32(4):983–997

66. Melo SA, Sugimoto H, O'Connell JT, Kato N, Villanueva A, Vidal A, Qiu L, Vitkin E, Perelman LT, Melo CA, Lucci A, Ivan C, Calin GA, Kalluri R (2014) Cancer exosomes perform cell-independent microRNA biogenesis and promote tumorigenesis. Cancer Cell 26(5):707–721
67. Joyce JA, Pollard JW (2009) Microenvironmental regulation of metastasis. Nat Rev Cancer 9:239–252
68. Martins VR, Dias MS, Hainaut P (2013) Tumor-cell-derived microvesicles as carriers of molecular information in cancer. Curr Opin Oncol 25:66–75
69. Al-Nedawi K, Meehan B, Micallef J, Lhotak V, May L, Guha A, Rak J (2008) Intercellular transfer of the oncogenic receptor EGFRvIII by microvesicles derived from tumour cells. Nat Cell Biol 10:619–624
70. Al-Nedawi K, Meehan B, Kerbel RS, Allison AC, Rak J (2009) Endothelial expression of autocrine VEGF upon the uptake of tumor-derived microvesicles containing oncogenic EGFR. Proc Natl Acad Sci U S A 106:3794–3799
71. Ciravolo V, Huber V, Ghedini GC, Venturelli E, Bianchi F, Campiglio M, Morelli D, Villa A, Della Mina P, Menard S, Filipazzi P, Rivoltini L, Tagliabue E, Pupa SM (2012) Potential role of HER2-overexpressing exosomes in countering trastuzumab-based therapy. J Cell Physiol 227:658–667
72. Kucharzewska P, Christianson HC, Welch JE, Svensson KJ, Fredlund E, Ringnér M, Mörgelin M, Bourseau-Guilmain E, Bengzon J, Belting M (2013) Exosomes reflect the hypoxic status of glioma cells and mediate hypoxia-dependent activation of vascular cells during tumor development. Proc Natl Acad Sci U S A 110:7312–7317
73. Aliotta JM, Pereira M, Li M, Amaral A, Sorokina A, Dooner MS, Sears EH, Brilliant K, Ramratnam B, Hixson DC, Quesenberry PJ (2012) Stable cell fate changes in marrow cells induced by lung-derived microvesicles. J Extracell Vesicles 10:3402
74. Demory Beckler M, Higginbotham JN, Franklin JL, Ham AJ, Halvey PJ, Imasuen IE, Whitwell C, Li M, Liebler DC, Coffey RJ (2013) Proteomic analysis of exosomes from mutant KRAS colon cancer cells identifies intercellular transfer of mutant KRAS. Mol Cell Proteomics 12:343–355
75. Peinado H, Alečković M, Lavotshkin S, Matei I, Costa-Silva B, Moreno-Bueno G, Hergueta-Redondo M, Williams C, García-Santos G, Ghajar C, Nitadori-Hoshino A, Hoffman C, Badal K, Garcia BA, Callahan MK, Yuan J, Martins VR, Skog J, Kaplan RN, Brady MS, Wolchok JD, Chapman PB, Kang Y, Bromberg J, Lyden D (2012) Melanoma exosomes educate bone marrow progenitor cells toward a pro-metastatic phenotype through MET. Nat Med 18:883–891
76. Corrado C, Raimondo S, Saieva L, Flugy AM, De Leo G, Alessandro R (2014) Exosome-mediated crosstalk between chronic myelogenous leukemia cells and human bone marrow stromal cells triggers an interleukin 8-dependent survival of leukemia cells. Cancer Lett 348(1–2):71–76
77. Roccaro AM, Sacco A, Maiso P, Azab AK, Tai YT, Reagan M, Azab F, Flores LM, Campigotto F, Weller E, Anderson KC, Scadden DT, Ghobrial IM (2013) BM mesenchymal stromal cell-derived exosomes facilitate multiple myeloma progression. J Clin Invest 123(4):1542–1555
78. Khan S, Aspe JR, Asumen MG, Almaguel F, Odumosu O, Acevedo-Martinez S, De Leon M, Langridge WH, Wall NR (2009) Extracellular, cell-permeable survivin inhibits apoptosis while promoting proliferative and metastatic potential. Br J Cancer 100(7):1073–1086
79. Kieran MW, Folkman J, Heymach J (2003) Angiogenesis inhibitors and hypoxia. Nat Med 9:1104; author reply 1104–1105
80. Hood JL, Pan H, Lanza GM, Wickline SA et al (2009) Paracrine induction of endothelium by tumor exosomes. Lab Invest 89:1317–1328
81. Park JE, Tan HS, Datta A, Lai RC, Zhang H, Meng W, Lim SK, Sze SK (2010) Hypoxic tumor cell modulates its microenvironment to enhance angiogenic and metastatic potential by secretion of proteins and exosomes. Mol Cell Proteomics 9:1085–1099

82. van Balkom BW, de Jong OG, Smits M, Brummelman J, den Ouden K, de Bree PM, van Eijndhoven MA, Pegtel DM, Stoorvogel W, Würdinger T, Verhaar MC (2013) Endothelial cells require miR-214 to secrete exosomes that suppress senescence and induce angiogenesis in human and mouse endothelial cells. Blood 121(3997–4006):S3991–S3915
83. Umezu T, Tadokoro H, Azuma K, Yoshizawa S, Ohyashiki K, Ohyashiki JH (2014) Exosomal miR-135b shed from hypoxic multiple myeloma cells enhances angiogenesis by targeting factor inhibiting HIF-1. Blood 124(25):3748–3757
84. Nazarenko I, Rana S, Baumann A, McAlear J, Hellwig A, Trendelenburg M, Lochnit G, Preissner KT, Zöller M (2010) Cell surface tetraspanin Tspan8 contributes to molecular pathways of exosome-induced endothelial cell activation. Cancer Res 70(4):1668–1678
85. Zhou W, Fong MY, Min Y, Somlo G, Liu L, Palomares MR, Yu Y, Chow A, O'Connor ST, Chin AR, Yen Y, Wang Y, Marcusson EG, Chu P, Wu J, Wu X, Li AX, Li Z, Gao H, Ren X, Boldin MP, Lin PC, Wang SE (2014) Cancer-secreted miR-105 destroys vascular endothelial barriers to promote metastasis. Cancer Cell 25(4):501–515
86. Umezu T, Ohyashiki K, Kuroda M, Ohyashiki JH (2013) Leukemia cell to endothelial cell communication via exosomal miRNAs. Oncogene 32(22):2747–2755
87. Tadokoro H, Umezu T, Ohyashiki K, Hirano T, Ohyashiki JH (2013) Exosomes derived from hypoxic leukemia cells enhance tube formation in endothelial cells. J Biol Chem 288(48):34343–34351
88. Gupta GP, Massague J (2006) Cancer metastasis: building a framework. Cell 127:679–695
89. Fidler IJ (2003) The pathogenesis of cancer metastasis: the 'seed and soil' hypothesis revisited. Nat Rev Cancer 3:453–458
90. Psaila B, Lyden D (2009) The metastatic niche: adapting the foreign soil. Nat Rev Cancer 9:285–293
91. Sceneay J, Parker BS, Smyth MJ, Moller A (2013) Hypoxia-driven immunosuppression contributes to the pre-metastatic niche. Oncoimmunology 2:e22355
92. Sceneay J, Smyth MJ, Moller A (2013) The pre-metastatic niche: finding common ground. Cancer Metastasis Rev 32(3–4):449–464
93. Aga M, Bentz GL, Raffa S, Torrisi MR, Kondo S, Wakisaka N, Yoshizaki T, Pagano JS, Shackelford J (2014) Exosomal HIF1alpha supports invasive potential of nasopharyngeal carcinoma-associated LMP1-positive exosomes. Oncogene 33(37):4613–4622
94. Ostenfeld MS, Jeppesen DK, Laurberg JR, Boysen AT, Bramsen JB, Primdal-Bengtson B, Hendrix A, Lamy P, Dagnaes-Hansen F, Rasmussen MH, Bui KH, Fristrup N, Christensen EI, Nordentoft I, Morth JP, Jensen JB, Pedersen JS, Beck M, Theodorescu D, Borre M, Howard KA, Dyrskjøt L, Ørntoft TF (2014) Cellular disposal of miR23b by RAB27-dependent exosome release is linked to acquisition of metastatic properties. Cancer Res 74(20):5758–5771
95. Atay S, Banskota S, Crow J, Sethi G, Rink L, Godwin AK (2014) Oncogenic KIT-containing exosomes increase gastrointestinal stromal tumor cell invasion. Proc Natl Acad Sci U S A 111(2):711–716
96. Luga V, Zhang L, Viloria-Petit AM, Ogunjimi AA, Inanlou MR, Chiu E, Buchanan M, Hosein AN, Basik M, Wrana JL (2012) Exosomes mediate stromal mobilization of autocrine Wnt-PCP signaling in breast cancer cell migration. Cell 151(7):1542–1556
97. Sung BH, Ketova T, Hoshino D, Zijlstra A (2015) Directional cell movement through tissues is controlled by exosome secretion. Nat Commun 6:7164
98. Costa-Silva B, Aiello NM, Ocean AJ, Singh S, Zhang H, Thakur BK, Becker A, Hoshino A, Mark MT, Molina H, Xiang J, Zhang T, Theilen TM, García-Santos G, Williams C, Ararso Y, Huang Y, Rodrigues G, Shen TL, Labori KJ, Lothe IM, Kure EH, Hernandez J, Doussot A, Ebbesen SH, Grandgenett PM, Hollingsworth MA, Jain M, Mallya K, Batra SK, Jarnagin WR, Schwartz RE, Matei I, Peinado H, Stanger BZ, Bromberg J, Lyden D (2015) Pancreatic cancer exosomes initiate pre-metastatic niche formation in the liver. Nat Cell Biol 17(6):816–826
99. Cai Z, Yang F, Yu L, Yu Z, Jiang L, Wang Q, Yang Y, Wang L, Cao X, Wang J (2012) Activated T-cell exosomes promote tumor invasion via Fas signaling pathway. J Immunol 188(12):5954–5961

100. Yang M, Chen J, Su F, Yu B, Su F, Lin L, Liu Y, Huang JD, Song E (2011) Microvesicles secreted by macrophages shuttle invasion-potentiating microRNAs into breast cancer cells. Mol Cancer 10:117
101. Wang M, Zhao C, Shi H, Zhang B, Zhang L, Zhang X, Wang S, Wu X, Yang T, Huang F, Cai J, Zhu Q, Zhu W, Qian H, Xu W (2014) Deregulated microRNAs in gastric cancer tissue-derived mesenchymal stem cells: novel biomarkers and a mechanism for gastric cancer. Br J Cancer 110(5):1199–1210
102. Fabbri M, Paone A, Calore F, Galli R, Gaudio E, Santhanam R, Lovat F, Fadda P, Mao C, Nuovo GJ, Zanesi N, Crawford M, Ozer GH, Wernicke D, Alder H, Caligiuri MA, Nana-Sinkam P, Perrotti D, Croce CM (2012) MicroRNAs bind to toll-like receptors to induce prometastatic inflammatory response. Proc Natl Acad Sci U S A 109(31):e2110–e2116
103. Valenzuela MM, Ferguson Bennit HR, Gonda A, Diaz Osterman CJ, Hibma A, Khan S, Wall NR (2015) Exosomes secreted from human cancer cell lines contain inhibitors of apoptosis (IAP). Cancer Microenviron 8(2):65–73. doi:10.1007/s12307-015-0167-9
104. Zomer A, Maynard C, Verweij FJ, Kamermans A, Schäfer R, Beerling E, Schiffelers RM, de Wit E, Berenguer J, Ellenbroek SI, Wurdinger T, Pegtel DM, van Rheenen J (2015) In vivo imaging reveals extracellular vesicle-mediated phenocopying of metastatic behavior. Cell 161(5):1046–1057
105. Grange C, Tapparo M, Collino F, Vitillo L, Damasco C, Deregibus MC, Tetta C, Bussolati B, Camussi G (2011) Microvesicles released from human renal cancer stem cells stimulate angiogenesis and formation of lung premetastatic niche. Cancer Res 71:5346–5356
106. Peng P, Yan Y, Keng S (2011) Exosomes in the ascites of ovarian cancer patients: origin and effects on anti-tumor immunity. Oncol Rep 25:749–762
107. Miller IV, Grunewald TG (2015) Tumour-derived exosomes: tiny envelopes for big stories. Biol Cell 107(9):287–305. doi:10.1111/boc.201400095
108. Szczepanski MJ, Szajnik M, Welsh A, Whiteside TL, Boyiadzis M (2011) Blast-derived microvesicles in sera from patients with acute myeloid leukemia suppress natural killer cell function via membrane-associated transforming growth factor-beta1. Haematologica 96:1302–1309
109. Xiang X, Poliakov A, Liu C, Liu Y, Deng ZB, Wang J, Cheng Z, Shah SV, Wang GJ, Zhang L, Grizzle WE, Mobley J, Zhang HG (2009) Induction of myeloid-derived suppressor cells by tumor exosomes. Int J Cancer 124:2621–2633
110. Valenti R, Huber V, Filipazzi P, Pilla L, Sovena G, Villa A, Corbelli A, Fais S, Parmiani G, Rivoltini L (2006) Human tumor-released microvesicles promote the differentiation of myeloid cells with transforming growth factor-beta-mediated suppressive activity on T lymphocytes. Cancer Res 66:9290–9298
111. Gabrilovich DI, Ostrand-Rosenberg S, Bronte V (2012) Coordinated regulation of myeloid cells by tumours. Nat Rev Immunol 12:253–268
112. Kim JW, Wieckowski E, Taylor DD, Reichert TE, Watkins S, Whiteside TL (2005) Fas ligand-positive membranous vesicles isolated from sera of patients with oral cancer induce apoptosis of activated T lymphocytes. Clin Cancer Res 11:1010–1020
113. Taylor DD, Gercel-Taylor C, Lyons KS, Stanson J, Whiteside TL (2003) T-cell apoptosis and suppression of T-cell receptor/CD3-zeta by Fas ligand-containing membrane vesicles shed from ovarian tumors. Clin Cancer Res 9:5113–5119
114. Liu C, Yu S, Zinn K, Wang J, Zhang L, Jia Y, Kappes JC, Barnes S, Kimberly RP, Grizzle WE, Zhang HG (2006) Murine mammary carcinoma exosomes promote tumor growth by suppression of NK cell function. J Immunol 176:1375–1385
115. Mrizak D, Martin N, Barjon C, Jimenez-Pailhes AS, Mustapha R, Niki T, Guigay J, Pancré V, de Launoit Y, Busson P, Moralès O, Delhem N (2014) Effect of nasopharyngeal carcinoma-derived exosomes on human regulatory T cells. J Natl Cancer Inst 107(1):363
116. Ye SB, Li ZL, Luo DH, Huang BJ, Chen YS, Zhang XS, Cui J, Zeng YX, Li J (2014) Tumor-derived exosomes promote tumor progression and T-cell dysfunction through the regulation of enriched exosomal microRNAs in human nasopharyngeal carcinoma. Oncotarget 5(14):5439–5452

117. Lundholm M, Schröder M, Nagaeva O, Baranov V, Widmark A, Mincheva-Nilsson L, Wikström P (2014) Prostate tumor-derived exosomes down-regulate NKG2D expression on natural killer cells and CD8+ T cells: mechanism of immune evasion. PLoS One 9(9):e108925
118. Lv LH, Wan YL, Lin Y, Zhang W, Yang M, Li GL, Lin HM, Shang CZ, Chen YJ, Min J (2012) Anticancer drugs cause release of exosomes with heat shock proteins from human hepatocellular carcinoma cells that elicit effective natural killer cell antitumor responses in vitro. J Biol Chem 287:15874–15885
119. Khan S, Jutzy JM, Aspe JR, McGregor DW, Neidigh JW, Wall NR (2011) Survivin is released from cancer cells via exosomes. Apoptosis 16:1–12
120. Shedden K, Xie XT, Chandaroy P, Chang YT, Rosania GR (2003) Expulsion of small molecules in vesicles shed by cancer cells: association with gene expression and chemosensitivity profiles. Cancer Res 63(15):4331–4337
121. Safaei R, Larson BJ, Cheng TC, Gibson MA, Otani S, Naerdemann W, Howell SB (2005) Abnormal lysosomal trafficking and enhanced exosomal export of cisplatin in drug-resistant human ovarian carcinoma cells. Mol Cancer Ther 4(10):1595–1604
122. Chen KG, Valencia JC, Lai B, Zhang G, Paterson JK, Rouzaud F, Berens W, Wincovitch SM, Garfield SH, Leapman RD, Hearing VJ, Gottesman MM (2006) Melanosomal sequestration of cytotoxic drugs contributes to the intractability of malignant melanomas. Proc Natl Acad Sci U S A 103(26):9903–9907
123. Yang C, Robbins PD (2011) The roles of tumor-derived exosomes in cancer pathogenesis. Clin Dev Immunol 2011:842849
124. Battke C, Ruiss R, Welsch U, Wimberger P, Lang S, Jochum S, Zeidler R (2011) Tumour exosomes inhibit binding of tumour-reactive antibodies to tumour cells and reduce ADCC. Cancer Immunol Immunother 60(5):639–648
125. Chen WX, Liu XM, Lv MM, Chen L, Zhao JH, Zhong SL, Ji MH, Hu Q, Luo Z, Wu JZ, Tang JH (2014) Exosomes from drug-resistant breast cancer cells transmit chemoresistance by a horizontal transfer of microRNAs. PLoS One 9:e95240
126. Ji R, Zhang B, Zhang X, Xue J, Yuan X, Yan Y, Wang M, Zhu W, Qian H, Xu W (2015) Exosomes derived from human mesenchymal stem cells confer drug resistance in gastric cancer. Cell Cycle 14:2473–2483
127. Taylor DD, Gercel-Taylor C (2008) MicroRNA signatures of tumor-derived exosomes as diagnostic biomarkers of ovarian cancer. Gynecol Oncol 110(1):13–21
128. Gallo A, Tandon M, Alevizos I, Illei GG (2012) The majority of microRNAs detectable in serum and saliva is concentrated in exosomes. PLoS One 7(3):e30679
129. Wang W, Chen Y (2014) Circulating miRNAs in cancer: from detection to therapy. J Hematol Oncol 7(1):86
130. Skog J, Würdinger T, van Rijn S, Meijer DH, Gainche L, Sena-Esteves M, Curry WT Jr, Carter BS, Krichevsky AM, Breakefield XO (2008) Glioblastoma microvesicles transport RNA and proteins that promote tumour growth and provide diagnostic biomarkers. Nat Cell Biol 10(12):1470–1476
131. Rabinowits G, Gercel Taylor C, Day JM, Taylor DD, Kloecker GH (2009) Exosomal microRNA: a diagnostic marker for lung cancer. Clin Lung Cancer 10(1):42–46
132. Lau C, Kim Y, Chia D, Spielmann N, Eibl G, Elashoff D, Wei F, Lin YL, Moro A, Grogan T, Chiang S, Feinstein E, Schafer C, Farrell J, Wong DT (2013) Role of pancreatic cancer-derived exosomes in salivary biomarker development. J Biol Chem 288(37):26888–26897
133. Nilsson J, Skog J, Nordstrand A, Baranov V, Mincheva-Nilsson L, Breakefield XO, Widmark A (2009) Prostate cancer-derived urine exosomes: a novel approach to biomarkers for prostate cancer. Br J Cancer 100(10):1603–1607
134. Corcoran C, Friel AM, Duffy MJ, Crown J, O'Driscoll L (2011) Intracellular and extracellular microRNAs in breast cancer. Clin Chem 57(1):18–32
135. Tanaka Y, Kamohara H, Kinoshita K, Kurashige J, Ishimoto T, Iwatsuki M, Watanabe M, Baba H (2013) Clinical impact of serum exosomal microRNA-21 as a clinical biomarker in human esophageal squamous cell carcinoma. Cancer 119(6):1159–1167

136. Arscott WT, Camphausen KA (2011) Exosome characterization from ascitic fluid holds promise for identifying markers of colorectal cancer. Biomark Med 5:821–822
137. Silva J, Garcia V, Rodriguez M, Compte M, Cisneros E, Veguillas P, Garcia JM, Dominguez G, Campos-Martin Y, Cuevas J, Peña C, Herrera M, Diaz R, Mohammed N, Bonilla F (2012) Analysis of exosome release and its prognostic value in human colorectal cancer. Genes Chromosomes Cancer 51:409–418
138. Madhavan B, Yue S, Galli U, Rana S, Gross W, Müller M, Giese NA, Kalthoff H, Becker T, Büchler MW, Zöller M (2015) Combined evaluation of a panel of protein and miRNA serum exosome biomarkers for pancreatic cancer diagnosis increases sensitivity and specificity. Int J Cancer 36:2616–2627
139. Lazar I, Clement E, Ducoux-Petit M, Denat L, Soldan V, Dauvillier S, Balor S, Burlet-Schiltz O, Larue L, Muller C, Nieto L (2015) Proteome characterization of melanoma exosomes reveals a specific signature for metastatic cell lines. Pigment Cell Melanoma Res 28:464–475
140. Alegre E, Sammamed M, Fernandez-Landazuri S, Zubiri L, Gonzalez A (2015) Circulating biomarkers in malignant melanoma. Adv Clin Chem 69:47–89
141. Chiam K, Wang T, Watson DI, Mayne GC, Irvine TS, Bright T, Smith L, White IA, Bowen JM, Keefe D, Thompson SK, Jones ME, Hussey DJ (2015) Circulating serum exosomal miRNAs as potential biomarkers for esophageal adenocarcinoma. J Gastrointest Surg 19:1208–1215
142. Zhou X, Zhu W, Li H, Wen W, Cheng W, Wang F, Wu Y, Qi L, Fan Y, Chen Y, Ding Y, Xu J, Qian J, Huang Z, Wang T, Zhu D, Shu Y, Liu P (2015) Diagnostic value of a plasma microRNA signature in gastric cancer: a microRNA expression analysis. Sci Rep 5:11251
143. Dutta S, Reamtong O, Pangvongsa W, Kitdumrongthum S, Janpipatkul K, Sangvanich P, Piyachaturawat P, Chairoungdua A (2015) Proteomics profiling of cholangiocarcinoma exosomes: a potential role of oncogenic protein transferring in cancer progression. Biochim Biophys Acta 1852:1989–1999
144. Gumireddy K, Li A, Chang DH, Liu Q, Kossenkov AV, Yan J, Korst RJ, Nam BT, Xu H, Zhang L, Ganepola GA, Showe LC, Huang Q (2015) AKAP4 is a circulating biomarker for non-small cell lung cancer. Oncotarget 6:17637–17647
145. Muller L, Muller-Haegele S, Mitsuhashi M, Gooding W, Okada H, Whiteside TL (2015) Exosomes isolated from plasma of glioma patients enrolled in a vaccination trial reflect antitumor immune activity and might predict survival. Oncoimmunology 4:e1008347
146. Melo SA, Luecke LB, Kahlert C, Fernandez AF, Gammon ST, Kaye J, LeBleu VS, Mittendorf EA, Weitz J, Rahbari N, Reissfelder C, Pilarsky C, Fraga MF, Piwnica-Worms D, Kalluri R (2015) Glypican-1 identifies cancer exosomes and detects early pancreatic cancer. Nature 523:177–182
147. Kogure T, Yan IK, Lin WL, Patel T (2013) Extracellular vesicle-mediated transfer of a novel long noncoding RNA TUC339: a mechanism of intercellular signaling in human hepatocellular cancer. Genes Cancer 4(7–8):261–272
148. Takahashi K, Yan IK, Kogure T, Haga H, Patel T (2014) Extracellular vesicle-mediated transfer of long non-coding RNA ROR modulates chemosensitivity in human hepatocellular cancer. FEBS Open Bio 4:458–467
149. Li Q, Shao Y, Zhang X, Zheng T, Miao M, Qin L, Wang B, Ye G, Xiao B, Guo J (2015) Plasma long noncoding RNA protected by exosomes as a potential stable biomarker for gastric cancer. Tumour Biol 36(3):2007–2012
150. Zhang Y, Liu D, Chen X, Li J, Li L, Bian Z, Sun F, Lu J, Yin Y, Cai X, Sun Q, Wang K, Ba Y, Wang Q, Wang D, Yang J, Liu P, Xu T, Yan Q, Zhang J, Zen K, Zhang CY (2010) Secreted monocytic miR-150 enhances targeted endothelial cell migration. Mol Cell 39:133–144
151. Bryniarski K, Ptak W, Jayakumar A, Püllmann K, Caplan MJ, Chairoungdua A, Lu J, Adams BD, Sikora E, Nazimek K, Marquez S, Kleinstein SH, Sangwung P, Iwakiri Y, Delgato E, Redegeld F, Blokhuis BR, Wojcikowski J, Daniel AW, Groot Kormelink T, Askenase PW (2013) Antigen-specific, antibody-coated, exosome-like nanovesicles deliver suppressor T-cell microRNA-150 to effector T cells to inhibit contact sensitivity. J Allergy Clin Immunol 132:170–181

152. Møller HG, Rasmussen AP, Andersen HH, Johnsen KB, Henriksen M, Duroux M (2013) A systematic review of microRNA in glioblastoma multiforme: micro-modulators in the mesenchymal mode of migration and invasion. Mol Neurobiol 47:131–144
153. Henriksen M, Johnsen KB, Andersen AP, Pilgaard L, Duroux M (2014) MicroRNA expression signatures determine prognosis and survival in glioblastoma multiforme—a systematic overview. Mol Neurobiol 50(3):896–913
154. Xin H, Li Y, Buller B, Katakowski M, Zhang Y, Wang X, Shang X, Zhang ZG, Chopp M (2012) Exosome-mediated transfer of miR-133b from multipotent mesenchymal stromal cells to neural cells contributes to neurite outgrowth. Stem Cells 30:1556–1564
155. Munoz JL, Bliss SA, Greco SJ, Ramkissoon SH, Ligon KL, Rameshwar P (2013) Delivery of functional anti-miR-9 by mesenchymal stem cell-derived exosomes to glioblastoma multiforme cells conferred chemosensitivity. Mol Ther Nucleic Acids 2:e126
156. Zitvogel L, Regnault A, Lozier A, Wolfers J, Flament C, Tenza D, Ricciardi-Castagnoli P, Raposo G, Amigorena S (1998) Eradication of established murine tumors using a novel cell-free vaccine: dendritic cell-derived exosomes. Nat Med 4(5):594–600
157. Yao Y, Chen L, Wei W, Deng X, Ma L, Hao S (2013) Tumor cell-derived exosome-targeted dendritic cells stimulate stronger CD8+ CTL responses and antitumor immunities. Biochem Biophys Res Commun 436:60–65
158. Tan A, De La Pena H, Seifalian AM (2010) The application of exosomes as a nanoscale cancer vaccine. Int J Nanomedicine 5:889–900
159. Escudier B, Dorval T, Chaput N, André F, Caby MP, Novault S, Flament C, Leboulaire C, Borg C, Amigorena S, Boccaccio C, Bonnerot C, Dhellin O, Movassagh M, Piperno S, Robert C, Serra V, Valente N, Le Pecq JB, Spatz A, Lantz O, Tursz T, Angevin E, Zitvogel L (2005) Vaccination of metastatic melanoma patients with autologous dendritic cell (DC) derived exosomes: results of the first phase I clinical trial. J Transl Med 3:10
160. Morse MA, Garst J, Osada T, Khan S, Hobeika A, Clay TM, Valente N, Shreeniwas R, Sutton MA, Delcayre A, Hsu DH, Le Pecq JB, Lyerly HK (2005) A phase I study of dexosome immunotherapy in patients with advanced non-small cell lung cancer. J Transl Med 3:9
161. Viaud S, Théry C, Ploix S, Tursz T, Lapierre V, Lantz O, Zitvogel L, Chaput N (2010) Dendritic cell-derived exosomes for cancer immunotherapy: what's next? Cancer Res 70:1281–1285
162. Rountree RB, Mandl SJ, Nachtwey JM, Dalpozzo K, Do L, Lombardo JR, Schoonmaker PL, Brinkmann K, Dirmeier U, Laus R, Delcayre A (2011) Exosome targeting of tumor antigens expressed by cancer vaccines can improve antigen immunogenicity and therapeutic efficacy. Cancer Res 71:5235–5244
163. Bu N, Wu H, Sun B, Zhang G, Zhan S, Zhang R, Zhou L (2011) Exosome loaded dendritic cells elicit tumor-specific CD8+ cytotoxic T cells in patients with glioma. J Neurooncol 104:659–667
164. Gehrmann U, Hiltbrunner S, Georgoudaki AM, Karlsson MC, Naslund TI, Gabrielsson S (2013) Synergistic induction of adaptive antitumor immunity by codelivery of antigen with alpha-galactosylceramide on exosomes. Cancer Res 73:3865–3876
165. Lee EY, Park KS, Yoon YJ, Lee J, Moon HG, Jang SC, Choi KH, Kim YK, Gho YS (2012) Therapeutic effects of autologous tumor-derived nanovesicles on melanoma growth and metastasis. PLoS One 7:e33330
166. Marleau AM, Chen CS, Joyce JA, Tullis RH (2012) Exosome removal as a therapeutic adjuvant in cancer. J Transl Med 10:134
167. Chalmin F, Ladoire S, Mignot G, Vincent J, Bruchard M, Remy-Martin JP, Boireau W, Rouleau A, Simon B, Lanneau D, De Thonel A, Multhoff G, Hamman A, Martin F, Chauffert B, Solary E, Zitvogel L, Garrido C, Ryffel B, Borg C, Apetoh L, Rébé C, Ghiringhelli F (2010) Membrane associated Hsp72 from tumor-derived exosomes mediates STAT3-dependent immunosuppressive function of mouse and human myeloid derived suppressor cells. J Clin Invest 120:457–471
168. Phuyal S, Hessvik NP, Skotland T, Sandvig K, Llorente A (2014) Regulation of exosome release by glycosphingolipids and flotillins. FEBS J 281:2214–2227

169. Trajkovic K, Hsu C, Chiantia S, Rajendran L, Wenzel D, Wieland F, Schwille P, Brügger B, Simons M (2008) Ceramide triggers budding of exosome vesicles into multivesicular endosomes. Science 319:1244–1247
170. Sioud M (2015) RNA interference: mechanisms, technical challenges, and therapeutic opportunities. Methods Mol Biol 1218:1–15
171. Vader P, Breakefield XO, Wood MJ (2014) Extracellular vesicles: emerging targets for cancer therapy. Trends Mol Med 20:385–393
172. Lima LG, Chammas R, Monteiro RQ, Moreira ME, Barcinski MA (2009) Tumor-derived microvesicles modulate the establishment of metastatic melanoma in a phosphatidylserine-dependent manner. Cancer Lett 283:168–175
173. van den Boorn JG, Dassler J, Coch C, Schlee M, Hartmann G (2013) Exosomes as nucleic acid nanocarriers. Adv Drug Deliv Rev 65(3):331–335
174. Hood JL, Scott MJ, Wickline SA (2013) Maximizing exosome colloidal stability following electroporation. Anal Biochem 448C:41–49
175. Koppers-Lalic D, Hogenboom MM, Middeldorp JM, Pegtel DM (2013) Virus-modified exosomes for targeted RNA delivery; a new approach in nanomedicine. Adv Drug Deliv Rev 65:348–356
176. Record M, Subra C, Silvente-Poirot S, Poirot M (2011) Exosomes as intercellular signalosomes and pharmacological effectors. Biochem Pharmacol 81:1171–1182
177. Subra C, Laulagnier K, Perret B, Record M (2007) Exosome lipidomics unravels lipid sorting at the level of multivesicular bodies. Biochimie 89:205–212
178. Zhuang X, Xiang X, Grizzle W, Sun D, Zhang S, Axtell RC, Ju S, Mu J, Zhang L, Steinman L, Miller D, Zhang HG (2011) Treatment of brain inflammatory diseases by delivering exosome encapsulated anti-inflammatory drugs from the nasal region to the brain. Mol Ther 19:1769–1779
179. Wahlgren J, De L, Karlson T, Brisslert M, Vaziri Sani F, Telemo E, Sunnerhagen P, Valadi H (2012) Plasma exosomes can deliver exogenous short interfering RNA to monocytes and lymphocytes. Nucleic Acids Res 40:130
180. Shtam TA, Kovalev RA, Varfolomeeva EY, Makarov EM, Kil YV, Filatov MV (2013) Exosomes are natural carriers of exogenous siRNA to human cells in vitro. Cell Commun Signal 11:88
181. Alvarez-Erviti L, Seow Y, Yin H, Betts C, Lakhal S, Wood MJA (2011) Delivery of siRNA to the mouse brain by systemic injection of targeted exosomes. Nat Biotechnol 29:341–345
182. Lin Q, Chen J, Zhang Z, Zheng G (2014) Lipid-based nanoparticles in the systemic delivery of siRNA. Nanomedicine (Lond) 9:105–120
183. Ozpolat B, Sood AK, Lopez-Berestein G (2013) Liposomal siRNA nanocarriers for cancer therapy. Adv Drug Deliv Rev 66:110–116
184. Yin W, Ouyang S, Li Y, Xiao B, Yang H (2013) Immature dendritic cell-derived exosomes: a promise subcellular vaccine for autoimmunity. Inflammation 36:232–240
185. Lee JK, Park SR, Jung BK, Jeon YK, Lee YS, Kim MK, Kim YG, Jang JY, Kim CW (2013) Exosomes derived from mesenchymal stem cells suppress angiogenesis by down-regulating VEGF expression in breast cancer cells. PLoS One 8(12):e84256
186. Tian Y, Li S, Song J, Ji T, Zhu M, Anderson GJ, Wei J, Nie G (2014) A doxorubicin delivery platform using engineered natural membrane vesicle exosomes for targeted tumor therapy. Biomaterials 35(7):2383–2390
187. Jang SC, Kim OY, Yoon CM, Choi DS, Roh TY, Park J, Nilsson J, Lötvall J, Kim YK, Gho YS (2013) Bioinspired exosome-mimetic nanovesicles for targeted delivery of chemotherapeutics to malignant tumors. ACS Nano 7:7678–7710
188. Tacar O, Sriamornsak P, Dass CR (2013) Doxorubicin: an update on anticancer molecular action, toxicity and novel drug delivery systems. J Pharm Pharmacol 65:157–170
189. Blaskovich MA, Sun J, Cantor A, Turkson J, Jove R, Sebti SM (2003) Discovery of JSI-124 (cucurbitacin I), a selective Janus kinase/signal transducer and activator of transcription 3 signaling pathway inhibitor with potent antitumor activity against human and murine cancer cells in mice. Cancer Res 63:1270–1279

190. Sun D, Zhuang X, Xiang X, Liu Y, Zhang S, Liu C et al (2010) A novel nanoparticle drug delivery system: the anti-inflammatory activity of curcumin is enhanced when encapsulated in exosomes. Mol Ther 18:1606–1614
191. Mizrak A, Bolukbasi MF, Ozdener GB, Brenner GJ, Madlener S, Erkan EP, Ströbel T, Breakefield XO, Saydam O (2013) Genetically engineered microvesicles carrying suicide mRNA/protein inhibit schwannoma tumor growth. Mol Ther 21:101–108
192. Hamstra DA, Lee KC, Tychewicz JM, Schepkin VD, Moffat BA, Chen M, Dornfeld KJ, Lawrence TS, Chenevert TL, Ross BD, Gelovani JT, Rehemtulla A (2004) The use of 19F spectroscopy and diffusion-weighted MRI to evaluate differences in gene-dependent enzyme prodrug therapies. Mol Ther 10:916–928
193. Blanc L, De Gassart A, Géminard C, Bette-Bobillo P, Vidal M (2005) Exosome release by reticulocytes—an integral part of the red blood cell differentiation system. Blood Cells Mol Dis 35:21–26
194. Johnstone RM, Bianchini A, Teng K (1989) Reticulocyte maturation and exosome release: transferrin receptor containing exosomes shows multiple plasma membrane functions. Blood 74:1844–1851
195. Qi H, Liu C, Long L, Ren Y, Zhang S, Chang X, Qian X, Jia H, Zhao J, Sun J, Hou X, Yuan X, Kang C (2016) Blood exosomes endowed with magnetic and targeting properties for cancer therapy. ACS Nano 10(3):3323–3333
196. Ge J, Hu Y, Biasini M, Beyermann WP, Yin Y (2007) Superparamagnetic magnetite colloidal nanocrystal clusters. Angew Chem Int Ed 46:4342–4345
197. ClinicalTrials.gov Identifier: NCT01159288
198. Dai S, Wei D, Wu Z, Zhou X, Wei X, Huang H, Li G (2008) Phase I clinical trial of autologous ascites-derived exosomes combined with GM-CSF for colorectal cancer. Mol Ther 16:782–790
199. ClinicalTrials.gov Identifier: NCT01550523
200. ClinicalTrials.gov Identifier: NCT01668849
201. ClinicalTrials.gov Identifier: NCT01294072

Targeting of EGFR Induced Signaling Network in Hepatocellular Carcinoma

Aliye Aras Perk, Riffat Batool, Sobia Kanwal, Edyta Pawlak-Adamska, Oskar Nowak, Muhammad Sheeraz Ahmad, Qaisar Mansoor, Mirna Azalea Romero, Madeeha Awan, Ammad Ahmad Farooqi, and Muhammad Ismail

Abstract Hepatocellular carcinoma is a multifaceted and genomically complex disease and rapidly emerging experimental evidence has started to shed light on wide ranging molecular mechanisms which underlie its development and progression. It is now known that Overexpression of oncogenes, inactivation of tumor suppressor genes, dysregulation of spatio-temporally controlled intracellular signaling cascades, genetic/epigenetic mutations, loss of apoptosis and intra-tumor

A.A. Perk
Botany Department, Faculty of Science, İstanbul University,
Suleymaniye, Istanbul 34460, Turkey

R. Batool
Department of Plant Sciences, Quaid e Azam University, Islamabad, Pakistan

S. Kanwal
Department of Zoology, PMAS-Arid Agriculture University, Rawalpindi, Pakistan

E. Pawlak-Adamska
Department of Experimental Therapy, Hirszfeld Institute of Immunology and Experimental Therapy, Polish Academy of Sciences, R. Weigl 12, Wroclaw 53-114, Poland

O. Nowak
Department of Human Evolutionary Biology, Institute of Anthropology, Adam Mickiewicz University, Umultowska 89, Poznan 61-614, Poland

M.S. Ahmad
Department of Biochemistry, PMAS-Arid Agriculture University, Rawalpindi, Pakistan

Q. Mansoor • A.A. Farooqi (✉) • M. Ismail
Institute of Biomedical and Genetic Engineering (IBGE),
G-9/1 Mauve Area, Islamabad, Pakistan
e-mail: ammadfarooqi@rlmclahore.com

M.A. Romero (✉)
Laboratorio de Investigación Clínica, Unidad Académica de Medicina, Universidad Autónoma de Guerrero, Av. Solidaridad S/N Col. Hornos Insurgentes, Acapulco, Guerrero, Mexico
e-mail: sonambul@yahoo.com.mx

M. Awan
UVAS, Lahore, Pakistan

A.A. Farooqi, M. Ismail (eds.), *Molecular Oncology: Underlying Mechanisms and Translational Advancements*, DOI 10.1007/978-3-319-53082-6_7

heterogeneity contribute significantly. Research over the years has gradually revealed intricate role of intracellular signaling cascades both in growth, development and cancer. Misrepresentation of EGFR induced intracellular signaling has been shown to fuel cancer development and progression. We partition this review into how EGFR modulates protein machinery in hepatocellular carcinoma and also summarize most recent updates on preclinical and clinical trials. Better and deeper understanding of the molecular mechanisms of HCC will be helpful in getting a step closer to individualized medicine.

Keywords Hepatocellular carcinoma • EGFR • MAPK • Lapatinib • Cetuximab • Signaling

Introduction

Landmark scientific report of Stanley Cohen in 1962 provided first clue of involvement of a salivary gland protein in modulation of tooth eruption and eye-lid opening in newborn mice. Subsequent studies revealed that this protein considerably enhanced proliferation potential of epithelial cells and was named epidermal growth factor (EGF) [1, 2]. Graham Carpenter made another breakthrough and identified the receptor for EGF. Research group suggested that EGFR was a 170 kDa membrane protein that transduced the signals intracellularly. Isolation, cloning and characterization of EGFR were conducted in 1984 from cancer cells and normal placental cells. EGFR (HER1 or ERBB1) is a member of ERBB family of cell-surface receptor tyrosine kinases. Interaction of EGF and EGFR induced homodimerization or heterodimerization of the receptor with other ERBB members. Ligand-receptor interaction induced autophosphorylation and activation of hierarchically organized network of proteins such as RAS–RAF–MEK–ERK– MAPK and PI3K–AKT–mTOR that fueled cancer development and progression [1, 2]. Shown in Fig. 1.

This chapter provides an overview of the most recent updates on EGF/EGFR signaling axis, how different proteins interact with this axis, how microRNAs tactfully modulate EGF/EGFR signaling. Last section deal with therapeutic strategies which are currently being used for efficient targeting of EGFR induced signaling in xenografted mice. After an overview of EGFR induced signaling, we focus our discussion on how it interacts with different oncogenic and tumor suppressor proteins.

Interaction of EGFR with Different Proteins

GOLM1: GOLPH2, a Golgi-related protein, encoded by GOLM1 was noted to be considerably upregulated in extra-hepatically metastasized HCC. Co-immunoprecipitation assay revealed that both endogenous and exogenous GOLM1 interacted with EGFR in

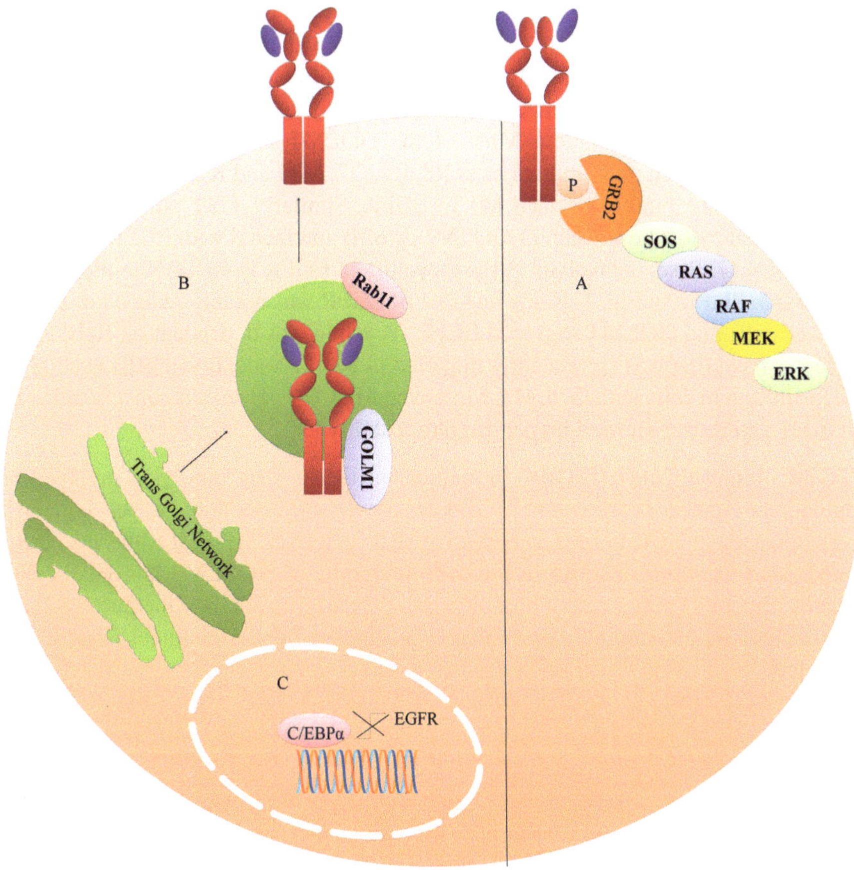

Fig. 1 Shows (**a**) EGF mediated transduction of signals intracellularly through EGFR. (**b**) Recycling of EGFR back to cell surface. (**c**) C/EBPα transcriptionally downregulated EGFR

PLC, MHCC-97H and Hep3B cells [3]. EGF-induced activation of both AKT and S6K were dramatically reduced in GOLM1 silenced cells, which was rescued by reconstitution of cells with shRNA-resistant GOLM1. EGF treatment promoted accumulation of both exogenous and endogenous GOLM1 within cytosol and formation of Rab5-positive vesicles. Results obtained from live-cell imaging also showed that interaction internalized EGFR dynamically interacted with one or more Rab5-positive GOLM1. Interference strategies indicated that constitutive endocytosis of EGFR was not impaired in GOLM1 silenced cells. However, notably enhanced EGFR degradation and a reduction in recycling rate of internalized EGFR to cell surface were noted in GOLM1 silenced cells [3]. Confocal co-localization analysis demonstrated that EGFR co-existed with Rab11^{+} recycling vesicles in EGF stimulated, shNT (short-hairpin non-target) treated MHCC-97H cells for 15 min but co-localized to a lesser extent with LAMP1 and LAMP2 (lysosome degradation markers) as compared to

MHCC-97H GOLM1 silenced cells. To further verify the role of GOLM1 and EGFR interaction in metastasis of HCC, researchers mapped the regions of EGFR and GOLM1 involved in structural interaction. A series of constructs encoding GOLM1 deletion mutants fused with FLAG tags were transfected into PLC and 293T cells following immunoprecipitation. Most of the GOLM1 fragments interacted with EGFR [3]. Moreover, point mutations at R8, R9, G7, M11 and K12 of GOLM1 notably abrogated the binding of GOLM1 to EGFR. Similarly, GST pull-down assays indicated that cytosolic domain of GOLM1 directly interacted with EGFR. Rab11, a well-known GTPase, is involved in the recycling of EGFR from TGN to the plasma membrane. Shown in Fig. 1. Recycling rate of EGFR was notably reduced in Rab11 silenced cells and GOLM1-triggered EGFR recycling was dependent on Rab11 [3]. Receptor recycling was significantly impaired in Rab11 knockdown cells even after reconstitution of cells with GOLM1. Moreover, MHCC-97H cells reconstructed with GOLM1 and Rab11 showed higher migration ability [3].

ITGB4: Integrin beta4 (ITGB4), a member of the integrin family, is involved in regulation of cancer progression. ITGB4 has previously been noted to be frequently overexpressed in HCC tissues and invasive HCC cell lines [4]. EGFR has also been noted to co-exist with ITGB4 in the cell membrane of HCCLM3 and HLF cells. Results obtained from western blot clearly indicated that ITGB4- mediated activation of AKT in anchorage independence was inhibited upon treatment with EGFR inhibitors [4]. ITGB4 and EGFR worked synchronously for activation of AKT by FAK in HCC cells. Gene silencing of either AKT1 or ITGB4 significantly inhibited HCC lung metastases however combinatorial gene silencing of AKT1 and ITGB4 did not enhance tumor inhibitory effects [4].

C/EBPα: CCAAT/enhancer-binding protein-α (C/EBPα) is involved in transcriptional regulation of different genes. C/EBPα binding site/s were identified within promoter region of β-catenin and EGFR as evidenced by ChIP-Seq analysis [5]. Shown in Fig. 1. Cells transfected with C/EBPα-short-activating RNAs (saRNA) showed strongly reduced levels of EGFR, p-EGFR, β-catenin and ADAM17. Moreover, both tumor size and intrahepatic metastasis were considerably reduced in mice intravenously injected with C/EBPα-saRNA [5].

Hepatocyte Growth Factor (HGF) transduced the signals intracellularly through c-Met, a high affinity receptor tyrosine kinase. It has been reported that c-Met inhibition induced an upregulation of EGFR (ErbB1) and ErbB3 in MHCC97-H cells [6]. PHA665752 effectively blocked phosphorylation of c-Met along with markedly reduced levels of phosphorylated Erk and Akt. However, ErbB3 expression was enhanced in the treated cancer cells. Cells combinatorially treated with TGF-α and PHA665752 revealed an active EGFR signaling cascade. p-EGFR, p-Akt, ErbB3 and p-Erk were notably enhanced in treated cancer cells. Gefitinib (EGFR inhibitor) decreased p-EGFR but did not exert inhibitory effects on p-Erk and p-Akt [6]. Data clearly suggested that cancer cells combinatorially treated with gefitinib and PHA665752 showed noteworthy inhibition of c-Met and EGFR signaling cascades.

Dynamin2: Dynamin2, a GTPase is involved in endocytosis of receptor tyrosine kinases (RTKs). Cell surface expression of EGFR was considerably higher in

Dynamin inhibitor treated HCC cells. In Huh7 and HCCLM3 cells, level of phosphorylated ERK1/2 was noted to be increased significantly after treatment with Dynamin inhibitor [7]. Astonishingly, there was a higher nuclear accumulation of p-ERK1/2 and activity persisted for a longer time period even after withdrawal of Dynamin inhibitor [7].

PTPRS: Protein tyrosine phosphatase receptor S (PTPRS), a tumor suppressor was found to be frequently down-regulated in HCC. Levels of phosphorylated EGFR and RET were considerably enhanced in SMMC7721 cells which had lower expression of PTPRS. However, levels of phosphorylated RET and EGFR were reduced in PTPRS overexpressing HCCLM3 cells. Phosphorylation levels of three amino acid residues (Tyr1068, Tyr 992 and Tyr1045) in EGFR were markedly reduced in PTPRS overexpressing cells [8].

Enoyl-coenzyme A hydratase short chain 1 (ECHS1): Enoyl-coenzyme A hydratase short chain 1 (ECHS1) is reportedly involved in tumor development. Phosphorylated EGFR, ERK1/2 (Thr202/Tyr204) and p-AKT were markedly decreased in ECHS1 silenced Hep and HuH7 cells [9].

GALNT1

N-acetylgalactosaminyltransferase 1 (GALNT1), a family member of Golgi resident polypeptide *N*-acetylgalactosamine (GalNAc)-transferases (GALNT) reportedly involved in regulation of mucin-type O-glycosylation [10]. GALNT1 was found to be frequently over-expressed in HCC and metastatic tumor nodules were not noted in NOD/SCID mice injected with GALNT1 knockdown cells. GALNT1 Knockdown dramatically reduced EGF-induced migration and invasion in PLC5 and HA22T cells. EGF-induced EGFR activation was markedly reduced and EGFR degradation rate increased remarkably in GALNT1 silenced cells [10]. EGFR co-localized with EEA1 at 3 min in both HA22T and PLC5 cells. Additionally, EGFR co-localization with LAMP1 was notably increased at 30 min and 10 min in GALNT1 silenced HA22T and PLC5 cells. VVA Lectin (*Vicia villosa*) has a binding affinity for EGFR O-glycans, however the binding affinity was substantially reduced in GALNT1 silenced cells [10].

UNC50: UNC50 is a protein present in Golgi apparatus membrane and frequently upregulated in HCC.

EGFR is endosomally-internalized and recycled to surface of cells even in the absence of ligands [11]. Endosomally retained EGFR provided a clue of cell surface EGFR amounts. UNC50 was noted to increase EGFR recycling, which resultantly increased cell surface EGFR amounts [11].

HuR: HBV-encoded X protein (HBx) was involved in increasing the levels of HER2 protein by stabilization of HER2 mRNA in HCC cells. HuR, a ubiquitously expressed RNA-binding protein was also found to be upregulated in Hep3Bx cells.

There was a notable decrease in the levels of HER2, however EGFR levels remained unchanged in HuR silenced cells [12].

CKAP4: Cytoskeleton-associated membrane protein 4 (CKAP4) negatively regulated EGFR in HCC cells. CKAP4 considerably inhibited EGF induced activation of EGFR in SMMC-7721 cells. However, EGF mediated activation of EGFR was evident in CKAP4 silenced SMMC-7721 cells [13].

S100A11: S100 calcium binding protein A11 (S100A11) was notably upregulated in EGFRvIII expressing Huh7 cells. STAT3 was found to be functionally active in EGFRvIII expressing Huh7 cells and inhibition of STAT3 significantly reduced expression of S100A11 [14].

Interplay of EGFR Induced Signaling, miRNAs and Long Non-coding RNAs in HCC

EGR1, a family member of early growth response (EGR) transcription factors is reportedly involved in transcriptional regulation of a tumor suppressor miRNA-203a. Interestingly, apoptotic rate was remarkably enhanced in SMMC-7721/Hep3B cells that overexpressed miR-203a [15, 16]. miR-203a quantitatively controlled an oncogene, HOXD3. Both EGFR and p-AKT were noted to be upregulated in HOXD3 expressing HCC cells. However gene silencing of HOXD3 also reduced the levels of EGFR and p-AKT in HCC cells. SMMC-7721 cells transduced with miR-203a expressing lentiviral vectors were subcutaneously injected into posterior flanks of nude mice. Tumor growth was markedly reduced in xenografted mice [15, 16].

NF90, a double-stranded RNA binding protein, heterodimerically complexed with NF45 to negatively regulate processing of pri-miRNA. NF90–NF45 complex has also been reported to negatively regulate miR-7 biogenesis [17]. NF90-NF45 positively modulated EGFR–AKT signaling by inhibiting miR-7 biogenesis. Shown in Fig. 2. Knockdown of NF90 or NF45 drastically reduced EGFR levels in treated cancer cells. Furthermore, levels of both EGFR and phosphorylated AKT were reduced in miR-7 mimic transfected HCC cells [17].

LINC01225, a lncRNA was frequently overexpressed in HCC. Use of interference strategy against LINC01225 notably reduced proliferation potential of SMCC7721 and MHCC97H cells [15, 16]. There is a direct piece of evidence highlighting an association of LINC01225 and EGFR protein. EGFR protein was noted to be reduced in LINC01225 depleted HCC cells [15, 16].

Cytoplasmic polyadenylation element binding protein 3 (CPEB3) is quantitatively controlled by miR-107. Subcutaneous injection of CPEB3 siRNA transfected HepG2 cells into the flank of nude mice induced development of HCC [18]. Expectedly, significantly enhanced tumor weight and size were noted in CPEB3 siRNA groups. Mechanistically it was shown that miR-107 mediated downregulation of CPEB3 facilitated an increase in the levels of EGFR and phosphorylated AKT [18]. Shown in Fig. 2.

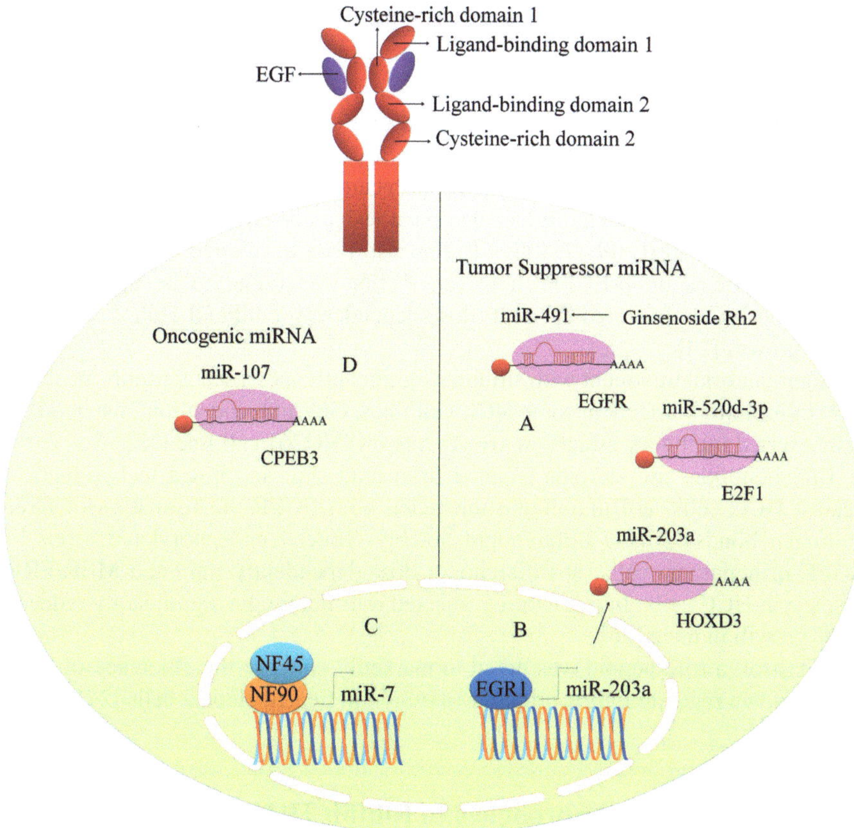

Fig. 2 Showing different structural components of EGFR. (**a**) miRNA mediated targeting of different genes. (**b**) EGR1 induced expression of miR-203a. miR-203a targeted HOXD3. (**c**) NF45 and NF90 induced downregulation of miR-7. (**d**) CPEB3 was targeted by miR-107

EGFR-AS1 located on chromosome 7 can undergo an oppositely directed transcription as lncRNA. EGFR-AS1 was upregulated in HCC tissues and correlated with poor prognosis. EGFR-AS1 and EGFR were noted to be considerably reduced in Growth hormone receptor (GHR)-siRNA-transfected cells. EGFR expression was remarkably reduced in EGFR-AS1 silenced cells [19].

Ginsenoside Rh2, a biologically active constituent isolated from red ginseng efficiently upregulated miR-491 in SMMC-7721 cells, which consequently inhibited EGFR mRNA level [20].

MiR-146a, a tumor suppressor miRNA is often downregulated in HCC and it has been shown that cells treated with miR-146a mimic demonstrated a higher apoptotic rate. Moreover, miR-146a mimic worked synergistically with cetuximab against HepG2, HepB3, and SNU449 cells [21].

Natural Products Mediated Targeting of EGFR

Actinidia chinensis root extract in combination with a prostaglandin E receptor 3 (EP3) antagonist considerably downregulated EGFR in HCC cells [22]. Wogonin, a flavonoid, isolated from Chinese herb, *Scutellaria baicalensis Georgi* had been shown to efficiently inhibit EGFR (Tyr845) phosphorylation in treated HCC cells [23].

Matrine, a sophora alkaloid has also been tested for efficacy and new matrine derivative, WM130 (C30N4H40SO5F) has also been developed. WM130 exerted inhibitory effects on p-EGFR, however, PTEN was found to be up-regulated. Intravenously administered WM130 dose-dependently inhibited Huh-7 xenograft tumor growth [24].

Combinatorial treatment with silibinin significantly increased gefitinib-mediated growth-inhibitory effects in some HCC cell lines. Gefitinib and silibinin synergistically exerted inhibitory effects on growth rate of SNU761 cell line [25].

Bufadienolides are steroids isolated from toad skin and noted to be effective against HCC cells. ψ-Bufarenogin interacted with EGFR via formation of three hydrogen bonds [26]. ψ-Bufarenogin notably reduced phosphorylated levels of EGFR in hepatoma cells. ψ-Bufarenogin dose-dependently inhibited MEK/ERK cascade in HCC cells. Intratumorally injected ψ-Bufarenogin significantly reduced HCC growth in mice [26].

Celastrol, a triterpenoid was noted to markedly enhance the efficiency of lapatinib to down regulate EGFR protein expression in treated HepG2 cells [27].

Nanotechnological Approaches to Inhibit HCC

Maternally expressed gene 3 (MEG3), a long non-coding RNA is a tumor suppressor gene. MS2 bacteriophage virus-like particles (VLPs) are biological agents which can carry RNA. However, because of their inability to pass through cell membrane, these molecules are cross-linked with different moieties to facilitate entry of the carriers into the cells [28]. In accordance with this approach, GE11 was used to crosslink VLPs to promote its entry into the cells. GE11 had the ability to interact with EGFR but did not trigger EGFR induced intracellular signaling in HCC cells. VLPs crosslinked with GE11 polypeptide were used to deliver MEG3 to EGFR overexpressing HCC cells. Tumor growth was significantly reduced in BALB/c nude mice treated with GE11-VLPs-MEG3 [28].

Microtubule destabilizing agents particularly, 2-methoxyestradiol (2ME) or combretastatin A4 (CA4) have shown remarkable efficacy against HCC. Interestingly encapsulation of these agents using poly(d,l-lactide-co-glycolide)-b-poly(ethylene glycol) (PLGA-b-PEG) further enhanced their killing activity [29]. Moreover, functionalization of these diblock co-polymeric coronas via surface modification using cetuximab, an anti-EGFR chimeric monoclonal antibody improved targeting of the encapsulated drugs [29].

Use of aptamer/s conjugation has been shown to facilitate the internalization of nanoparticles because of selective binding to specified receptors on cancer cells. A15, an RNA aptamer binds to CD133 and facilitates targeted and effective internalization of drug loaded nanoparticles. CL4, another RNA aptamer exclusively interacted with EGFR overexpressing cancer cells. Therefore researchers used poly(lactic-co-glycolic acid) nanoparticles for loading of salinomycin and later conjugated with both A15 and CL4 aptamers for efficient targeting of HCC cells [30].

Tyrphostins are protein tyrosine kinase inhibitors and reported to be effective against different cancers. Tyrphostin AG-1478 loaded in nanostructured lipid carriers showed remarkable activity against HCC cells [31].

Clinical Trials

Ganetespib (STA-9090), an Hsp90 inhibitor has been studied to effectively downregulate c-MET, VEGFR , HER2, EGFR, and different Hsp90 client proteins contributory in hepatocarcinogenesis. Phase I of ganetespib has recently been conducted and results revealed a manageable safety profile in patients with advanced HCC who had progressed on at least one line of systemically administered therapy [32]. Fifty-one patients were enrolled in a phase II study to evaluate efficacy and tolerability in this Asian cohort and results revealed that patients treated with erlotinib plus Bevacizumab showed modest activity and good tolerability [33].

Preclinical Studies

Lapatinib, an orally administered small-molecule significantly targeted EGFR and considerably reduced tumor growth in xenografted mice. Moreover, detailed mechanistic insights indicated that lapatinib induced autophagy in hepatoma cells as evidenced by increase in autophagy-related proteins and detection of autophagic LC3-II conversion [34].

EGFR variant III has been observed to impair sensitivity of HCC cells to chemotherapeutic drugs. Mechanistically it has been shown that EGFRvIII induced downregulation of miR-520d-3p (tumor suppressor miRNA) in EGFRvIII overexpressing cells. E2F1, a transcription factor was a direct target of miR-520d-3p and transfection of Huh7-EGFRvIII cells with miR-520d-3p mimic markedly reduced E2F1. Shown in Fig. 2. However, E2F1 levels were notably higher in Huh7-EGFRvIII cells. Thymidylate synthase (TS) gene expression was regulated by the E2F-1 and both worked synchronously to induce resistance against different therapeutics. CH12, a monoclonal antibody directed against EGFRvIII, worked synergistically with 5-FU and remarkably reduced tumor growth in mice xenografted with EGFRvIII^{+} HCC cells [35].

Interestingly, expression levels of HER3 and EGFR were considerably reduced in HCC cells combinatorially treated with Sorafenib and gefitinib [36].

LZ8, a medicinal peptide purified from the herb Lingzhi efficiently inhibited functionally active EGFR in HCC329 cancer cells [37].

Pseudomonas aeruginosa mannose-sensitive haemagglutinin (PA-MSHA) was found to be an effective anticancer agent. PA-MSHA had an affiliation for mannose oligosaccharides present on surface of cancer cells. PA-MSHA concentration-dependently inhibited NF-κβ expression and activity in treated cancer cells [38]. Despite the fact that basal levels of unphosphorylated and phosphorylated Iκβ were both significantly increased by PAMSHA, the rate of basally phosphorylated Iκβ to unphosphorylated Iκβ was much higher in PA-MSHA treated cells. After PA-MSHA treatment, the MHCC97L tumors and HepG2 tumors were significantly smaller as compared to control group and the lung metastasis was completely inhibited in PA-MSHA treated cells [38].

Conclusion

Rapidly emerging scientific information has deepened our understanding of the dysregulations of EGF/EGFR signaling axis. EGF mediated signaling cross-talks with a plethora of proteins to trigger HCC development and progression. Rapid breakthroughs made in the medicine field using different strategies to target EGFR in different cancers are encouraging. In accordance with this concept, development and approval of four EGFR inhibitors (gefitinib, cetuximab, erlotinib, and panitumumab) from FDA for clinical use in a very short time substantiates the role of EGFR as a molecular target involved in regulation of tumor cell behavior and treatment response.

Different combinatorial strategies are also being investigated for possible synergistic effects. Tyrosine Kinase inhibitors (TKIs) in combination with EGFR-targeted antibodies, dual EGFR-targeted antibodies and dual TKIs are being tested for efficacy and evaluation of off target effects. EGFR-targeted antibody mixtures are also being tested clinically for efficacy. Sym004 (mixture of two monoclonal antibodies) and MM-151 (mixture of three monoclonal antibodies) are currently in various phases of clinical trials. Studies have shown that TKI dual therapy significantly enhanced cell-surface appearance of EGFR however, antibody combination therapy reduced overcrowding of EGFRs on cell surface. Natural products mediated targeting of EGFR in different cancer cell lines and xenografted mice has also generated encouraging results. Different phytochemicals have been shown to either degrade EGFR or inhibit the activation of EGFR. miRNAs mediated quantitative regulation of EGFR is also an area of current research. EGFR targeting miRNAs have been identified and use of their mimics or upregulation of these miRNAs using different synthetic or natural agents will be helpful in improving the efficacy of therapeutics.

References

1. Chong CR, Jänne PA (2013) The quest to overcome resistance to EGFR-targeted therapies in cancer. Nat Med 19(11):1389–1400. doi:10.1038/nm.3388
2. Wheeler DL, Dunn EF, Harari PM (2010) Understanding resistance to EGFR inhibitors-impact on future treatment strategies. Nat Rev Clin Oncol 7(9):493–507. doi:10.1038/nrclinonc.2010.97
3. Ye QH, Zhu WW, Zhang JB, Qin Y, Lu M, Lin GL, Guo L, Zhang B, Lin ZH, Roessler S, Forgues M, Jia HL, Lu L, Zhang XF, Lian BF, Xie L, Dong QZ, Tang ZY, Wang XW, Qin LX (2016) GOLM1 modulates EGFR/RTK cell-surface recycling to drive hepatocellular carcinoma metastasis. Cancer Cell 30(3):444–458
4. Leng C, Zhang ZG, Chen WX, Luo HP, Song J, Dong W, Zhu XR, Chen XP, Liang HF, Zhang BX (2016) An integrin beta4-EGFR unit promotes hepatocellular carcinoma lung metastases by enhancing anchorage independence through activation of FAK-AKT pathway. Cancer Lett 376(1):188–196
5. Huan H, Wen X, Chen X, Wu L, Liu W, Habib NA, Bie P, Xia F (2016) C/EBPα short-activating RNA suppresses metastasis of hepatocellular carcinoma through inhibiting EGFR/β-catenin signaling mediated EMT. PLoS One 11(4):e0153117
6. Steinway SN, Dang H, You H, Rountree CB, Ding W (2015) The EGFR/ErbB3 pathway acts as a compensatory survival mechanism upon c-Met inhibition in human c-Met$^+$ hepatocellular carcinoma. PLoS One 10(5):e0128159
7. Gong C, Zhang J, Zhang L, Wang Y, Ma H, Wu W, Cui J, Wang Y, Ren Z (2015) Dynamin2 downregulation delays EGFR endocytic trafficking and promotes EGFR signaling and invasion in hepatocellular carcinoma. Am J Cancer Res 5(2):702–713
8. Wang ZC, Gao Q, Shi JY, Guo WJ, Yang LX, Liu XY, Liu LZ, Ma LJ, Duan M, Zhao YJ, Wu YN, Gao DM, Wang XY, Shi GM, Ding ZB, Ke AW, Tang QQ, Cao Y, Zhou J, Fan J (2015) Protein tyrosine phosphatase receptor S acts as a metastatic suppressor in hepatocellular carcinoma by control of epithermal growth factor receptor-induced epithelial-mesenchymal transition. Hepatology 62(4):1201–1214
9. Lin BY, Xiao CX, Zhao WX, Xiao L, Chen X, Li P, Wang XM (2015) Enoyl-coenzyme A hydratase short chain 1 silencing attenuates the proliferation of hepatocellular carcinoma by inhibiting epidermal growth factor signaling in vitro and in vivo. Mol Med Rep 12(1):1421–1428
10. Huang MJ, Hu RH, Chou CH, Hsu CL, Liu YW, Huang J, Hung JS, Lai IR, Juan HF, Yu SL, Wu YM, Huang MC (2015) Knockdown of GALNT1 suppresses malignant phenotype of hepatocellular carcinoma by suppressing EGFR signaling. Oncotarget. 6(8):5650–5665
11. Fang Z, Zhou L, Jiang S, Cao L, Yu L (2015) UNC50 prompts G1/S transition and proliferation in HCC by regulation of epidermal growth factor receptor trafficking. PLoS One 10(3):e0119338
12. Hung CM, Huang WC, Pan HL, Chien PH, Lin CW, Chen LC, Chien YF, Lin CC, Leow KH, Chen WS, Chen JY, Ho CY, Hou PS, Chen YJ (2014) Hepatitis B virus X upregulates HuR protein level to stabilize HER2 expression in hepatocellular carcinoma cells. Biomed Res Int 2014:827415
13. Li SX, Liu LJ, Dong LW, Shi HG, Pan YF, Tan YX, Zhang J, Zhang B, Ding ZW, Jiang TY, Hu HP, Wang HY (2014) CKAP4 inhibited growth and metastasis of hepatocellular carcinoma through regulating EGFR signaling. Tumour Biol 35(8):7999–8005
14. Luo X, Xie H, Long X, Zhou M, Xu Z, Shi B, Jiang H, Li Z (2013) EGFRvIII mediates hepatocellular carcinoma cell invasion by promoting S100 calcium binding protein A11 expression. PLoS One 8(12):e83332
15. Wang L, Sun H, Wang X, Hou N, Zhao L, Tong D, He K, Yang Y, Song T, Yang J, Huang C (2016) EGR1 mediates miR-203a suppress the hepatocellular carcinoma cells progression by targeting HOXD3 through EGFR signaling pathway. Oncotarget 7(29):45302–45316. doi:10.18632/oncotarget.9605

16. Wang X, Zhang W, Tang J, Huang R, Li J, Xu D, Xie Y, Jiang R, Deng L, Zhang X, Chai Y, Qin X, Sun B (2016) LINC01225 promotes occurrence and metastasis of hepatocellular carcinoma in an epidermal growth factor receptor-dependent pathway. Cell Death Dis 7:e2130. doi:10.1038/cddis.2016.26
17. Higuchi T, Todaka H, Sugiyama Y, Ono M, Tamaki N, Hatano E, Takezaki Y, Hanazaki K, Miwa T, Chin See LS, Morisawa K, Tsuda M, Taniguchi T, Sakamoto S (2016) Suppression of miR-7 biogenesis by NF90-NF45 controls cell proliferation in hepatocellular carcinoma. J Biol Chem 291(40):21074–21084. doi:10.1074/jbc.M116.748210
18. Zou CD, Zhao WM, Wang XN, Li Q, Huang H, Cheng WP, Jin JF, Zhang H, Wu MJ, Tai S, Zou CX, Gao X (2016) MicroRNA-107: a novel promoter of tumor progression that targets the CPEB3/EGFR axis in human hepatocellular carcinoma. Oncotarget. 7(1):266–278
19. Qi HL, Li CS, Qian CW, Xiao YS, Yuan YF, Liu QY, Liu ZS (2016) The long noncoding RNA, EGFR-AS1, a target of GHR, increases the expression of EGFR in hepatocellular carcinoma. Tumour Biol 37(1):1079–1089
20. Chen W, Qiu Y (2015) Ginsenoside Rh2 targets EGFR by up-regulation of miR-491 to enhance anti-tumor activity in hepatitis B virus-related hepatocellular carcinoma. Cell Biochem Biophys 72(2):325–331
21. Huang S, He R, Rong M, Dang Y, Chen G (2014) Synergistic effect of MiR-146a mimic and cetuximab on hepatocellular carcinoma cells. Biomed Res Int 2014:384121
22. Fang T, Hou J, He M, Wang L, Zheng M, Wang X, Xia J (2016) *Actinidia chinensis* Planch root extract (acRoots) inhibits hepatocellular carcinoma progression by inhibiting EP3 expression. Cell Biol Toxicol 32(6):499–511
23. Liu X, Tian S, Liu M, Jian L, Zhao L (2016) Wogonin inhibits the proliferation and invasion, and induces the apoptosis of HepG2 and Bel7402 HCC cells through NF-κB/Bcl-2, EGFR and EGFR downstream ERK/AKT signaling. Int J Mol Med 38(4):1250–1256
24. Qian L, Liu Y, Xu Y, Ji W, Wu Q, Liu Y, Gao Q, Su C (2015) Matrine derivative WM130 inhibits hepatocellular carcinoma by suppressing EGFR/ERK/MMP-2 and PTEN/AKT signaling pathways. Cancer Lett 368(1):126–134
25. Gu HR, Park SC, Choi SJ, Lee JC, Kim YC, Han CJ, Kim J, Yang KY, Kim YJ, Noh GY, No SH, Jeong JH (2015) Combined treatment with silibinin and either sorafenib or gefitinib enhances their growth-inhibiting effects in hepatocellular carcinoma cells. Clin Mol Hepatol 21(1):49–59
26. Ding J, Wen W, Xiang D, Yin P, Liu Y, Liu C, He G, Cheng Z, Yin J, Sheng C, Zhang W, Nan F, Ye W, Zhang X, Wang H (2015) ψ-Bufarenogin, a novel anti-tumor compound, suppresses liver cancer growth by inhibiting receptor tyrosine kinase-mediated signaling. Oncotarget 6(13):11627–11639
27. Yan YY, Guo Y, Zhang W, Ma CG, Zhang YX, Wang C, Wang HX (2014) Celastrol enhanced the anticancer effect of lapatinib in human hepatocellular carcinoma cells in vitro. J BUON 19(2):412–418
28. Chang L, Wang G, Jia T, Zhang L, Li Y, Han Y, Zhang K, Lin G, Zhang R, Li J, Wang L (2016) Armored long non-coding RNA MEG3 targeting EGFR based on recombinant MS2 bacteriophage virus-like particles against hepatocellular carcinoma. Oncotarget. 7(17):23988–24004
29. Poojari R, Kini S, Srivastava R, Panda D (2015) A chimeric cetuximab-functionalized corona as a potent delivery system for microtubule-destabilizing nanocomplexes to hepatocellular carcinoma cells: a focus on EGFR and tubulin intracellular dynamics. Mol Pharm 12(11):3908–3923
30. Jiang J, Chen H, Yu C, Zhang Y, Chen M, Tian S, Sun C (2015) The promotion of salinomycin delivery to hepatocellular carcinoma cells through EGFR and CD133 aptamers conjugation by PLGA nanoparticles. Nanomedicine (Lond) 10(12):1863–1879
31. Bondì ML, Azzolina A, Craparo EF, Botto C, Amore E, Giammona G, Cervello M (2014) Entrapment of an EGFR inhibitor into nanostructured lipid carriers (NLC) improves its antitumor activity against human hepatocarcinoma cells. J Nanobiotechnol 12:21. doi:10.1186/1477-3155-12-21
32. Goyal L, Wadlow RC, Blaszkowsky LS, Wolpin BM, Abrams TA, McCleary NJ, Sheehan S, Sundaram E, Karol MD, Chen J, Zhu AX (2015) A phase I and pharmacokinetic study of ganetespib (STA-9090) in advanced hepatocellular carcinoma. Invest New Drugs 33(1):128–137

33. Hsu CH, Kang YK, Yang TS, Shun CT, Shao YY, Su WC, Sandoval-Tan J, Chiou TJ, Jin K, Hsu C, Cheng AL (2013) Bevacizumab with erlotinib as first-line therapy in Asian patients with advanced hepatocellular carcinoma: a multicenter phase II study. Oncology 85(1):44–52
34. Chen YJ, Chi CW, Su WC, Huang HL (2014) Lapatinib induces autophagic cell death and inhibits growth of human hepatocellular carcinoma. Oncotarget. 5(13):4845–4854
35. Jiang H, Dong Q, Luo X, Shi B, Wang H, Gao H, Kong J, Zhang J, Li Z (2014) The monoclonal antibody CH12 augments 5-fluorouracil-induced growth suppression of hepatocellular carcinoma xenografts expressing epidermal growth factor receptor variant III. Cancer Lett 342(1):113–120
36. Blivet-Van Eggelpoël MJ, Chettouh H, Fartoux L, Aoudjehane L, Barbu V, Rey C, Priam S, Housset C, Rosmorduc O, Desbois-Mouthon C (2012) Epidermal growth factor receptor and HER-3 restrict cell response to sorafenib in hepatocellular carcinoma cells. J Hepatol 57(1):108–115
37. Wu JR, Hu CT, You RI, Ma PL, Pan SM, Lee MC, Wu WS (2015) Preclinical trials for prevention of tumor progression of hepatocellular carcinoma by LZ-8 targeting c-Met dependent and independent pathways. PLoS One 10(1):e0114495
38. Li T, Dong ZR, Guo ZY, Wang CH, Zhi XT, Zhou JW, Li DK, Chen ZT, Chen ZQ, Hu SY (2015) Mannose-mediated inhibitory effects of PA-MSHA on invasion and metastasis of hepatocellular carcinoma via EGFR/Akt/IκBβ/NF-κB pathway. Liver Int 35(4):1416–1429

Targeting of Heat Shock Proteins by Natural Products in Cancer

Evren Önay Uçar, Murat Pekmez, and Nazlı Arda

Abstract Initially discovered as a group of proteins showing significantly higher expression in response to heat stress, Heat shock proteins (HSPs) have gained considerable appreciation. Overwhelmingly increasing scientific evidence has highlighted the role of these proteins as molecular chaperones which trigger protein holding and folding thus facilitating freshly synthesized protein/s to achieve mature and biologically active conformation. It is becoming progressively more understandable that HSPs are involved in post-translational modification of proteins of signaling cascades, modulation of apoptosis related proteins, assembly and disassembly of transcriptional machinery. Recently emerging functional and structural data has provided new insights related to biochemical regulation of HSPs and the structural dynamics used by these proteins to act on a diverse client repertoire.

Different strategies are currently being tested to effectively inhibit/downregulate HSPs in cancer cells. Wide ranging natural products, particularly, antioxidant compounds, prevent HSP expression and induce apoptosis in tumor cells. Besides, these compounds help to reduce off-target effects of radio- or chemotherapies in many types of cancers.

Plethora of information has considerably improved our understanding of the molecular and cellular basis of HSP induced regulation of myriad of proteins and these insights may lead to the development of efficient therapeutic agents. The current chapter focuses on suppression of HSPs by using natural compounds in cancer cells.

Keywords Cancer • Heat shock proteins • Phytochemicals • Natural products • Therapeutic target • HSP

E. Önay Uçar (✉) • M. Pekmez • N. Arda
Department of Molecular Biology and Genetics, Faculty of Science, Istanbul University, Vezneciler, Istanbul 34134, Turkey
e-mail: evrenonay@istanbul.edu.tr

A.A. Farooqi, M. Ismail (eds.), *Molecular Oncology: Underlying Mechanisms and Translational Advancements*, DOI 10.1007/978-3-319-53082-6_8

Abbreviations

17-AAG	17-allylamino-17-demethoxygeldanamycin
7-KC	7-Ketocholestrol
ALS	Amyotrophic lateral sclerosis
CDDP	Cisplatin
CML	Chronic myelogenous leukemia
DMC	Demethoxycurcumin
Dox	Doxorubicin
EGCG	Epigallocatechin-3-gallate
HSF	Heat shock factor
HSP	Heat shock protein
HSR	Heat shock response
PEITC	Phenethyl isothiocyanate
siRNA	Small interfering RNA
TF	Theaflavin
TR	Thearubigin

Introduction

Cancer is a life threatening disease. In 2008 alone, 14 million people suffered from cancer and 8.2 million of them died [1]. Radiotherapy, chemotherapy and surgery are used for cancer therapy, but unfortunately these treatments combined or alone are not convincingly effective against different cancers. Therefore, cancer researchers have been trying to establish new therapeutic strategies for improving cancer treatments. Heat shock proteins (HSPs) or stress proteins are one of the new targets in cancer therapy.

Evolutionarily conserved HSPs are important components of the cytoplasmic network responsible for maintaining protein homeostasis in the cell. They are categorized in distinct families with respect to their molecular weights: HSP100, HSP90, HSP70, HSP60, HSP40 and small HSPs [2, 3]. These proteins can be expressed either constitutively or inducibly in the cells. When an organism is exposed to environmental or physiological stress such as heat, inflammation, oxidative stress, radiation, or ischemia etc., HSPs can be overexpressed in that organism to protect it from potential hazardous effects of stress. Overexpressed HSPs are involved in regulation of the refolding or degradation of damaged proteins in the stress-exposed cells [4, 5]. HSPs not only have chaperone functions, but also have a role in cell viability and death, cell division, metastasis, and inhibition of apoptosis [6, 7].

Rapidly accumulating experimental evidences have helped us in developing a better understanding of different roles of HSPs [8–10]. Many studies have presented the relation between frequently overexpressed HSPs and cancer types [11–15]. Therefore, these proteins are regarded as remarkable therapeutic targets for cancer therapy. In this respect, there have been a lot of studies examining the relationship between natural compounds and HSPs. A variety of natural compounds and plant extracts have been shown to downregulate HSP expression in some tumor types [16–22]. In this chapter, we review HSP suppression by several natural compounds from medicinal plants and discuss the role of these compounds in inhibiting/down-regulating HSPs as a strategy of cancer therapy.

HSP and Cancer

The intimate relationship between HSPs and cancer has been known for some years. Different HSPs are known to be altered in different cancer types [23].

Some HSPs are frequently overexpressed in cancer cells as compared to normal cells. It has been shown that some specific HSPs are augmented in different cancer types. For example: Hsp105 is increased in colon cancer [13], Hsp90 in lung cancer [12], Hsp70 in hepatocellular carcinoma [15], Hsp60 in colorectal carcinoma [11], and Hsp27 in gastric cancer [14]. Therefore these proteins have been accepted as "biomarkers" for some cancer types [9, 11, 13, 14, 24, 25]. Elevated HSPs in cancer cells are also proposed to be responsible for greater resistance to chemo/radio-therapy and poor prognosis [12, 26, 27]. Several studies have emphasized on a tight correlation between chemotherapy resistance and HSPs in tumor cells [8–10, 28–30].

Hsp105 has been shown to be significantly augmented in colorectal and pancreatic cancer patients [13, 31]. Overexpression of Hsp90 has been determined in bladder and hepatocellular carcinomas, breast and lung cancers, and in leukemia [12, 24, 32–34]. Hsp70 is found to be remarkably overexpressed in prostate cancer patients, when compared with normal individuals [35]. It is known that Hsp60 levels are increased in colorectal, lung, and prostate cancers [11, 36, 37]. Elevated Hsp27 has been determined in metastatic hepatocarcinoma and gliomas in comparison to non-metastatic tissue [38, 39]. Upregulated Hsp27 has been proposed as a potential diagnostic biomarker for breast cancer [25]. Correlative results were also found in other tumor types [38, 40–44].

Researchers have reported a remarkable association between overexpression of HSPs, drug resistance [45] and gradual loss of apoptosis [46]. A number of reports have demonstrated that overexpressed HSPs in cancer cells can promote drug resistance [9, 47–52], or the lethal effects of gamma radiation [29, 48, 53].

Yamamoto et al. [10] showed that Hsp27 and Hsp70 are linked with drug (Cisplatin, CDDP) resistance in ovarian cancer cell line. Supporting results were also provided in breast cancer. Several researchers have found a correlation between resistance against chemotherapeutic drugs (Doxorubicin) and increased Hsp27/Hsp70 expression [9, 28, 49, 54–56]. Overexpressed Hsp27 has been shown to decrease response of breast cancer cells to Herceptin [50]. Inhibition of Hsp70 has been shown to activate apoptosis in breast cancer [30]. There is a remarkable correlation between weak prognosis and upregulated Hsp70 in several cancer types [7, 15, 57]. Besides, Hsp27 expression is correlated with aggressiveness and progression of prostate cancer [25]. Overexpressed Hsp27 and Hsp70 have generated resistance against apoptosis and chemotherapy in human prostate cancer [8, 58]. Downregulation of Hsp72 decreased the resistance against radiotherapy or chemotherapy in a prostate cancer cell line (PC-3 cells) [59]. Additionally, some studies had indicated that suppression of Hsp70 in various tumor cells induced cell death [30]. It is well known that some upregulated HSPs hamper caspase-dependent apoptosis in cancer cells [60–63].

Consequently, better understanding of the structures and conformational changes of HSPs and modes of interaction with client proteins will be helpful in development of effective therapeutics against different HSPs.

In the upcoming section we comprehensively discuss about different natural products found to be effective against HSPs.

Targeting of HSPs by Plant Natural Compounds

Medicinal plants have been used in the treatment of different diseases since ancient times. Natural compounds, which are isolated from plants, serve as supplemental products in cancer therapy. Nowadays, researchers focus on the inhibition/reduction of HSPs in cancer cells as an important therapeutic target [64]. Therefore, some natural products, antisense oligonucleotides, siRNAs (small interfering RNAs) have been used to suppress HSPs in cancer therapy [65]. These HSP inhibitors have been tested either alone or with chemotherapeutic agents for treatment. A detailed list of plant extracts and natural compounds that alter HSP expression is given in Table 1 (revised from [23]). In this section, some natural compounds and plant extracts will be evaluated in detail as potential HSP inhibitors. The structures of these naturally occurring compounds are shown in Fig. 1.

Lycopene

Lycopene, a major carotenoid has been reported to exert wide ranging biological effects. It is present particularly in tomatoes (*Solanum lycopersicum*) and is known to have beneficial effects on human health, especially against cancer and cardiovascular diseases [98]. There are various beneficial effects of this molecule. It has an antioxidant activity [99], it was found to be effective against on inflammation and mutagenesis [100], it increases cell-cell communication [101], diminishes tumor cell proliferation [102] and enhances programmed cell death [99, 103]. It is suggested that the metabolites or oxidation products of lycopene are responsible for its activities [104–106]. Palozza and co-workers showed that lycopene prevents 7-ketocholesterol (7-KC)-mediated oxidative stress, cell cycle arrest and programmed cell death (apoptosis) in human macrophages [107]. 7-KC is one of the oxysterols which is also involved in the initiation and progression of atherosclerosis [108]. Palozza and co-workers evaluated whether lycopene could counteract the

Table 1 Altered HSPs by use of natural compound/plant extract in different cancer cells/types (revised from [23])

Plant extract/natural compound	Cancer cell/type	Findings	References
Betulin	Lung cancer cell line (A549)	Hsp90 ↓	[66]
Boesenbergin A	T4 Lymphoblastoid cells	Hsp70 ↓, apoptosis ↑	[21]
Cimicifuga foetida extract	Breast cancer cells (MCF-7 cell line)	Hsp27 ↓	[67]
Deguelin	Head and neck squamous cell carcinoma	Hsp90 ↓, apoptosis ↑, autophagy ↑	[68, 69]
	Non-small cell lung cancer cell line (NSCLC)	Hsp90 ↓, antiangiogenic activity ↑	[70]
Demethoxycurcumin (DMC)	Human prostate cancer cell lines	Hsp70 ↓, apoptosis ↑	[71]
Ellagitannin geraniin	HeLa and Jurkat cell lines	Hsp90 ↓	[72]
Epigallocatechin-3-gallate (EGCG)	Breast cancer cells (MCF-7 cell line)	Hsp70 ↓, Hsp90 ↓	[73]
	Urinary bladder carcinoma	Hsp27 ↓, apoptosis ↑	[74]
Gedunin	Breast cancer cell lines	Hsp90 ↓	[75]
Ginkgo biloba extract (EGb761)	Non-small cell lung cancer cell line (NSCLC)	Hsp27 ↓, migration ability ↓	[76]
Green tea extract	Human pancreatic ductal adenocarcinoma cells (HPAF-II)	Hsp27 ↓, Hsp75 ↓, Hsp90 ↓, apoptosis ↑	[77]
Kaempferol	Leukemia cell line (HL-60)	Hsp27 ↓, Hsp70↓	[78]
Lycopene	Acute monocytic leukemia cell	Hsp70 ↓, Hsp90 ↓	[79]
Phenethyl isothiocyanate (PEITC)	Breast cancer cell	Hsp27 ↓, Hsp70 ↓, Hsp90 ↓, HSF-1 ↓	[80]
Quercetin	Breast cancer	Dox efficacy↑	[81]
	Glioblastoma cell lines (U251 and U87)	Hsp27 ↓, t-AUCB efficacy ↑	[82]
	Glioma cell line (MOGGCCM)	Hsp27 ↓, Hsp72 ↓, temozolomid efficacy ↑, apoptosis ↑	[83]
	HeLa cell line	Hsp27 ↓, Hsp70 ↓, CDDP-induced apoptosis ↑	[84, 85]
	Leukemia cell line (HL-60)	Hsp27 ↓, Hsp70 ↓	[78]
	Lung cancer cell line (A549)	Hsp27 ↓, CDDP and gemcitabine efficacy ↑	[86]
	Neuroblastoma and Ewing's sarcoma	Hsp27 ↓, Dox efficacy ↑	[87]
	Neuroblastoma cell line	Hsp27 ↓, Hsp70 ↓, apoptosis ↑	[88]
	Oral squamous cell carcinoma	Hsp27 ↓, apoptosis ↑, CDDP efficacy↑	[89]
	Pancreatic cancer cells	Hsp70 ↓	[90]
	Prostate cancer	Hsp70 ↓, apoptosis ↑	[16, 19, 20]
	Prostate cancer	Hsp90 ↓, apoptosis ↑	[91]

(continued)

Table 1 (continued)

Plant extract/natural compound	Cancer cell/type	Findings	References
Resveratrol	Breast cancer cells (MCF-7 cell line)	Hsp27 ↓, apoptosis ↑, Dox efficacy↑	[17]
Taxifolin, isorhamnetin	Leukemia cell line (HL-60)	Hsp70↓	[78]
Taxol	Ovarian and uterine cancer cells	Hsp27↓, etoposide, colcemid and vincristine efficacy↑	[92]
Theaflavin and thearubigin	Leukemia cell lines (U937 and K562)	Hsp90 ↓, apoptosis ↑	[93]
Triptolide	HeLa cell line	Hsp70↓	[94]
Vinca alkaloid (vincristine)	Breast cancer cells (MCF-7 cell line)	Hsp27↓, apoptosis ↑	[95]
Viscum album extract	Glioma cell line	Hsp27 ↓ , 14-3-3 β ↓ , ζ ↓, γ ↓, apoptosis ↑	[22]
Withaferin A	Pancreatic cancer	Hsp90 ↓	[96]
Zerumbone	Lung adenocarcinoma cells	Hsp27↓, radiosensitization ↑	[97]

(↑: upregulation, ↓: downregulation)

expression of the inducible forms of Hsp70 and Hsp90 induced by 7-KC. They found that lycopene completely downregulated Hsp70 and Hsp90 expression [107]. Uppala et al. [109] treated a breast cancer cell line (MCF-7) and a immortalized breast cell line (MCF-10) with different concentrations of lycopene, and identified the variation of protein expression using MALDI-TOF/TOF. Hsp27 was amongst the proteins exhibiting differential expression. The expression level of Hsp27 was found to be significantly higher in breast cancer cells compared with normal breast cells at a range of different lycopene concentrations. Catalano et al. [79] investigated the antioxidant activities of lycopene and its metabolites (apo-10′-lycopenic acid and apo-14′-lycopenic acid) in human macrophages. The study utilised H_2O_2 and cigarette smoke extract-treated THP-1 macrophages and showed that Hsp70 and Hsp90 proteins were upregulated after H_2O_2-induced oxidative stress. The expression levels of these proteins were measured in cells treated with lycopene and its metabolites, followed by exposure to 0.1 μM H_2O_2 for 3 h. Prooxidant addition downregulated the expression of Hsp70 and Hsp90 compared with the control cells. Expression of both Hsp70 and Hsp90 was reduced by using lycopene and apo-14′-lycopenic acid more than by using apo-10′-lycopenic acid [79].

Quercetin

Quercetin (3,3′,4′,5,7-pentahydroxyflavone), one of the key secondary plant metabolites, is a flavonoid found in many edible fruits, vegetables, nuts and beverages from plants including tea, coffee, and red wine [110, 111]. As an inherent flavonoid, quercetin is a common dietary component with multiple medicinal properties. This

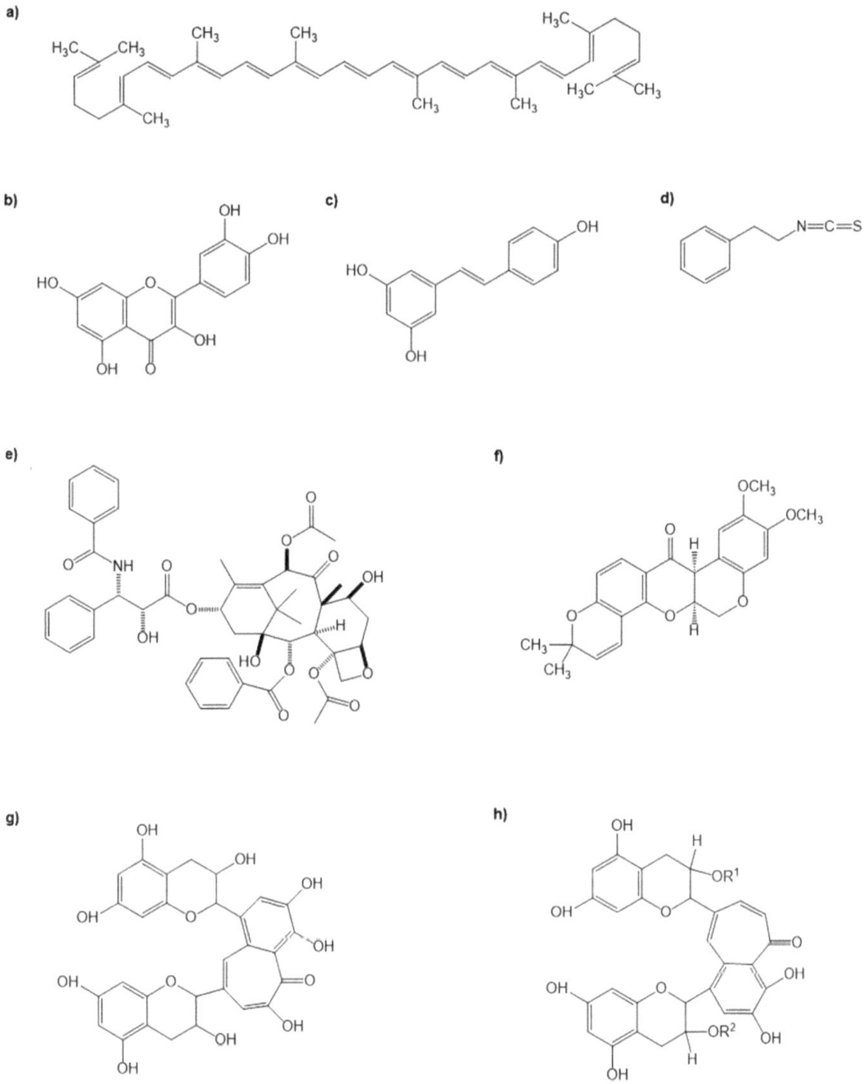

Fig. 1 Chemical structure of some naturally occurring potential HSP inhibitors. (**a**) Lycopene, (**b**) Quercetin, (**c**) Resveratrol, (**d**) PEITC, (**e**) Taxol (Paclitaxel), (**f**) Deguelin, (**g**) Theaflavins, (**h**) Thearubigins (R = gallate or other groups)

molecule is known to possess a wide range of biological and pharmacological effects [110, 112]. Quercetin has anti-allergic, anticancer, antioxidant, antiproliferative, antithrombotic, antiviral, and cardioprotective properties [111, 113]. The ability to act as an antioxidant is the best described property of quercetin [111]. Another important feature of quercetin is in the induction of apoptosis by caspase activation and release of cytochrome c [84, 114]. In addition, quercetin is a well-known inhibitor of HSP expression [84].

In many studies, quercetin is reported to reduce HSP expression in different tumor cells. According to the results of Jakubowicz-Gil and co-workers, quercetin induces programmed cell death (apoptosis) and silences Hsp27 and Hsp72 expression in glioma and HeLa cells [83–85, 88, 115]. Hyun and co-workers reported the inhibitory effect of quercetin on Hsp70 expression in pancreatic cancer cells [90]. A number of studies showed that Hsp70 inhibition by using quercetin, antisense oligonucleotide or siRNA enhanced programmed cell death in prostate cancer cells [19, 25]. Similarly, it has been shown that quercetin induced apoptosis in prostate cancer cells by downregulating Hsp90 levels [91]. This molecule also inhibited the heat dependent overexpressed Hsp70 in myeloid and lymphoid-leukemia cell lines [116, 117] and increased the number of apoptotic leukemic cells [117]. As an HSP inhibitor, quercetin downregulates some heat shock induced-stress proteins; such as Hsp70 expression in prostate cancer cells [16, 19, 20]; Hsp27 and Hsp70 expression in HeLa cells [84]; Hsp27 and Hsp70 expression in leukemia cells [78].

Many studies have reported that quercetin exhibits a synergistic antitumor effect with chemotherapeutic agents [85, 118]. The suppression of Hsp27 and Hsp72 expression following quercetin treatment sensitized against cisplatin-mediated apoptosis in HeLa cells [85]. Treatment with a combination quercetin and temozolomide at high concentrations caused apoptosis through inhibition of Hsp27 and Hsp72 expression in glioma cells [83]. Quercetin was found to enhance Doxorubicin (Dox) efficacy in breast cancer and to assist in a decrease of the toxic side effects of the drug in normal cells [81]. It is known that Dox resistance is enhanced by the overexpression of HSPs. Quercetin treatment was found to produce a reduction in HSP expression in neuroblastoma and Ewing's sarcoma cells; consequently, the cells became more sensitive to Dox [87]. In addition, quercetin has been found to diminish Hsp27 expression in lung cancer cells and its combination with chemotherapeutic agents (cisplatin or gemcitabine) caused the decrease of survival rate of lung cancer stem cells by 20% and 30%, respectively compared to that of the chemotherapy alone [86].

Although it has not yet been completely clarified, there is a plausible explanation for the effect of quercetin on HSP suppression. Quercetin downregulates the heat-induced expression of HSPs in many different cell types by acting on heat shock factor 1 (HSF1) [61, 119, 120]. It diminishes HSF1 dependent induction of *hsp* gene expression at the transcription level [16, 20, 84, 119, 121] and inhibits heat shock response (HSR) by blocking the generation of HSF trimers [120]. Quercetin acts on the early steps of HSP synthesis by preventing post-translational modifications required for HSFs activation and by suppressing its interaction with other DNA-binding proteins in the promoter region of the related gene [84, 122].

Resveratrol

Resveratrol (3,4′,5-trans-trihydroxystilbene) is a natural polyphenol found in several plants such as fruits, vegetables and medicinal plants, that exhibits chemopreventive and antitumor effects. Resveratrol was initially used for cancer therapy, but also in several degenerative and cardiovascular diseases like aging, atherosclerosis, diabetes, heart failure, hypertension, ischemia/reperfusion, and obesity [123]. Investigations into the health-promoting effects of resveratrol have revealed several molecular targets. Interaction with estrogen receptors [124], phosphodiesterase [125], protein deacetylases [126], protein kinases [127], stress proteins (e.g. Hsp25, [128]) have been reported. Han et al. [128] investigated whether resveratrol may inhibit the motor neuron degeneration in a transgenic model of amyotrophic lateral sclerosis (ALS). They used transgenic mice overexpressing G93A-SOD1 (a mutant superoxide dismutase). Intraperitoneal injection of resveratrol retarded the onset of ALS disease and increased survival of the transgenic mice. Levels of Hsp25 and Hsp70 were elevated in resveratrol-treated G93A mice, while HSF1 acetylation levels decreased in these mice. According to their data, resveratrol may protect motor neurons from the mutant SOD1-induced neurotoxicity [128]. Şahin et al. [129] investigated how resveratrol affects HSPs, transcription factors and antioxidative enzymes in the liver of quail under heat stress. According to their results, resveratrol has a protective effect against heat stress, and this protection is connected to the reduction of lipid peroxidation, inhibition of HSPs and NF-KB (Nuclear Factor Kappa B) expressions, and activation of Nrf2 expression [129].

Chronic myelogenous leukemia (CML) is a myeloproliferative disease. Leukemia biology has been extensively studied and different oncoproteins have been reported to contribute in leukemogenesis. BCR-ABL is a fused onco-protein and tactfully rewires intracellular signaling cascades to promote leukemia. As a result of the disease, Bcr-Abl protein (a protein tyrosine-kinase) is expressed. There are several treatment methods involving tyrosine kinase inhibitors, but after the treatment, drug resistance is encountered in the cells. High endogenous Hsp70 levels lead to drug resistance in CML. Chakraborty et al. [130] studied the chemotherapeutic effects and mode of action of resveratrol on chronic myelogenous leukemia cells (K562 cells). It was shown that resveratrol caused apoptosis, and induced suppression of Hsp70 both in mRNA and protein levels in K562 cells. Resveratrol was also shown to inhibit Hsp70 levels significantly via blocking of HSF1 activity and to increase the pro-apoptotic effects of Hsp90 inhibitor (17-allylamino-17-demethoxygeldana mycin, 17-AAG).

Diaz-Chavez et al. [17] showed that treatment with resveratrol evoked Hsp27 inhibition and stimulated programmed cell death in breast cancer cells (MCF-7). Additionally, the usage of siRNA for Hsp27 inhibition also augmented Dox efficacy in MCF-7 cells.

Phenethyl Isothiocyanate (PEITC)

Isothiocyanates (also known as mustard oils) are found in Brassica and other vegetables of Cruciferae (Brassicaceae) family. There are many reports that isothiocyanates may inhibit carcinogenesis and tumorigenesis, and they are used as chemo-preventive agents against the development and progression of cancer [44,

131, 132]. These types of compounds are also known to induce apoptosis in certain cancer cell lines. Phenethyl isothiocyanate (PEITC) is an isothiocyanate that exhibits chemo-preventive activity and little toxicity. PEITC potentially inhibits Phase I enzymes and induces Phase II enzymes, including glutathione S-transferase and quinone reductase, that inactivate carcinogens [133]. Moon and co-workers showed that PEITC treatment (3 μM) efficiently upregulated tumor suppressor genes and simultaneously downregulated oncogenes in human breast cancer cells. They reported the activation of ATF-2, BRCA2, CYP19, Hsp27, IL-2, p53 and p57 genes by PEITC for the first time [134]. Sarkars et al. [80] worked with two different breast cancer cell lines (MCF-7 and MDA-MB-231) to determine the effect of PEITC on different HSPs (Hsp27, Hsp70 and Hsp90) and HSF1. According to their results, PEITC significantly inhibited the expression of Hsp27, Hsp70, Hsp90 and HSF1 in a concentration-dependent manner.

Taxol

Taxol (paclitaxel), a bark extract of *Taxus brevifolia,* is a tubulin depolymerization inhibitor, and is commonly used for the treatment of a variety of cancers such as ovarian, breast, lung etc. [135]. Tanaka et al. [92] conducted a study to determine whether paclitaxel inhibits the expression of Hsp27. They used two different gynecologic cancer cell lines (BG-1 ovarian and HeLa uterine cancer cells) and compared the action of antineoplastic agents having different cytotoxic mechanisms. They found that paclitaxel inhibited Hsp27 expression, while the other agents (colcemid and vincristine) increased it. Paclitaxel has been found to diminish HSP expression in breast cancer cells (MCF-7 and MDA-MB-435 cell lines). Paclitaxel dramatically reduced Hsp27 levels in Hsp27 over-expressing breast cancer cells and made them more sensitive to Doxorubicin [136]. Vydra et al. [137] have investigated the sensitivity of mouse (B16F10) and human (WM793B and 1205Lu) melanoma cells, which overexpressed HSF1 to different chemotherapeutic agents. HSF1 overexpression did not influence the survival of the cells treated with cisplatin, vinblastine or bortezomib. However, Doxorubicin or paclitaxel significantly enhanced the survival of the cells. As a result, HSF1-overexpressing melanoma cells were noted to be more resistant to doxorubicin or paclitaxel.

Deguelin

Deguelin is a rotenoid, and it can be extracted from several plants of the legume family. This compound is potential chemo-preventive agent and reported to be effective against various cancer types. Oh et al. [68] showed that deguelin inhibited chaperone activity of Hsp90, resulting in the ubiquitin-mediated degradation of Hsp90 client proteins in xenografted mice. Yang et al. [69] also showed that deugelin isolated from *Mundulea sericea* had anticancer activity against different human xenografts tumors such as head and neck, lung, prostate and stomach cancers. In addition, induction of both apoptosis and autophagy by deugelin has been shown in cultured head and neck squamous cell carcinoma (HNSCC) cells. This action is generated by inhibition of Akt signaling, and downregulation of cyclin-dependent kinase 4 (Cdk4) and survivin, disrupting their association with Hsp-90.

Tea Polyphenols (Theaflavins and Thearubigins)

Tea (*Camellia sinensis*) is effective against many cancer types. Many studies in various test systems have revealed that theaflavins (TFs) and thearubigins (TRs), polyphenols of black tea, have chemo-preventive effects [138]. Halder et al. [93] used human leukemic cell lines (U937 and K562 cells) to investigate the molecular mechanisms involved in the arrest of cell-cycle dynamics by TFs and TRs. They also evaluated the effects of these compounds on PKB/Akt signaling. The first finding of this study was the suppression of Hsp90 by TFs and TRs, which caused blocking of cell-cycle. In addition, TF- and TR-mediated Hsp90 suppression reduced Akt signaling reduced the level of CDK2, downregulated cell proliferation and increased apoptosis in the cells [93].

Green tea is one of the widely used beverages all over the World. The major constituents in green tea are catechins, which are natural polyphenols. They have a number of biological activities. Epigallocatechin-3-gallate (EGCG), is found in green tea as a major catechin, and is known as a chemotherapeutic agent for several cancers. Tran et al. [73] examined the effect of EGCG on the expression of various HSPs and the suppression of different tumors. They used the MCF-7 breast cell line and found that EGCG treatment decreased cell proliferation and colony formation. Hsp70 and Hsp90 expression was specifically inhibited by EGCG. The sensitivity of MCF-7 cells against heat shock and oxidative stress was increased by pretreatment with EGCG. Moreover, it was found that EGCG treatment (10 mg/kg) retarded tumor incidence, decreased the tumor size, and downregulated the expression of Hsp70 and Hsp90 in a xenograft model. Data clearly suggested that both Hsp70 and Hsp90 were potential targets of EGCG [73]. Chen et al. [74] demonstrated that EGCG induced apoptosis in human urinary carcinoma cell line (TSGH-8301) by Hsp27 downregulation. In another study, Zhang and co-workers identified the cellular targets of green tea by exposing human pancreatic ductal adenocarcinoma (HPAF-II) cells to green tea extract. The expression levels of 32 proteins were found to be altered in the green tea extract-treated cells and these proteins were related to detoxification, drug resistance, gene regulation, motility, and metabolism of the cancer cells. It was shown that green tea extract significantly inhibited molecular chaperones Hsp90, Hsp75 and Hsp27, and induced apoptosis in pancreatic adenocarcinoma cells [77].

On the other hand, green tea polyphenols also reduced Hsp27 and Hsp90 levels in mouse kidney and liver [139].

Plant Extracts

Different plant extracts exert their biological effects through the modulation of diverse cellular and physiological pathways. Recent studies showed that some plant extracts inhibited the growth and induced apoptosis in HSPs overexpressing cancer cells [22, 67]. Our own group investigated the HSP inhibitory effect of *Viscum album* (mistletoe) extract in glioma cells. It is known that various commercial *V. album* extracts are widely used as complementary cancer therapies in European countries [140–143]. Our studies revealed that antioxidant *Viscum album* extract reduced the expression level of some 14-3-3 proteins (β, γ and ζ isoforms) and Hsp27 in C6 rat glioma cells, and increased apoptosis via caspase-3 activation in heat shocked and extract-treated cells [22].

Cimicifuga foetida has long been used as traditional Chinese medicine. Soler and co-workers showed that *C. foetida* extract downregulated the level of Hsp27 expression in breast cancer cells [67]. Since *Ginkgo biloba* has a great antioxidant potential, the extracts from the leaves have been also used in China and Western countries. EGb761 is the commercial leaf extract of *G. biloba* and some of its components are flavonoids (22–27%) and terpenoids (5–7%). Tsai et al. [76] investigated the effects of EGb761 on HSP expression in non-small cell lung cancer (NSCLC) cell lines. Normally, Hsp27 is upregulated in NSCLC tissue versus normal lung tissue. It was found that EGb761 suppressed the level of Hsp27 expression and migration of cancer cells (A549/H441). The authors concluded that Hsp27 is a poor prognostic factor of NSCLC, but that EGb761 extract can be utilized in complementary therapy for NSCLC treatment since it has an inhibitory effect on Hsp27 expression level [76]. *Garcinia oblongifolia* is also used as traditional Chinese medicinal herb. Fu et al. [144] have performed a study with hepatocellular carcinoma (HCC) cells investigating the suppression of Hsp27 with xanthones isolated from *G. oblongifolia*. They found down-regulation of Hsp27 and increased caspase-mediated apoptosis in xanthone-treated cells.

Perspectives and Conclusions

According to the statistical data, cancer is a major cause of death throughout the world. Recent studies have shown enhanced expression of HSPs in many tumor cell types, allowing these cells to evade the apoptotic process. The suppression of some HSPs allows the programmed cell death in the tumor cells. Hence the suppression of HSPs is considered as a conventional therapy for cancer treatment. Currently, 50 active clinical trials relating to HSPs are in progress, most of these relating to the treatment of different cancer types. Among the ongoing studies, 3 are for Hsp27, 3 for Hsp40, 8 for Hsp70, 16 for Hsp90 and 3 for Hsp110 (https://clinicaltrials.gov/). Some plant extracts or phytochemicals isolated from plants represent potent novel HSP inhibitors. The use of these natural compounds in combination with common chemotherapeutic agents promotes drug sensitivity in tumor cells. Several studies have been conducted that emphasize that some natural compounds, mostly antioxidants, downregulate or inhibit HSPs expression and improve the responsiveness of cancer cells to different therapeutics. As described in this chapter, some plant products possessing HSP suppression activity are promising agents for the treatment of cancer. In the future, new compounds from medicinal plants are expected to be evaluated for their HSP-inhibiting/suppressing activity.

Acknowledgements The authors wish to dedicate this chapter to the memory of Professor Alastair Aitken for his invaluable motivation and great contribution to their knowledge and experience, both in science and in life. The authors also thank to Michele Learmonth and Gökçe Ünar for helpful suggestions. This study was supported by the Research Fund of Istanbul University (Project no. T-746/13092005, 22649 and 27484).

References

1. Ferlay J, Shin HR, Bray F, Forman D, Mathers CD, Parkin D (2010) GLOBOCAN 2008, Cancer incidence and mortality worldwide: IARC CancerBase No. 10 [Internet]. International Agency for Research on Cancer, Lyon, France. http://globocan.iarc.fr
2. Benjamin IJ, McMillan DR (1998) Stress (heat shock) proteins molecular chaperones in cardiovascular biology and disease. Circ Res 83:117–132
3. Snoeckx LHEH, Cornelussen RN, Van Nieuwenhoven FA, Reneman RS, Van der Vusse GJ (2001) Heat shock proteins and cardiovascular pathophysiology. Physiol Rev 81(4):1461–1497
4. Alberts B, Johnson A, Lewis J, Raff M, Roberts K, Walter P (2002) Molecular biology of the cell, 4th edn. Garland Science, New York. ISBN: 0-8153-4072-9
5. Papp E, Nardai G, Söti C, Csermely P (2003) Molecular chaperons, stress proteins and redox homeostasis. Biofactors 17:249–257
6. Lanneau D, Thonel A, Maurel S, Didelot C, Garrido C (2007) Apoptosis versus cell differentiation: role of heat shock proteins HSP90, HSP70 and HSP27. Prion 1(1):53–60
7. Sarto C, Binz PA, Mocarelli P (2000) Heat shock proteins in human cancer. Electrophoresis 21(6):1218–1226
8. Andrieu C, Taieb D, Baylot V, Ettinger S, Soubeyran P, De-Thonel A, Nelson C, Garrido C, So A, Fazli L, Bladou F, Gleave M, Iovanna JL, Rocchi P (2010) Heat shock protein 27 confers resistance to androgen ablation and chemotherapy in prostate cancer cells through eIF4E. Oncogene 29:1883–1896
9. Oesterreich S, Weng CN, Qiu M, Hilsenbeck SG, Osborne CK, Fuqua SA (1993) The small heat shock protein hsp27 is correlated with growth and drug resistance in human breast cancer cell lines. Cancer Res 53(19):4443–4448
10. Yamamoto K, Okamoto A, Isonishi S, Ochiai K, Ohtake Y (2001) Heat shock protein 27 was up-regulated in cisplatin resistant human ovarian tumor cell line and associated with the cisplatin resistance. Cancer Lett 168(2):173–181

11. Capello F, Bellafiore M, Palma A, David S, Marciano V, Bartolotta T, Sciume C, Modica G, Farina F, Zummo G, Bucchieri F (2003) 60Kda chaperonin (HSP60) is over-expressed during colorectal carcinogenesis. Eur J Histochem 47(2):105–110
12. Didelot C, Lanneau D, Brunet M, Joly AL, De Thonel A, Chiosis G, Garrido C (2007) Anti-cancer therapeutic approaches based on intracellular and extracellular heat shock proteins. Curr Med Chem 14:2839–2847
13. Kai M, Nakatsura T, Egami H, Senju S, Nishimura Y, Ogawa M (2003) Heat shock protein 105 is overexpressed in a variety of human tumors. Oncol Rep 10(6):1777–1782
14. Ryu JW, Kim HJ, Lee YS, Myong NH, Hwang CH, Lee GS, Yom HC (2003) The proteomics approach to find biomarkers in gastric cancer. J Korean Med Sci 18(4):505–509
15. Takashima M, Kuramitsu Y, Yokoyama Y, Iizuka N, Toda T, Sakaida I, Okita K, Oka M, Nakamura N (2003) Proteomic profiling of heat shock protein 70 family members as biomarkers for hepatitis C virus-related hepatocellular carcinoma. Proteomics 3(12):2487–2493
16. Asea A, Ara G, Teicher BA, Stevenson MA, Calderwood SK (2001) Effects of the flavonoid drug quercetin on the response of human prostate tumors to hyperthermia *in vivo*. Int J Hyperthermia 17:347–356
17. Diaz-Chavez J, Fonseca-Sanchez MA, Arechaga-Ocampo E, Flores-Perez A, Palacios-Rodriguez Y, Dominguez-Gomez G, Marchat LA, Fuentes-Mera L, Mendoza-Hernandez G, Gariglio P, Lopez-Camarillo C (2013) Proteomic profiling reveals that resveratrol inhibits HSP27 expression and sensitizes breast cancer cells to doxorubicin therapy. PLoS One 8(5):e64378
18. Gorman AM, Heavey B, Creagh E, Cotter TG, Samali A (1999) Antioxidant-mediated inhibition of the heat shock response leads to apoptosis. FEBS Lett 445:98–102
19. Jones EL, Zhao MJ, Stevenson MA, Calderwood SK (2004) The 70 kilodalton heat shock protein is an inhibitor of apoptosis in prostate cancer. Int J Hyperthermia 20(8):835–849
20. Kagaya A, Okada A, Jitsuiki H, Tawara Y, Inagaki M, Takebayashi M, Saeki T, Nishida A, Nakata Y, Yamawaki S (2000) Effect of heat stress on serotonin-2A receptor-mediated intracellular calcium mobilization in rat C6 glioma cells. J Neural Transm 107:919–929
21. Ng KB, Bustamam A, Sukari MA, Abdelwahab SI, Mohan S, Buckle MJC, Kamalidehghan B, Nadzri NM, Anasamy T, Hadi AHA, Rahman HS (2013) Induction of selective cytotoxicity and apoptosis in human T4-lymphoblastoid cell line (CEMss) by boesenbergin a isolated from *Boesenbergia rotunda* rhizomes involves mitochondrial pathway, activation of caspase 3 and G2/M phase cell cycle arrest. BMC Complement Altern Med 13:41
22. Önay-Uçar E, Arda N, Aitken A (2012) An extract from mistletoe, *Viscum album* L. reduces Hsp27 and 14-3-3 proteins expression and induces apoptosis in C6 rat glioma cells. Genet Mol Res 11(3):2801–2813
23. Önay-Uçar E (2015) Heat shock protein-based therapies. In: Asea AAA (ed) Heat shock proteins, Chapter 3: Heat shock proteins and cancer: plant based therapy, vol 9. Springer, Switzerland, pp 27–48
24. Ischia J, So AI (2013) The role of heat shock proteins in bladder cancer. Nat Rev Urol 10:386–395
25. So A, Hadaschik B, Sowery R, Gleave M (2007) The role of stress proteins in prostate cancer. Curr Genomics 8: 252–261.
26. Garrido C, Brunet M, Didelot C, Zermati Y, Schmitt E, Kroemer G (2006) Heat shock proteins 27 and 70: anti-apoptotic proteins with tumorigenic properties. Cell Cycle 5(22):2592–2601
27. Nakajima M, Kuwano H, Miyazaki T, Masuda N, Kato H (2002) Significant correlation between expression of heat shock proteins 27, 70 and lymphocyte infiltration in esophageal squamous cell carcinoma. Cancer Lett 178(1):99–106
28. Ciocca DR, Calderwood SK (2005) Heat shock proteins in cancer: diagnostic, prognostic, predictive, and treatment implications. Cell Stress Chaperones 10(2):86–103
29. Lee SJ, Choi SA, Lee KH, Chung HY, Kim TH, Cho CK, Lee YS (2001) Role of inducible heat shock protein in radiation- induced cell death. Cell Stress Chaperones 6(3):273–281

30. Nylandsted J, Brand K, Jaatela M (2000) Heat shock protein 70 is required for the survival of cancer cells. Ann N Y Acad Sci 926:122–125
31. Nakatsura T, Senju S, Yamada K, Jotsuka T, Ogawa M, Nishimura Y (2001) Gene cloning of immunogenic antigens overexpressed in pancreatic cancer. Biochem Biophys Res Commun 281:936–944
32. Lim SO, Park SG, Yoo JH, Park YM, Kim HJ, Jang KT, Cho JW, Yoo BC, Jung GH, Park CK (2005) Expression of heat shock proteins (HSP27, HSP60, HSP70, HSP90, GRP78, GRP94) in hepatitis B virus-related hepatocellular carcinomas and dysplastic nodules. World J Gastroenterol 11(14):2072–2079
33. Pick E, Kluger Y, Giltnane JM, Moeder C, Camp RL, Rimm DL, Kluger HM (2007) High HSP90 expression is associated with decreased survival in breast cancer. Cancer Res 67:2932–2937
34. Zackova M, Mouckova D, Lopotova T, Ondrackova Z, Klamova H, Moravcova J (2013) Hsp90—a potential prognostic marker in CML. Blood Cells Mol Dis 50:184–189
35. Abe M, Manola J, Oh WK, Parslow DL, George DJ, Austin CL, Kantoff PW (2004) Plasma levels of heat shock protein 70 in patients with prostate cancer: a potential biomarker for prostate cancer. Clin Prostate Cancer 3(1):49–53
36. Capello F, Rappa F, David S, Anzalone R, Zummo G (2003) Immunohistochemical evaluation of PCNA, p53, HSP60, HSP10 and MUC-2 presence and expression in prostate carcinogenesis. Anticancer Res 23(2B):1325–1331
37. Rubporn A, Srisomsap C, Subhasitanont P, Chokchaichamnankit D, Chiablaem K, Svasti J, Sangvanich P (2009) Comparative proteomic analysis of lung cancer cell line and lung fibroblast cell line. Cancer Genomics Proteomics 6:229–238
38. Liang S, Shen G, Liu Q, Xu Y, Zhou L, Xiao S, Xu Z, Gong F, You C, Wei Y (2009) Isoform-specific expression and characterization of 14-3-3 proteins in human glioma tissues discovered by stable isotope labeling with amino acids in cell culture-based proteomic analysis. Proteomics Clin Appl 3:743–753
39. Song HY, Liu YK, Feng JT, Cui JF, Dai Z, Zhang LJ, Feng JX, Shen HL, Tang ZY (2006) Proteomic analysis on metastasis-associated proteins of human hepatocellular carcinoma tissues. J Cancer Res Clin Oncol 132:92–98
40. Cao WD, Zhang X, Zhang JN, Yang ZJ, Zhen HN, Cheng G, Li B, Gao DK (2006) Immunocytochemical detection of 14-3-3 in primary nervous system tumors. J Neurooncol 77:125–130
41. Cao L, Cao WD, Zhang W, Lin H, Yang X, Zhen H, Cheng J, Dong W, Huo J, Zhang X (2008) Identification of 14-3-3 protein isoforms in human astrocytoma by immunohistochemistry. Neurosci Lett 432:94–99
42. Chen J, Kahne T, Rocken C, Gotze T, Yu J, Sung JJ, Chen M, Hu P, Malfertheiner P, Ebert MP (2004) Proteome analysis of gastric cancer metastasis by two-dimensional gel electrophoresis and matrix assisted laser desorption/ionization-mass spectrometry for identification of metastasis-related proteins. J Proteome Res 3:1009–1016
43. Pei HP, Ge H, Jiang R, Zhu H (2010) Expression and clinical significance of 14-3-3 sigma and heat shock protein 27 in colorectal cancer. Zhonghua Wei Chang Wai Ke Za Zhi 13(3):213–215
44. Zhang Y, Tang L, Gonzalez V (2003) Selected isothiocyanates rapidly induce growth inhibition of cancer cells. Mol Cancer Ther 2:1045–1052
45. Ciocca DR, Oesterreich S, Chamness GC, McGuire WL, Fuqua SA (1993) Biological and clinical implications of heat shock protein 27,000 (Hsp27): a review. J Natl Cancer Inst 85(19):1558–1570
46. Bruey JM, Paul C, Fromentin A, Hilpert S, Arrigo AP, Solary E, Garrido C (2000) Differential regulation of HSP27 oligomerization in tumor cells grown *in vitro* and *in vivo*. Oncogene 19(42):4855–4863
47. Garrido C, Mehlen P, Fromentin A, Hammann A, Assem M, Arrigo AP, Chauffert B (1996) Inconstant association between 27-kDa heat-shock protein (Hsp27) content and doxorubicin

resistance in human colon cancer cells. The doxorubicin-protecting effect of Hsp27. Eur J Biochem 237:653–659
48. Guttmann DM, Koumenis C (2011) The heat shock proteins as targets for radiosensitization and chemosensitization in cancer. Cancer Biol Ther 12(12):1023–1031
49. Hansen RK, Parra I, Lemieux P, Oesterreich S, Hilsenbeck SG, Fuqua SA (1999) Hsp27 overexpression inhibits doxorubicin-induced apoptosis in human breast cancer cells. Breast Cancer Res Treat 56:187–196
50. Kang SH, Kang KW, Kim KH, Kwon B, Kim SK, Lee HY, Kong SY, Lee ES, Jang SG, Yoo BY (2008) Upregulated HSP27 in human breast cancer cells reduces Herceptin susceptibility by increasing Her2 protein stability. BMC Cancer 8:286
51. Rocchi P, So A, Kojima S, Signaevsky M, Beraldi E, Fazli L (2004) Heat shock protein 27 increases after androgen ablation and plays a cytoprotective role in hormone-refractory prostate cancer. Cancer Res 64:6595–6602
52. Verrills NM, Liem NL, Liaw TY, Hood BD, Lock RB, Kavallaris M (2006) Proteomic analysis reveals a novel role for the actin cytoskeleton in vincristine resistant childhood leukemia—an *in vivo* study. Proteomics 6:1681–1694
53. Park SH, Lee SJ, Chung HY, Kim TH, Cho CK, Yoo SY, Lee YS (2000) Inducible heat shock protein 70 involved in the radioadaptive response. Radiat Res 153(3):318–326
54. Calderwood S (2007) Heat shock proteins in extracellular signaling. Methods 43(3):167
55. Calderwood SK, Ciocca DR (2008) Heat shock proteins: stress proteins with Janus-like properties in cancer. Int J Hyperthermia 24(1):31–39
56. Kim LS, Kim JH (2011) Heat shock protein as molecular targets for breast cancer therapeutics. J Breast Cancer 14(3):167–174
57. Chuma M, Sakamoto M, Yamazaki K, Ohta T, Ohki M, Asaka M, Hirohashi S (2003) Expression profiling in multistage hepatocarcinogenesis: identification of HSP70 as a molecular marker of early hepatocellular carcinoma. Hepatology 37(1):198–207
58. Bauer K, Nitsche U, Slotta-Huspenina J, Drecoll E, von Weyhern CH, Rosenberg R, Höfler H, Langer R (2012) High HSP27 and HSP70 expression levels are independent adverse prognostic factors in primary resected colon cancer. Cell Oncol 35:197–205
59. Gabai VL, Budagova KR, Sherman MY (2005) Increased expression of the major heat shock protein Hsp72 in human prostate carcinoma cells is dispensable for their viability but confers resistance to a variety of anticancer agents. Oncogene 24:3328–3338
60. Bruey JM, Ducasse C, Bonniaud P, Ravagnan L, Susin SA, Diaz-Latoud C, Gurbuxani S, Arrigo AP, Kroemer G, Solary E, Garrido C (2000) Hsp27 negatively regulates cell death by interacting with cytochrome C. Nat Cell Biol 2:645–652
61. Ciocca DR, Arrigo AP, Calderwood SK (2013) Heat shock proteins and heat shock factor 1 in carcinogenesis and tumor development: an update. Arch Toxicol 87:19–48
62. Concannon CG, Gorman AM, Samali A (2003) On the role of Hsp27 in regulating apoptosis. Apoptosis 8(1):61–70
63. Jaatella M (1999) Escaping cell death: survival proteins in cancer. Exp Cell Res 248(1):30–43
64. Jego G, Hazoumé A, Seigneuric R, Garrido C (2013) Targeting heat shock proteins in cancer. Cancer Lett 332(2):275–285
65. McConnell JR, McAlpine SR (2013) Heat shock proteins 27, 40, and 70 as combinational and dual therapeutic cancer targets. Bioorg Med Chem Lett 23:1923–1928
66. Pyo JS, Roh SH, Kim DK, Lee JG, Lee YY, Hong SS, Kwon SW, Park JH (2009) Anticancer effect of betulin on a human lung cancer cell line: a pharmacoproteomic approach using 2D SDS PAGE coupled with nano-HPLC tandem mass spectrometry. Planta Med 75:127–131
67. Soler MC, Molina JL, Díaz HA, Pinto VC, Barrios YL, He K, Roller M, Weinstein-Oppenheimer CR (2011) Effect of the standardized *Cimicifuga foetida* extract on Hsp 27 expression in the MCF-7 cell line. Biol Res 44(3):243–249
68. Oh SH, Woo JK, Yazıcı YD, Myers JN, Kim WY, Jin Q, Hong SS, Park HJ, Suh YG, Kim KW, Hong WK, Lee HY (2007) Structural basis for depletion of heat shock protein 90 client proteins by deguelin. J Natl Cancer Inst 90(12):949–961

69. Yang YL, Ji C, Bi ZG, Lu CC, Wang R, Gu B, Cheng L (2013) Deguelin induces both apoptosis and autophagy in cultured head and neck squamous cell carcinoma cells. PLoS One 8(1):e54736
70. Chang DJ, An H, Kim K, Kim HH, Jung J, Lee JM, Kim NJ, Han YT, Yun H, Lee S, Lee G, Lee S, Lee JS, Cha JH, Park JH, Park JW, Lee SC, Kim SG, Kim JH, Lee HY, Kim KW, Suh YG (2012) Design, synthesis, and biological evaluation of novel deguelin-based heat shock protein 90 (HSP90) inhibitors targeting proliferation and angiogenesis. J Med Chem 55:10863–10884
71. Hung CM, Su YH, Lin HY, Lin JN, Liu LC, Ho CT, Way TD (2012) Demethoxycurcumin modulates prostate cancer cell proliferation via AMPK-induced down-regulation of HSP70 and EGFR. J Agric Food Chem 60:8427–8434
72. Vassallo A, Vaccaro MC, De Tommasi N, Dal Piaz F, Leone A (2013) Identification of the plant compound geraniin as a novel Hsp90 inhibitor. PLoS One 8(9):e74266. doi:10.1371/journal.pone.0074266
73. Tran P, Kim SA, Choi HS, Yoon JH, Ahn SG (2010) Epigallocatechin-3-gallate suppresses the expression of HSP70 and HSP90 and exhibits anti-tumor activity *in vitro* and *in vivo*. BMC Cancer 10:276
74. Chen NG, Lu CC, Lin YH, Shen WC, Lai CH, Ho YJ, Chun JG, Lin TH, Lin YC, Yang JS (2011) Proteomic approaches to study epigallocatechin gallate-provoked apoptosis of TSGH-8301 human urinary bladder carcinoma cells: roles of AKT and heat shock protein 27-modulated intrinsic apoptotic pathways. Oncol Rep 26:939–947
75. Brandt GE, Schmidt MD, Prisinzano TE, Blagg BS (2008) Gedunin, a novel hsp90 inhibitor: semisynthesis of derivatives and preliminary structure-activity relationships. J Med Chem 51:6495–6502. doi:10.1021/jm8007486
76. Tsai JR, Liu PL, Chen YH, Chou SH, Yang MC, Cheng YJ, Hwang JJ, Yin WH, Chong IW (2014) *Ginkgo biloba* extract decreases non-small cell lung cancer cell migration by down-regulating metastasis-associated factor heat-shock protein 27. PLoS One 9:e91331. doi:10.1371/journal.pone.0091331
77. Zhang L, Pang E, Loo RR, Rao J, Go VL, Loo JA, Lu QY (2011) Concomitant inhibition of HSP90, its mitochondrial localized homologue TRAP1 and HSP27 by green tea in pancreatic cancer HPAF-II cells. Proteomics 11(24):4638–4647
78. Rusak G, Gutzeit HO, Ludwig-Müller J (2002) Effects of structurally related flavonoids on hsp gene expression in human promyeloid leukaemia cells. Food Technol Biotechnol 40(4):267–273
79. Catalano A, Simone RE, Cittadini A, Reynaud E, Caris-Veyrat C, Palozza P (2013) Comparative antioxidant effects of lycopene, apo-10′-lycopenoic acid and apo-14′-lycopenoic acid in human macrophages exposed to H_2O_2 and cigarette smoke extract. Food Chem Toxicol 51:71–79
80. Sarkars R, Mukherjee S, Roy M (2013) Targeting heat shock proteins by phenethyl isothiocyanate results in cell-cycle arrest and apoptosis of human breast cancer cells. Nutr Cancer 65(3):480–493
81. Staedler D, Idrizi E, Kenzaoui BH, Juillerat-Jeanneret L (2011) Drug combinations with quercetin: doxorubicin plus quercetin in human breast cancer cells. Cancer Chemother Pharmacol 68:1161–1172
82. Li J, Tang C, Li L, Li J, Fan Y (2016) Quercetin blocks t-AUCB-induced autophagy by Hsp27 and Atg7 inhibition in glioblastoma cells *in vitro*. J Neurooncol 129:39–45
83. Jakubowicz-Gil J, Langner E, Wertel I, Piersiak T, Rzeski W (2010) Temozolomide, quercetin and cell death in the MOGGCCM astrocytoma cell line. Chem Biol Interact 188:190–203
84. Jakubowicz-Gil J, Rzymowska J, Gawron A (2002) Quercetin, apoptosis, heat shock. Biochem Pharmacol 64:1591–1595
85. Jakubowicz-Gil J, Paduch R, Piersiak T, Glowniak K, Gawron A, Kandefer-Szerszen M (2005) The effect of quercetin on pro-apoptotic activity of cisplatin in HeLa cells. Biochem Pharmacol 69:1343–1350

86. Hsu HS, Lin JH, Huang WC, Hsu TW, Su K, Chiou SH, Tsai YT, Hung SC (2011) Chemoresistance of lung cancer stemlike cells depends on activation of Hsp27. Cancer 117:1516–1528
87. Zanini C, Giribaldi G, Mandili G, Carta F, Crescenzio N, Bisaro B, Doria A, Foglia L, di Montezemolo LC, Timeus F, Turrini F (2007) Inhibition of heat shock proteins (HSP) expression by quercetin and differential doxorubicin sensitization in neuroblastoma and Ewing's sarcoma cell lines. J Neurochem 103:1344–1354
88. Jakubowicz-Gil J, Rzeski W, Zdzisińska B, Piersiak T, Weiksza K, Głowniak K, Gawron A (2008) Different sensitivity of neurons and neuroblastoma cells to quercetin treatment. Acta Neurobiol Exp 68:463–476
89. Chen SF, Nieh S, Jao SW, Liu CL, Wu CH, Chang YC, Yang CY, Lin YS (2012) Quercetin suppresses drug-resistant spheres via the p38 MAPK–Hsp27 apoptotic pathway in oral cancer cells. PLoS One 7(11):e49275. doi:10.1371/journal.pone.0049275
90. Hyun JJ, Lee HS, Keum B, Seo YS, Jeen YT, Chun HJ, Um SH, Kim CD (2013) Expression of heat shock protein 70 modulates the chemoresponsiveness of pancreatic cancer. Gut Liver 7(6):739–746
91. Aalinkeel R, Bindukumar B, Reynolds JL, Sykes DE, Mahajan SD, Chadha KC, Schwartz SA (2008) The dietary bioflavonoid, quercetin, selectively induces apoptosis of prostate cancer cells by down-regulating the expression of heat shock protein 90. Prostate 68:1773–1789
92. Tanaka Y, Fujiwara K, Tanaka H, Maehata K, Kohno I (2004) Paclitaxel inhibits expression of heat shock protein 27 in ovarian and uterine cancer cells. Int J Gynecol Cancer 14:616–620
93. Halder B, Gupta SD, Gomes A (2012) Black tea polyphenols induce human leukemic cell cycle arrest by inhibiting Akt signaling possible involvement of Hsp90, Wnt/b-catenin signaling and FOXO1. FEBS J 279:2876–2891
94. Westerheide SD, Kawahara TLA, Orton K, Morimoto RI (2006) Triptolide, an inhibitor of the human heat shock response that enhances stress-induced cell death. J Biol Chem 281(14):9616–9622
95. Casado P, Zuazua-Villar P, del Valle E, Martinez-Campa C, Lazo PS, Ramos S (2007) Vincristine regulates the phosphorylation of the antiapoptotic protein HSP27 in breast cancer cells. Cancer Lett 247:273–282
96. Yu Y, Hamza A, Zhang T, Gu M, Zou P, Newman B, Li Y, Gunatilaka AAL, Whitesell L, Zhan CG, Sun D (2010) Withaferin A targets heat shock protein 90 in pancreatic cancer cells. Biochem Pharmacol 79(4):542–551
97. Choi SH, Lee YJ, Seo WD, Lee HJ, Nam JW, Lee YJ, Kim J, Seo EK, Lee YS (2011) Altered cross-linking of HSP27 by zerumbone as a novel strategy for overcoming HSP27-mediated radioresistance. Int J Radiat Oncol Biol Phys 79(4):1196–1205
98. Rao AV, Rao LG (2007) Carotenoids and human health. Pharmacol Res 55:207–216
99. Palozza P, Parrone P, Simone R, Catalano A (2011) Role of lycopene in the control of ROS-mediated cell growth: implications in cancer prevention. Curr Med Chem 18:1846–1860
100. Palozza P, Parrone P, Catalano A, Simone R (2010) Tomato lycopene and inflammatory cascade: basic interactions and clinical implications. Curr Med Chem 17:2547–2563
101. Zhang LX, Cooney RV, Bertram JS (1991) Carotenoids enhance gap junctional communication and inhibit lipid peroxidation in C3H/10T1/2 cells: relationship to their cancer chemopreventive action. Carcinogenesis 12:2109–2114
102. Nahum A, Zeller L, Danilenko M, Prall OW, Watts CK, Sutherland RL, Levy J, Sharoni Y (2006) Lycopene inhibition of IGF-induced cancer cell growth depends on the level of cyclin D1. Eur J Nutr 45:275–282
103. Liu C, Russell RM, Wang XD (2006) Lycopene supplementation prevents smoke induced changes in p53, p53 phosphorylation, cell proliferation and apoptosis in gastric mucosa of ferrets. Cancer Res 63:3138–3144
104. Linnewiel K, Ernst H, Caris-Veyrat C, Ben-Dor A, Kampf A, Salman H, Danilenko M, Levy J, Sharoni Y (2009) Structure activity relationship of carotenoid derivatives in activation of

the electrophile/antioxidant response element transcription system. Free Radic Biol Med 47:659–667
105. Mein JR, Wang XD (2008) Biologic activity of lycopene metabolites: implications for cancer prevention. Nutr Rev 66:667–683
106. Nagao A (2004) Oxidative conversion of carotenoids to retinoids and other products. J Nutr 134:237S–240S
107. Palozza P, Simone R, Catalano A, Boninsegna A, Böhm V, Fröhlich K, Mele MC, Monego G, Ranelletti FO (2010) Lycopene prevents 7-ketocholesterol-induced oxidative stress, cell cycle arrest and apoptosis in human macrophages. J Nutr Biochem 21:34–46
108. Brown AJ, Jesup W (1999) Oxysterols and atheresclerosis. Atherosclerosis 142:1–28
109. Uppala PT, Dissmore T, Lau BHS, Andacht T, Rajaram S (2013) Selective inhibition of cell proliferation by lycopene in MCF-7 breast cancer cells in vitro: a proteomic analysis. Phytother Res 27:595–601
110. Bischoff SC (2008) Quercetin: potentials in the prevention and therapy of disease. Curr Opin Clin Nutr Metab Care 11(6):733–740
111. Gupta C, Vikram A, Tripathi DN, Ramarao P, Jena GB (2010) Antioxidant and antimutagenic effect of quercetin against DEN induced hepatotoxicity in rat. Phytother Res 24(1):119–128
112. Madaan K, Lather V, Pandita D (2015) Evaluation of polyamidoamine dendrimers as potential carriers for quercetin, a versatile flavonoid. Drug Deliv 21:1–9
113. Inal M, Kahraman A (2000) The protective effect of flavonol quercetin against ultraviolet a induced oxidative stress in rats. Toxicology 154(1–3):21–29
114. Ramos S (2007) Effects of dietary flavonoids on apoptotic pathways related to cancer chemoprevention. J Nutr Biochem 18(7):427–442
115. Jakubowicz-Gil J, Langner E, Bądziul D, Wertel I, Rzeski W (2013) Silencing of Hsp27 and Hsp72 in glioma cells as a tool for programmed cell death induction upon temozolomide and quercetin treatment. Toxicol Appl Pharmacol 273(3):580–589
116. Elia G, Santoro MG (1994) Regulation of heat shock protein synthesis by quercetin in human erythroleukaemia cells. Biochem J 300:201–209
117. Wei YQ, Zhao X, Kariya Y, Fukata H, Teshigawara K, Uchida A (1994) Induction of apoptosis by quercetin: involvement of heat shock protein. Cancer Res 54:4952
118. Cipak L, Novotny L, Cipakova I, Rauko P (2003) Differential modulation of cisplatin and doxorubicin efficacies in leukemia cells by flavonoids. Nutr Res 23:1045–1057
119. Hosokawa N, Hirayoshi K, Kudo H, Takechi H, Aoike A, Kawai K, Nagata K (1992) Inhibition of the activation of heat shock factor in vivo and in vitro by flavonoids. Mol Cell Biol 12:3490–3498
120. Nagai N, Nakai A, Nagata K (1995) Quercetin suppresses heat shock response by downregulation of HSF1. Biochem Biophys Res Commun 208(3):1099–1105
121. Hosokawa N, Hirayoshi K, Nakai A, Hosokawa Y, Marui N, Yoshida M, Sakai T, Nishino H, Aoike A, Kawai K, Nagata K (1990) Flavonoids inhibit the expression of heat shock proteins. Cell Struct Funct 15:393–401
122. Hansen RK, Oesterreich S, Lemieux P, Sarge KD, Fuqua SAW (1997) Quercetin inhibits heat shock protein induction but not heat shock factor DNA-binding in human breast carcinoma cells. Biochem Biophys Res Commun 239:851–856
123. Cucciolla V, Borriello A, Oliva A, Galletti P, Zappia V, Ragione FD (2007) Resveratrol: from basic science to the clinic. Cell Cycle 6(20):2495–2510
124. Gehm BD, Mcandrews JM, Chien PY, Jameson JL (1997) Resveratrol, a polyphenolic compound found in grapes and wine, is an agonist for the estrogen receptor. Proc Natl Acad Sci U S A 94:14138–14143
125. Park SJ, Ahmad F, Philp A, Baar K, Williams T, Luo H, Ke H, Rehmann H, Taussig R, Brown A, Kim MK, Beavewn MA, Burgin AB, Manqaniello V, Chung JH (2012) Resveratrol ameliorates aging-related metabolic phenotypes by inhibiting cAMP phosphodiesterases. Cell 148(3):421–433
126. Hu Y, Liu J, Wang J, Liu Q (2011) The controversial links among calorie restriction. SIRT1 and resveratrol. Free Radic Biol Med 51:250–256

127. Dasgupta B, Milbrandt J (2007) Resveratrol stimulates AMP kinase activity in neurons. Proc Natl Acad Sci U S A 104(17):7217–7222
128. Han S, Choi JR, Soon Shin K, Kang SJ (2012) Resveratrol upregulated heat shock proteins and extended the survival of G93A-SOD1 mice. Brain Res 5(1483):112–117
129. Şahin K, Akdemir F, Orhan C, Tuzcu M, Hayırli A, Şahin N (2010) Effects of dietary resveratrol supplementation on egg production and antioxidant status. Poult Sci 89:1190–1198
130. Chakraborty PK, Mustafi SB, Ganguly S, Chatterjee M, Raha S (2008) Resveratrol induces apoptosis in K562 (chronic myelogenous leukemia) cells by targeting a key survival protein, heat shock protein 70. Cancer Sci 99(6):1109–1116
131. Jakubikova J, Bao Y, Sedlak J (2005) Isothiocyanates induce cell cycle arrest, apoptosis and mitochondrial potential depolarization in HL-60 and multidrug-resistant cell lines. Anticancer Res 25:3375–3386
132. Wu X, Zhou QH, Xu K (2009) Are isothiocyanates potential anti-cancer drugs? Acta Pharmacol Sin 30:501–512
133. Zhang Y, Talalay P (1994) Anticarcinogenic activities of organic isothiocyanates: chemistry and mechanisms. Cancer Res 54(7):1976–1981
134. Moon YJ, Brazeau DA, Morris ME (2011) Dietary phenethyl isothiocyanate alters gene expression in human breast cancer cells. Evid Based Complement Alternat Med. doi:10.1155/2011/462525
135. Priyadarshini K, Keerthi AU (2012) Paclitaxel against cancer: a short review. Med Chem 2(7):139–141
136. Shi P, Wang MM, Jiang LY, Liu HT, Sun JZ (2008) Paclitaxel-doxorubicin sequence is more effective in breast cancer cells with heat shock protein 27 overexpression. Chin Med J (Engl) 121:1975–1979
137. Vydra N, Toma A, Glowala-Kosinska M, Gogler-Piglowska A, Widlak W (2013) Overexpression of heat shock transcription factor 1 enhances the resistance of melanoma cells to doxorubicin and paclitaxel. BMC Cancer 13:504–514
138. Halder B, Pramanik S, Mukhopadyay S, Giri AK (2005) Inhibition of benzo[a]pyrene induced mutagenicity and genotoxicity by black tea polyphenols theaflavins and thearubigins in multiple test systems. Food Chem Toxicol 43:591–597
139. Inoue H, Akiyama S, Maeda-Yamamoto M, Nesumi A, Tanaka T, Murakami A (2011) High-dose green tea polyphenols induce nephrotoxicity in dextran sulfate sodium-induced colitis mice by down-regulation of antioxidant enzymes and heat-shock protein expressions. Cell Stress Chaperones 16(6):653–662
140. Ernst E, Schmidt K, Steuer-Vogt MK (2003) Mistletoe for cancer? A systematic review of randomised clinical trials. Int J Cancer 107:262–267
141. Grossarth-Maticek R, Ziegler R (2007) Prospective controlled cohort studies on long-term therapy of ovarian cancer patients with mistletoe (*Viscum album* L.) extracts iscador. Arzneimittelforschung 57(10):665–678
142. Kienle GS, Kiene H (2010) Influence of *Viscum album* L. (European mistletoe) extracts on quality of life in cancer patients: a systematic review of controlled clinical studies. Integr Cancer Ther 9:142–157
143. Tröger W, Galun D, Reif M, Schumann A, Stankovic N, Milićević M (2013) *Viscum album* [L.] extract therapy in patients with locally advanced or metastatic pancreatic cancer: a randomised clinical trial on overall survival. Eur J Cancer 49(18):3788–3797
144. Fu WM, Zhang JF, Wang H, Xi ZC, Wang WM, Zhuang P, Zhu X, Chen SC, Chan TM, Leung KS, Lu G, Xu HX, Kung HF (2012) Heat shock protein 27 mediates the effect of 1,3,5-trihy droxy-13,13-dimethyl-2H-pyran [7,6-b] xanthone on mitochondrial apoptosis in hepatocellular carcinoma. J Proteomics 75:4833–4843

The Immunobiology of Cancer: From Tumor Escape to Cancer Immunoediting Towards Immunotherapy in Gynecologic Oncology

Maria Luisa Gasparri, Ilary Ruscito, Katayoun Taghavi, Ammad Ahmad Farooqi, Andrea Papadia, Chiara Focaccetti, Vincenzo Barnaba, Pierluigi Benedetti Panici, and Michael D. Mueller

Abstract The immune system is known to play a pivotal role in cancer pathogenesis. In a dynamic balance between immune system and cancer cells, the first one recognizes the second as non-self and effectively clears them from the system. This phenomenon, called *immune surveillance*, is based on the interaction between antigen presenting cells and T lymphocytes that get activated eliciting a specific and enduring response. In certain circumstances, tumor cells are able to evade this mechanism allowing the tumor to develop. This mechanism is called *tumor escape.*

The role of immunotherapy is to restore a balance between immune system and tumor cells by boosting the former. In the past, drugs that work on the immune system in various malignancies have shown striking result, in both response rates and survival, which has led to their FDA approval. The use of these new drugs is currently being investigated with promising results in various other settings, including gynecological malignancies.

M.L. Gasparri, M.D. (✉)
Department of Gynecology and Obstetrics, "Sapienza" University of Rome, Rome, Italy

Department of Gynecology and Obstetrics, University Hospital of Berne, Berne, Switzerland
e-mail: marialuisa.gasparri@uniroma1.it

I. Ruscito • P.B. Panici
Department of Gynecology and Obstetrics, "Sapienza" University of Rome, Rome, Italy

K. Taghavi • A. Papadia • M.D. Mueller
Department of Gynecology and Obstetrics, University Hospital of Berne, Berne, Switzerland

A.A. Farooqi
Laboratory for Translational Oncology and Personalized Medicine, Rashid Latif Medical College, Lahore, Pakistan

C. Focaccetti • V. Barnaba
Laboratory of Cellular and Molecular Immunology, "Sapienza" University of Rome, Rome, Italy

The Laboratory of Proteomics, Department of Internal Medicine, "Sapienza" University of Rome, Rome, Italy

A.A. Farooqi, M. Ismail (eds.), *Molecular Oncology: Underlying Mechanisms and Translational Advancements*, DOI 10.1007/978-3-319-53082-6_9

The definition of immunotherapy encompasses various treatment strategies that include tumor antigen–targeted monoclonal antibodies, immunological checkpoint inhibitors, cytokines, and therapeutic cancer vaccines. These treatments differ as they use distinct mechanisms of actions. However, they all share the fact that their anti-tumor effect is exerted through a boost or a restoration of the immune system.

Owing to its potential to affect mutating cancer cells through the dynamic interplay between cancer and the immune system, immunotherapy offers the potential for durable clinical effects and synergy with subsequent therapies.

Keywords Gynecologic malignancies • Tumor escape • Immuno-editing • Immunotherapy • Monoclonal antibodies • Cancer vaccines • Checkpoint inhibitors • Cytokines

The Basis of Immunity

The main function of the immune system is to protect the body against diseases of both exogenous and endogenous origin. Ideally, it has the ability to identify a variety of threats, distinguishing them from the body's own healthy tissue and eliminate them. This is how the immune system preserves bodily integrity and homeostasis.

The immune system's ability to distinguish between *self* and *non-self* is central to its ability to carry out this task. This is a phenomenon called immune surveillance. Non-self is fundamentally different to self in terms of biochemistry, including the arrangement and make-up of glycoproteins on cells and the composition of DNA. Therefore, even the smallest non-self particles or antigens can be identified and contested. The sequence of steps that takes place to eliminate antigens is known as the immune response.

The first line of immunity, called innate immunity, is effective from the time of birth and present before any exposure to pathogens. This general immunity is composed of physical barriers such as the skin and mucous membranes, as well as physiological parameters such as temperature, pH, and oxygen levels. More complex but still nonspecific in terms of antigen recognition are the phagocytic and cytotoxic cells [1]. Cytokines, or local chemical messengers, are also important in this line of defense as they mediate multiple immune functions [2, 3]. For example, Interleukins 1, 6, and 12 activate macrophages, natural-killer cells, and stimulate the elevation of the body temperature [4, 5]. Interferons work by interfering with DNA and RNA or protein synthesis [6]. The nonspecific immune system quickly recognizes non-self and mounts a generalized attack designed to eliminate the pathogen by undermining its replicative capacity.

If the threat is capable of resisting these initial defenses, the immune system can utilize more specific defenses that generate a targeted response. Acquired immunity develops only after exposure to non-self agents including microbes, toxins, or tumors. Lymphocytes are triggered to develop a very specific response to the target, thereby eliminating the pathogen [7]. Lymphocytes that mature in the thymus are called T cells, which are further classified into T helper and cytotoxic varieties. Lymphocytes that mature in bone marrow are called B cells. Lymphocytes can also be characterized by cell surface markers as well as their specific functions [8].

B cells are known as the antibody factories of the immune system. They also function as antigen-presenting cells (APCs) for the T helper cells. The T helper cells in turn secrete various cytokines to help mediate the reaction. The cytotoxic T cells function to eliminate the pathogens specifically by targeting markers or proteins on target cells, or cells that have been altered by microbial invasion or cancer. Targeted cells then undergo apoptosis (organized cell death) preventing any further pathogenesis.

The important properties of acquired immunity can be described in four stages; specificity, trafficking, adaptability, and memory. The specificity of the immune response refers to the property that ensures that a distinct antigen will elicit a specific response. For example, infection with a virus that causes the common cold triggers a response by a different set of cells than infection with tuberculosis. Trafficking refers to the ability of activated immune cells to mobilize and migrate to specific target sites throughout the body. Adaptability allows the immune system to respond to additional antigens on a pathogen or tumor by a process called antigen spreading. When a tumor-specific T cell initiates lysis of a tumor, additional fragments are taken up by the APCs and this allows the activation of the immune system by additional antigens. The final and main differentiating feature of acquired immunity is the mechanism of immunological memory or the enduring response. This describes the immune response to a threatening molecule that has previously been encountered. It describes the ability of T cells to continue to recognize an antigen over time and mount a faster and heightened response upon re-exposure. This is the mechanism of action in vaccination.

Cancer Pathogenesis

In normal cells, genes regulate growth, maturity, and death of the cells. Cells that are no longer needed or are a threat to the organism are destroyed by a tightly regulated cell suicide process known as programmed cell death, or apoptosis [9]. The fundamental abnormality resulting in the development of cancer is the continual, unregulated proliferation of cancer cells. Rather than responding appropriately to the signals that control normal cell behavior, cancer cells grow and divide in an uncontrolled manner, invading normal tissues and organs and eventually spreading throughout the body [10].

Genetic changes underpin these abnormalities and can occur at many levels. Genome instability and mutations may lead to disturbance of gene expression. The broad categories of genetic mutations involved include the activation of oncogenes (tumor promoter or cancer-causing genes) or inactivation of tumor suppressor genes (these genes normally inhibit cell division and prevent survival of cells that have damaged DNA). Oncogenes may be normal genes that are expressed at inappropriately high levels in patients with cancers or mutations of normal genes. Tumor suppressor genes, on the other hand, can be disabled in patients with cancer. This is caused by cancer-promoting genetic changes. Mutations can lead to a gain or loss of entire chromosomes or a single point mutation affecting a single (important) DNA nucleotide. Typically, changes in many genes are required to transform a normal cell into a cancer cell.

Genetic and cellular changes in turn lead to eight hallmark functions that are commonly described in cancer pathogenesis. They include sustaining proliferative signaling, evading growth suppressors, resisting cell death, enabling replicative immortality, inducing angiogenesis, activating invasion and metastasis, reprogramming of energy metabolism, and evading immune destruction. All these events lead to cancer develop and progression.

Immune Response against Cancer

Cancer cells can also be recognized by the immune system. Although tumor cells are self in origin, their biochemistry and behavior differ from their healthy counterparts [11]. This requires the detection of altered self. Furthermore, it is now understood that tumor growth can be explained in terms of its relationship with the immune system [12]. This interaction is dynamic. Tumor growth can be either blocked or promoted (tumor evasion) by the immune system [13]. The notion of immune control of neoplastic disease was first introduced by Burnet and Thomas in 1964, and is now a concept that is widely acknowledged. Over time, cancer cells develop mechanisms to escape control by the immune system, leading to the progression of disease.

Tumor Escape and Cancer Immunoediting

The regulation of tumor growth represents a dynamic state balanced by immune protection when the immune system is able to eradicate or contain the cancer cells and immune evasion when it is not. This can be simplified to three stages defined by processes of elimination, equilibrium, and escape [14].

Elimination refers to the stage in which cancer cells are identified and effectively eliminated by the immune system. This is generally thought to be the state operating in early and undetectable tumors. The equilibrium phase describes the state when the immune system is not able to eliminate all cancer cells but can control or prevent spread or invasion. This is also thought to be the longest of the three stages and may persist for many years. The escape phase is characterized by the spread of cancer cells. During this stage, the immune system is overloaded and no longer able to contain the growth of cells. It may also be linked to the ability of tumors to actively suppress immunity [15]. It may also result from the acquisition of genetic mutations that suppress the immune system [16].

Rational of the Immunotherapy

Immunotherapy is defined as treatment to enhance or restore the ability of the immune system to fight disease [16]. Reviewing the framework above, it is understood that innate immunity is limited in its contribution to secretion of cytokines that recruit immune cells [17]. On the other hand, the adaptive immune system plays a central role in the antitumor immune response, due to its capacity to process and specifically target non-self cells. Many techniques have been developed through deepened understanding of the interplay between cancer and the immune system. Those demonstrating the most promising results in the medical literature include: vaccination, cytokines, monoclonal antibodies, and checkpoint inhibitors. These treatments all advance immune function in some manner through different mechanisms that are classified according to how they interact with the hosts immunity. Some stimulate an immune response directly against the tumor, for example, as in cancer vaccinations, and this is called active immunotherapy. This line of treatment can result in immunologic memory and have a long-lasting effect. On the other hand, passive immunity works by enhancing a pre-existing immune response, for example, as with monoclonal antibodies and cytokines. These are short lived and require chronic administration to have an effect. They do not generate immunologic memory. These treatments can also be classified as specific versus non-specific. Using this classification, monoclonal antibodies used in immunotherapy produce a specific response to a particular antigen whereas cytokines produce a wide range of antitumor effects and are therefore non-specific.

Immunotherapy is generally associated with a delay in generating an immune response; as such, it may not be associated with an immediate reduction in tumor size or associated tumor markers. However, because of the potential to stimulate immunologic memory, the benefits of sustained immune enhancement, even after treatment is discontinued, may result in significant improvements in survival [4].

Immunotherapy Approaches in Gynecologic Oncology

There have been many advances in immunotherapeutic approaches to gynecologic malignancies in recent years. These breakthroughs come as a result of mutual learning: as immune cells teach researchers more about the intricacies of the immune system and its interplay with cancer cells, researchers are teaching immune cells ways to modulate or optimize their function to more effectively target tumors. The principles of common approaches are cancer vaccines, monoclonal antibodies, cytokines, and checkpoint inhibitors.

The general principle of cancer vaccines is to expose the body to a recombinant protein comprised of a tumor antigen [18–20]. Once exposed, APCs process the antigen and express fragments on their surface for presentation by T cells. This in turn stimulates a T cell driven immune response. An important distinction to note between cancer vaccines and traditional vaccines is that cancer vaccines are designed to treat cancers that already exist in the host. They intend to delay or stop cell growth leading to tumor shrinkage, prolonged remission, or to work synergistically with other treatment modalities. Cancer vaccination trials often aimed to activate CD8(+) cytotoxic T-cell (CTL) responses with short peptides and targeted CD4(+) helper T cells with HLA class II-binding longer peptides that were derived from tumor antigens, furthermore short peptide vaccine is able to activate a specific CD4(+) T-cell repertoire, facilitating a strong combined CD4(+)/CD8(+) T-cell response [21].

Monoclonal antibodies are identical antibodies produced by a single clone of cells. They are designed to target specific sites, such as tumor cells. When bound, they can elicit a direct or indirect immune response that leads to cell death. This can be achieved by the interference of pathways required for tumor growth, blocking angiogenesis, or initiation of an immune mediated cytotoxic response. Now in third phase clinical trials, this method has shown promise for increasing overall survival rates a variety of different cancers.

Cytokines are messenger molecules that mediate immune responses. They have a specific effect on the interactions between cells, on communications between cells, or on the behavior of cells. They enhance the immune response rather than generating a specific antigenic one. These pro-inflammatory cytokines have shown promise in pre-clinical models and partial efficacy in clinical trials of cancer patients.

Checkpoint inhibitors activity is linked to the principle that tumors can actively suppress immunity. Checkpoint blockades prevent this suppression and have been found to significantly enhance anti-cancer immunity. The checkpoint targets that have been tested to date include CTLA4, PD1. These are checkpoint molecules expressed on T lymphocyte cells. Monoclonal anti-bodies have been used to inhibit these checkpoints and to revert a state of immune quiescence tumor induced. Although studies have found promising results using this strategy, the extent of the tumor burden and the suppressive effect of the tumor microenvironment are known to affect its potency [22].

Immunotherapy in Ovarian Cancer

Ovarian cancer is currently the leading cause of death among gynecological malignancies [23]. This tumor is an optimal candidate to study the efficacy of immune activation strategies performed in immunotherapy experimental programs, since this cancer usually shows a short progression free survival, is confined to the peritoneal cavity and paradigmatically represents an immunosuppressive tumor. For this reason, ovarian cancer immunotherapy is a promising approach to be developed in conjunction with conventional treatments, in order to control/eliminate immunosuppressive and immune evasive mechanisms.

Up to now, several immunotherapy approaches have been attempted in ovarian cancer setting [24], mostly adopting peptide- or protein-based vaccinations, oncolytic viruses, anti-idiotypic antibodies, dendritic cells or retargeted lymphocytes, and more recently, checkpoint inhibitors.

Peptide-Based Vaccination

The rationale to vaccine ovarian cancer patients with tumor associate- or tumor specific- peptides is that these molecules, overexpressed or exclusively expressed in cancer tissue, can be recognized by patients' dendritic cells thus eliciting a T-cell specific response against tumor. The advantages of peptide-based vaccines are specificity, stability, a good toxicity profile and the ability to be manufactured to increase their immunogenicity. The major disadvantage is that each peptide contains epitopes which are HLA-restricted (this means that vaccinated patients should express the same HLA, e.g. HLA-A2, in order to experience an immune activation against the peptide). To be immunogenic, manufactured peptides should be administered together with inflammatory substances, which can act as second signal (co-stimulation) to guarantee an effective adaptive immune response towards the vaccine. The pro-inflammatory substances contained in peptide-based vaccines (e.g. KLH or Montanide-ISA) are known as "adjuvants". Up to now, several peptides have been tested in terms of immunogenicity among ovarian cancer patients and the most significant experiences were reported employing peptides derived from Her2/neu, NY-ESO, MAGE-1 and MUC1. In several cases, vaccination with single peptide or multi-peptide mixtures showed the in vivo induction of T cell response specific for other epitopes, a phenomenon known as "epitope spreading". Epitope spreading may occur thanks to the "molecular mimicry".

Oncolytic Viruses

Oncolytic viruses are genetically modified viruses that preferentially infect and kill tumor cells. The mechanisms of action of this immunotherapy approach include the direct lysis of infected cell and the activation of a cancer-specific immune response elicited by epitopes released by destroyed tumor cells. Oncolytic viruses derive their tumor-specific action by binding cancer cell surface receptor or exploiting gene expression aberrations occurring in tumor cells.

Different types of viruses including adenovirus, measles and herpes simplex have been tested as oncolytic agents. In October 2015, the Food and Drug Administration (FDA) approved an oncolytic virus (T-VEC) for the treatment of inoperable melanoma, thus being the first approved oncolytic agent of the western world.

Several clinical trials employing oncolytic viruses administered intraperitoneally have been carried out in ovarian cancer [25]. In most of them the treatment was well tolerated and a considerable percentage of patients showed stable durable disease.

Dendritic Cell-Based Vaccines

Immunotherapy strategies, which employ autologous dendritic cells (DCs), generally provides three distinct clinico-laboratory steps: in the first one, patients' immature dendritic cells are collected from peripheral blood by apheresis; after isolation, DCs maturation and activation is induced ex vivo in presence of tumor lysate or in presence of specific tumor associated antigens; finally, activated DCs pulsed with tumor-specific or tumor associated peptides are re-infused in the patient to present the processed epitopes to naïve T cells, thus stimulating an in vivo T cell-specific anti-tumor response.

Up to now, different clinical trials adopting autologous pulsed DCs as tumor vaccine were carried out on ovarian cancer patients. In most cases, DCs have been pulsed with immunogenic peptides derived from Her2/neu, MUC1, folate-receptor-α, WT1; in other cases DCs have been pulsed with tumor lysate. Encouraging results show that DCs-based vaccinations are more effective in inducing a durable TCD8+ cytotoxic response and a measurable clinical effect compared to peptide-based vaccination [26].

Lymphocytes-Based Vaccines

The administration of lymphocyte-based vaccines to cancer patients is a type of passive immunotherapy due to the fact that autologous T cells, after in vitro incubation with IL2 or other stimulating factors, are re-infused into the patient to be directed against the tumor, thus exerting their killer activity. Some experiences with lymphocyte based vaccine in ovarian cancer patients have been carried out in the middle nineties but, being a passive immunotherapy strategy, their clinical use has been conditioned by the frequent need of re-boosts.

Checkpoint Inhibitors

It has been largely demonstrated that tumors can acquire immune escape mechanisms by exploiting immunosuppressive co-signaling on T cell via programmed cell death 1 (PD-1) and PD-1 ligand 1 (PD-1/PD-L1) and/or via CTLA-4 and B7 (CTLA-4/B7). These two pivotal immune checkpoints have been recently targeted with two monoclonal antibodies, which inhibit the two immune checkpoint systems, thus resulting in a strong aspecific T cell activation against tumor cells. In particular, anti-CTLA-4 antibody (Ipilimumab/Tremelimumab) blocks CTLA-4 binding with B7-1 or B7-2 and inhibits antigen-specific T-cell recognition in the lymph nodes, whereas anti-PD-1 antibody (Nivolumab) and anti-PD-L1 antibody (Atezolizumab) block signaling through PD-1 and the PD-1 ligands (PD-L1 and PD-L2) and inhibit T-cell activation within the tumor microenvironment. After exciting randomized phase III trial showing over 50% in survival benefits, Ipilimumab and Nivolumab are currently standard of care in metastatic melanoma and lung cancer, respectively [27, 28]. In ovarian cancer setting, published phase I/II trials with checkpoint inhibitors evidenced that the clinical responses, although measurable, did not reach the rates reported in melanoma or lung cancer, thus suggesting that there is an urgent need to define patient selection methods based on predictive biomarkers of anti-tumor response in order to maximize the clinical benefit of this novel and very promising immunotherapy strategy in ovarian cancer.

Immunotherapy in Cervical Cancer

Cervical cancer is the fourth neoplasm affecting women worldwide, after breast, lung and colorectal cancer, and the fourth cause of female deaths from tumor [23].

The rational of immunotherapy in cervical cancer is that this malignancy has a viral pathogenesis, being HPV responsible for cell transformation and progression, and viral proteins are non-self components that act as potent inducers of antitumor immune responses. As a consequence, vaccination strategies include mainly HPV E6/E7 long or short peptides-based vaccines, HPV E6/E7 peptides-pulsed autologous dendritic cell-based vaccines and virus or plasmid encoding HPV16/18 E6 and/or E7 proteins.

E6/E7 Protein and Peptides Based Vaccination

In cervical epithelial cells infected by HPV, the combined expression of high-risk HPV E6 and E7 proteins causes inactivation of the pRB and p53 tumor suppressor pathways and induces cell transformation.

Preclinical studies carried out in mice showed that immunotherapy with synthetic peptides derived from HPV 16 E7 protein were capable of eradicating HPV 16+ tumors [29]. In humans, a E6/E7 specific-T cell activation has been elicited with different formulations of E6/E7 short or long peptides in association with adjuvants but a detailed analysis of T cell subpopulations showed that the vaccine is also able to induce immunosuppressive T regulatory cells [30].

Dendritic Cell-Based Vaccines

Limited experiences have been carried out in cervical cancer patients with DCs pulsed with high risk HPV E6 and E7 peptides. Although in some cases an antibody response against E6 and E7 together with E6/E7-specific T cell response has been reported, few clinical responses have been observed.

Checkpoint Inhibitors

In cervical cancer, anti-CTLA4 monoclonal antibody (ipilimumab) treatment after chemoradiation is currently under evaluation in Phase I clinical trial (NCT01711515) in patients with locally advanced or metastatic cervical cancer. Furthermore, other trials are now testing agents directed against the PDL1-PD1 pathway (NCT02257528) in patients with advanced or recurrent cervical and head and neck cancers. In the near future we will be able to establish if checkpoint inhibitors applied to cervical cancer patients are effective in inducing a clinically relevant anti-tumor immune activation.

Immunotherapy in Endometrial Cancer

Endometrial cancer is the most common gynecologic malignancy in developed countries. Although often diagnosed at a low stage disease, the prognosis for patients with advanced stage and high-risk histological subtypes is still poor.

Immunotherapy in endometrial cancer has been largely limited to small series of patients treated with peptide-based vaccine and dendritic cell vaccines. The advent of immune checkpoint inhibitors has recently induced researchers to test these agents also in endometrial cancer. Of particular interest is the observation that approximately 20–30% of endometrial cancers report by high microsatellite instability due to genetic or epigenetic defects in the DNA mismatch repair pathway (associated to Lynch Syndrome, which include increased risk of hereditary endometrial cancer) [31]. Surprisingly, patients affected by mismatch repair defects seems to be more responsive to checkpoint inhibitors, due to the fact that their tumors are characterized by high expression of immune checkpoints. Phase I/II trials of checkpoint inhibitors in endometrial cancer are currently ongoing.

References

1. Candeias SM, Gaipl US (2016) The immune system in cancer prevention, development and therapy. Anticancer Agents Med Chem 16:101–107
2. Dunn GP et al (2005a) Interferon-gamma and cancer immunoediting. Immunol Res 32:231–245
3. Dunn GP et al (2005b) A critical function for type I interferons in cancer immunoediting. Nat Immunol 6:722–729
4. Smyth MJ, Taniguchi M, Street SE (2000) The anti-tumor activity of IL-12: mechanisms of innate immunity that are model and dose dependent. J Immunol 165:2665–2670
5. Street SE et al (2002) Suppression of lymphoma and epithelial malignancies effected by interferon gamma. J Exp Med 196:129–134
6. Shankaran V et al (2001) IFNgamma and lymphocytes prevent primary tumour development and shape tumour immunogenicity. Nature 410:1107–1111
7. Smyth MJ, Dunn GP, Schreiber RD (2006) Cancer immunosurveillance and immunoediting: the roles of immunity in suppressing tumor development and shaping tumor immunogenicity. Adv Immunol 90:1–50
8. Dunn GP, Koebel CM, Schreiber RD (2006) Interferons, immunity and cancer immunoediting. Nat Rev Immunol 6:836–848
9. Finn OJ (2008) Cancer immunology. N Engl J Med 358:2704–2715
10. Dunn GP et al (2002) Cancer immunoediting: from immunosurveillance to tumor escape. Nat Immunol 3:991–998
11. Schreiber RD, Old LJ, Smyth MJ (2011) Cancer immunoediting: integrating immunity's roles in cancer suppression and promotion. Science 331:1565–1570
12. Page DB et al (2014) Immune modulation in cancer with antibodies. Annu Rev Med 65:185–202
13. Zitvogel L, Tesniere A, Kroemer G (2006) Cancer despite immunosurveillance: immunoselection and immunosubversion. Nat Rev Immunol 6:715–727
14. Dunn GP, Old LJ, Schreiber RD (2004) The three Es of cancer immunoediting. Annu Rev Immunol 22:329–360
15. Gravitz L (2013) Cancer immunotherapy. Nature 504:S1
16. Lizee G et al (2013) Harnessing the power of the immune system to target cancer. Annu Rev Med 64:71–90
17. De Felice F et al (2015) Immunotherapy of ovarian cancer: the role of checkpoint inhibitors. J Immunol Res 191832
18. De Vries J, Figdor C (2016) Immunotherapy: cancer vaccine triggers antiviral-type defences. Nature 534:329–331
19. Kepp O, Senovilla L, Vitale I, Vacchelli E, Adjemian S, Agostinis P, Apetoh L, Aranda F, Barnaba V et al (2014) Consensus guidelines for the detection of immunogenic cell death. Oncoimmunology 3
20. Palombo F, Focaccetti C, Barnaba V (2014) Therapeutic implications of immunogenic cell death in human cancer. Front Immunol 4:503
21. Gross S, Lennerz V, Gallerani E, Mach N, Böhm S, Hess D, von Boehmer L, Knuth A, Ochsenbein A, Gnad-Vogt U, Forssmann U, Woelfel T, Kaempgen E (2016) Short peptide vaccine induces CD4+ T helper cells in patients with different solid cancers cancer. Immunol Res 4:18–25
22. Pardoll DM (2012) The blockade of immune checkpoints in cancer immunotherapy. Nat Rev Cancer 12:252–264
23. Torre LA et al (2015) Global cancer statistics 2012. CA Cancer J Clin 65:87–108
24. Bellati F, Napoletano C, Ruscito I, Visconti V, Antonilli M, Gasparri ML, Zizzari IG, Rahimi H, Palaia I, Rughetti A, Benedetti Panici P, Nuti M (2013) Past, present and future strategies of immunotherapy in gynecological malignancies. Curr Mol Med 13:1–22

25. Galanis E et al (2010) Phase I trial of intraperitoneal administration of an oncolytic measles virus strain engineered to express carcinoembryonic antigen for recurrent ovarian cancer. Cancer Res 70:875–882
26. Coosemans A et al (2013) Dendritic cell-based immunotherapy in ovarian cancer. Oncoimmunology. 2:e27059
27. Brahmer J et al (2015) Nivolumab versus docetaxel in advanced squamous-cell non–small-cell lung cancer. N Engl J Med 373:123–135
28. Hodi FS et al (2010) Improved survival with ipilimumab in patients with metastatic melanoma. N Engl J Med 363:711–723
29. Zwaveling S et al (2001) Established human papillomavirus type 16-expressing tumors are effectively eradicated following vaccination with long peptide. J Immunol 69:350–358
30. Welters MJ et al (2008) Induction of tumor-specific CD4+ and CD8+ T-cell immunity in cervical cancer patients by a human papillomavirus type 16 E6 and E7 long peptides vaccine. Clin Cancer Res 14:178–187
31. Howitt BE et al (2015) Association of polymerase e-mutated and microsatellite-instable endometrial cancers with neoantigen load, number of tumor-infiltrating lymphocytes, and expression of PD-1 and PD-L1. JAMA Oncol 1:1319–1323

Investigation of Androgen Receptor Signaling Pathways with Epigenetic Machinery in Prostate Cancer

Ken-ichi Takayama and Satoshi Inoue

Abstract Androgen receptor (AR) is a ligand-dependent transcription factor reportedly involved in regulation of wide ranging target genes. Rapidly emerging experimental evidence has provided detailed information related to 3D crystal structures of the ligand binding domain (LBD) and DNA binding domain (DBD) of AR.

Targeting of AR induced signaling cascade is assumed to be effective for treating castration-resistant prostate cancer (CRPC), which possesses resistance to the general anti-androgen therapy. The aggressiveness of cancer cells is induced by the interplay of multiple signal pathways, transcription factors and epigenetic machinery. To investigate how AR modulates transcriptional networks in prostate cancer cells, global analyses determining AR binding sites and androgen-regulated transcripts including coding and non-coding genes have been performed. In addition, diverse regulations of epigenetics such as histone modification and DNA methylation were found to be linked with the activation and repression of enhancers and promoters with AR recruitments. These regulatory mechanisms are interconnected strongly and regulate the gene expression in prostate cancer cells. In recent studies, many androgen-regulated genes have been shown to have important roles in the development of prostate cancer and clinical relevance as new biomarkers and therapy targets. In this chapter, we highlight those epigenetic mechanisms for AR activation by various factors, especially long non-coding RNA (lncRNA) and microRNA (miRNA). We also describe the molecular mechanism through which AR downstream signals induce tumor growth and inhibit apoptosis for developing CRPC.

Keywords Androgen receptor • Prostate cancer • Epigenetic regulation • lncRNA • Non-coding RNA • miRNA

K.-i. Takayama
Department of Functional Biogerontology, Tokyo Metropolitan Institute of Gerontology, 35-2 Sakae-cho, Itabashi-ku, Tokyo 173-0015, Japan

S. Inoue (✉)
Department of Functional Biogerontology, Tokyo Metropolitan Institute of Gerontology, 35-2 Sakae-cho, Itabashi-ku, Tokyo 173-0015, Japan

Division of Gene Regulation and Signal Transduction, Research Center for Genomic Medicine, Saitama Medical University, Hidaka, Saitama 350-1241, Japan
e-mail: sinoue@tmig.or.jp

A.A. Farooqi, M. Ismail (eds.), *Molecular Oncology: Underlying Mechanisms and Translational Advancements*, DOI 10.1007/978-3-319-53082-6_10

Molecular Mechanisms of Androgen Receptor (AR)

AR has an important role in androgen signaling in prostate by functioning as a nuclear receptor [1, 2]. Nuclear receptors including AR have multiple domains called DNA binding domain, a ligand-binding domain (LBD), and an N-terminal domain (NTD) [3–5]. In the NTD, the transcriptional activation function 1 (AF1) domain promotes transcriptional activation with or without ligand binding [6–8], which is associated with enhanced AR function in aggressive prostate cancer. In the LBD, the binding of androgen hormone to AR is promoted. Testosterone is the most abundant circulating androgen (~90%) produced in the testes. 5α-reductase converts testosterone to dihydrotestosterone (DHT), which binds to the receptor more tightly [9] in prostate cells. AF2 domain in the LBD interacts with co-regulators with LXXLL motif [10]. Point mutations mapped to the LBD have been identified to have relevance with the treatment-resistance to drugs targeting AR [11–13].

In the absence of hormone, AR forms a complex with the heat shock protein (Hsp) family that functions as molecular chaperones and co-chaperone and AR localizes in the cytoplasm. By binding to androgen, a conformational change of AR-Hsp complex is induced and then AR can translocate to the nucleus. In the nucleus, AR recognizes and binds to the genomic regions including sequence motifs called androgen responsive elements (AREs) as a dimer. Most of AR binding sites (ARBSs) have been identified in the promoter/enhancer regions of target genes [14]. AR regulates the epigenetic condition of ARBSs and promotes enhancer activity (Fig. 1a) [15].

Hormone therapy is a first-line and useful strategy for treating advanced prostate cancer. Blocking AR activity by castration or using antagonists of AR elicits a favorable response. However, most of these tumors relapse and progress to hormone therapy resistant prostate cancer (HRPC) or CRPC due to enhanced AR downstream signals caused by aberrant activation of AR variants (particularly AR-Vs), hypersensitivity to androgens, overexpression of AR or intratumoral steroidogenesis [16–19]. AR mRNA is alternatively spliced to AR-Vs and results in prematurely termination of the full AR protein. Most AR-Vs are missing LBD, however, retain the NTD to drive transcription androgen-independently. Among these variants, AR-V7 is expressed in HRPC/CRPCs most frequently and could be the therapeutic target of tumors resistant to existing therapies directed to androgen/AR [20, 21]. Thus, it is critical to investigate AR downstream-signaling or regulatory mechanisms by AR to understand how CRPC develop among the patients [22].

Studying AR Downstream Signals with High-Throughput Methods

The new technology rapidly developed for detecting transcription factor binding sites has changed the studies in the research field of nuclear receptors. Chromatin immunoprecipitation (ChIP) analysis is the basis for these technologies. In ChIP

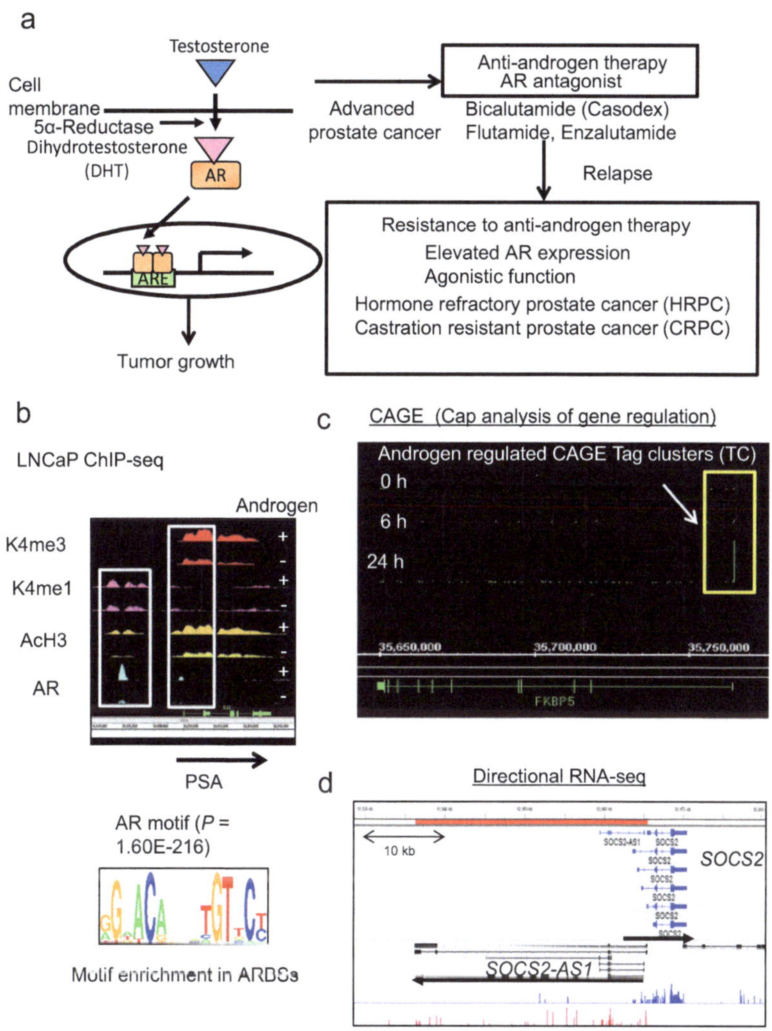

Fig. 1 Investigation of AR dependent transcriptional network. (**a**) Action of AR for prostate cancer progression. (**b**) ChIP-seq analysis of AR and histone modification. Histone H3 lysine 4 (H3K4) methylation (H3K4me1, H3K4me3) and histone H3 acetylation were analyzed. *Prostate specific antigen (PSA)* is the representative AR target gene. AR motif was highly enriched within ARBSs. (**c**) Cap analysis of gene expression (CAGE) and directional RNA-seq were performed for identifying comprehensive androgen-mediated transcripts. *FKBP5*, *SOCS2* and *SOCS2-AS1* are androgen regulated genes. (**d**) Directional RNA-seq for SOCS2-SOCS2-AS1 region

experiment, cells are fixed by formaldehyde treatment to strengthen the protein and chromatin associations before lysis and then chromatin is segmented by ultrasound. An antibody which is specific to the transcription factors of interest is added for immunoprecipitation. DNA obtained by ChIP contains enriched transcription factor binding regions.

A combined analysis using ChIP samples and genome tiling array (chip) have been developed to analyze a comprehensive transcription factor binding sites. We performed ChIP-chip analysis by small types of genome tiling array, the ENCODE array containing 1% of human genome and the array containing chromosome 21 and 22 sequences [23, 24] in AR positive prostate cancer LNCaP cells. We validated ARBSs identified by these studies and found AR-target genes including cadherin-2 (*CDH2*) and amyloid precursor protein (APP). By exploring the function and clinical significance in prostate cancer, we identified APP is correlated with prostate cancer progression. Another study [25] analyzed AR-dependent signals in a CRPC cell model, LNCaP-abl cells which was established from LNCaP cells. They found that AR is involved in CRPC development by activating of cell cycle related genes, mainly mitotic phase related gene expressions.

Next, ChIP-sequence (ChIP-seq) analyses using next-generation sequencers have been developed as a high-throughput strategy to identify transcription factor binding regions (Fig. 1b) [26]. In the regions in which probes could not be prepared, it was impossible to find binding sites by ChIP-chip. However, ChIP-seq could detect unbiased binding regions because sequencing whole genome. For instance, AR ChIP-seq was performed in two LNCaP-derived prostate cancer cell lines with higher AR expression [27]. Interestingly, more ARBSs were obtained in these cell lines when they were treated with low concentrations of androgen. Moreover, the strength of AR binding is also associated with AR expression level. These data indicate that the higher expression of AR sensitizes the receptor binding to genome, thus illustrating the mechanism that the AR signaling pathway is enhanced in CRPC. Furthermore, binding sites of AR-associated transcription partners such as forkhead box protein A1 (FOXA1) [28], GATA2 [29], Oct1 [30], RUNX1 [31, 32] and NKX3-1 [28] have been mapped to the prostate cancer genome and these studies suggested the global role of these factor to activate AR-driven transcriptional program.

Integrative Analysis to Identify Global Signals Regulated by Androgen

Sequencing method is also used to analyze the transcriptome and epigenetic condition of prostate cancer cells. Although microarray analysis detects only the gene expression levels binding to probes, sequence analysis can determine the unbiased expression profiles. Cap analysis of gene expression (CAGE) analysis can reveal the gene expression and promoter usage by identifying transcription start sites (TSS) using high throughput technique [33] (Fig. 1c). The initial 20 nucleotides at the 5′ ends of mRNAs were cleaved and ligated for sequencing in CAGE study. The frequency of CAGE tags is positively associated with results in other analyses using microarray. Therefore, CAGE analysis was performed to determine all androgen-regulated transcripts. We combined the result with that of ChIP-chip analysis which identified global ARBSs and activated histone marker (acetylated histone H3) in prostate cancer cells [34]. This integrated high-throughput analyses presented useful information to explain the AR-mediated transcriptional program that accelerates the progression of prostate cancer. In CAGE study, 13,110 significant androgen-regulated TSSs (10 nM R1881 treatment for 24 h) were identified. By referencing the publicly available gene expression data in clinical prostate cancer samples, we demonstrated that many androgen-induced genes with ARBSs and CAGE tag clusters in the adjacent regions were activated signals in prostate cancer cells.

Recent analysis by sequencing human genome revealed that more than 90% is actively transcribed [35]. Interestingly, the non-coding RNAs (ncRNAs) occupy the majority of such expressed transcripts and only 2% of these transcripts are protein-coding genes [36]. Generally we classify ncRNAs into long (>200 nt) and short (<200 nt) transcripts [37]. Our CAGE analysis also found that both short RNAs including miRNA and long non-coding RNA (lncRNAs) were included in AR-targeted transcripts. In addition, we also performed a comprehensive sequence study of mRNAs, directional RNA-sequence analysis (Fig. 1d), to investigate androgen-regulated transcripts in AR-positive prostate cancer cell lines and castration-resistant model cells derived from them. This study revealed comprehensive androgen-regulated coding and non-coding RNAs and important molecules activated in CRPC. In addition, by combining this result with ARBSs, co-regulator recruitments and histone modification patterns obtained by ChIP-seq. AR-mediated regulation of these downstream signals could be visualized. We showed androgen-dependent transcripts expressed widely in the genome including the antisense (AS) regions of protein-coding genes [34, 38]. Interestingly, several pairs of sense/antisense transcripts regulated by androgen were newly identified, indicating AS non-coding RNA and sense protein-coding genes have a role of mutual transcriptional regulation.

Epigenetic Regulations by Androgen-Mediated miRNAs

DNA, histones and other chromatin proteins formed chromatin as a highly ordered structure. Histones form a unit called the nucleosome consisting of a histone octamer (H2A, H2B, H3 and H4, two pairs of each) around which DNA is wrapped for a tight DNA packaging in all eukaryotic cells. Conformational changes of the chromatin induce the rapid and reversible regulation of gene expression and subsequent biological events such as hormone action without altering genomic sequences. This process is called epigenetic control and is promoted by post-translational modifications of histone tails and DNA modifications [39–41].

DNA methylation is the representative epigenetic mark adding a methyl group to the 5′ position of cytosine (5-mC). DNA methylation is added or removed in a spatially and temporally defined context throughout the genome including enhancer or non-CpG regions. DNA methyltransferases (DNMTs) is responsible for the process as enzymes. DNMTs include DNMT3A/DNMT3B for de novo and DNMT1 for maintenance of methylation [42]. The ten-eleven translocation (TET) family proteins catalyzed the production of 5-hydroxymethylcytosine (5-hmC), an oxidation product of 5-mC [43]. Several studies have demonstrated that 5-hmC is not only an intermediate product of a demethylation process, but can also act as an epigenetic mark stably. Recently several studies have shown that TET-mediated 5-hmC production regulates the activity of these elements and 5-hmC modifications can be highly enriched at poised and active enhancers [44].

miRNA, a class of short ncRNAs, plays important roles in gene expression by post-transcriptionally modifying targeted mRNA [45]. Generally miRNAs binds to the 3′ untranslated region (UTR) of mRNAs to inhibit their translation. Dysregulation of miRNA expression profiles during the progression of prostate cancer have been discussed. For examples, miR-21, miR-29a/b, miR-32, miR-99a, miR-148a, miR-125b and miR-141 were found to be androgen-regulated miRNAs ([46], Table 1). Recent studies have shown that these miRNA expressions have critical meanings in prostate cancer biology. Upregulated miR-21 enhanced AR-dependent cell proliferation and associated with development of CRPC [56, 57]. The miR-21 repressed the expression level of MARCKS (myristoylated alanine rich protein kinase C substrate), which modulates cell motility [51], BTG2 (B-cell translocation gene 2) and PTEN [52]. Another androgen regulated miRNA, miR-125b targets apoptosis inducing factors regulated by p53 (PUMA and BAK1) [49]. Thus, by repressing these genes, overexpression of miR-125b in tumors collapses the balance between pro- and anti-apoptotic processes. We have reported that miR-148a is also regulated by androgen and highly induced in AR positive prostate cancer cells. We showed that miR-148a targetscullin-associated and neddylation dissociated 1 (CAND1), a cell cycle regulator, to promote cell proliferation [48]. Moreover, miR-32 inhibits apoptosis by targeting BIM, a pro-apoptotic member of the BCL2 family [55, 58]. Both miR-32 and miR-148a were overexpressed in CRPC tissues, indicating that these miRNAs have important roles in the promotion of castration-resistance [55].

We have demonstrated that miR-29 family and miR-22 are highly induced by androgen in bicalutamide (anti-androgen drug)-resistant prostate cancer cells that we established from LNCaP cells. The roles of miR-29 family in cancer are still

Table 1 Summary of androgen-regulated miRNAs in prostate cancer (Reviewed in [46])

miRNA	Mechanism/signaling pathway	Target genes
miR-141	Cell proliferation/AR activation	Small heterodimer partner (Shp) [47]
miR-148a	Cell proliferation/Cell cycle	CAND1 [48]
miR-29a/b, miR-22	Epigenetic	TET2 [31, 32]
miR-125b	Anti-apoptosis	BAK1 [49]
miR-99a	Growth inhibition	PSA mTOR [50]
miR-21	Cell proliferation	MARCKS [51], BTG2, PTEN [52], PDCD4 [53]
miR-221	CRPC development	HECTD2 RAB1A [54]
miR-32	Cell proliferation	BIM BTG2 [55]

controversial because their expressions are reduced in several cancer tissues in comparison with normal [59, 60]. However, it was reported that they promote breast cancer metastasis [61–63] and enhance hepatoma cell migration [64]. Additionally, their overexpression inhibits apoptosis in lung cancer as oncogenic miRNAs [65]. In prostate cancer our analysis using clinical samples revealed that the expression level of miR-29a/b is negatively associated with that of TET2. Importantly, our in situ hybridization (ISH) study indicated that miR-29a/b is highly expressed in a subset of prostate cancers with poor prognoses. In vitro, miR-29a/b upregulates cell motility and cell cycle-associated genes and enhanced cell proliferation and migration of hormone-refractory prostate cancer cells. Moreover, inhibition of miR-29a/b expression increased TET2 expression level and retarded hormone-refractory prostate cancer cell growth. We further demonstrated that miR-29a/b promotes tumor growth using several in vivo hormone-refractory prostate cancer models. Mechanistically TET2 repression decreased 5-hmC levels and enhanced FOXA1 transcriptional activity. FOXA1 activation induced expressions of prostate cancer related genes. We found that one of such 5-hmC regulated gene was mammalian target of rapamycin (mTOR) (Fig. 2). Our experimental and clinical data suggested a novel oncogenic role of miR-29 family in prostate cancer progression [31, 32]. In addition to androgen-signaling, exome sequencing analysis revealed that somatic mutations of TET2 exon are involved in metastatic CRPC development [66]. Rare variation in TET2 is also associated with the development of prostate cancer [67]. Thus, the role of TET2 and 5-hmC modification in prostate cancer deserves additional analysis and may define a subset of metastatic disease.

Targeting Histone Modification by AR for Treating CRPC

In addition to DNA methylation, histone modification patterns have also been investigated in prostate cancer. Histone modifications affect the interaction of DNA with histones, transcription factors or other proteins binding to DNA, thus playing a role in the epigenetic control of biological events. Lysine, arginine, serine and threonine residues enriched in N-terminal histone tails serve as substrates for post-translational modifications such as acetylation, phosphorylation, methylation, ubiquitination, sumoylation and deamination. Histone H3, one of the major histones, is most important for epigenetic regulation. The methylation of lysine on position 9 (H3K9) and H3K27 is an epigenetic mark of condensed chromatin and silent loci, while the methylation of H3K4 and H3K36 is generally correlated with open chromatin structures. Acetylation of lysine residues of H3 is also associated with activated enhancer and promoter. Alterations in these modifications induce carious pathological conditions [68]. AR is involved in the modification changes ligand dependently by interacting with many co-regulators including various histone-modifying enzymes (Fig. 3) [69].

Methylations of H3K4 (mono-, di- or tri-methylation) indicate the active promoter or enhancer regions and promoted by the SET1/MLL histone methyltransfer-

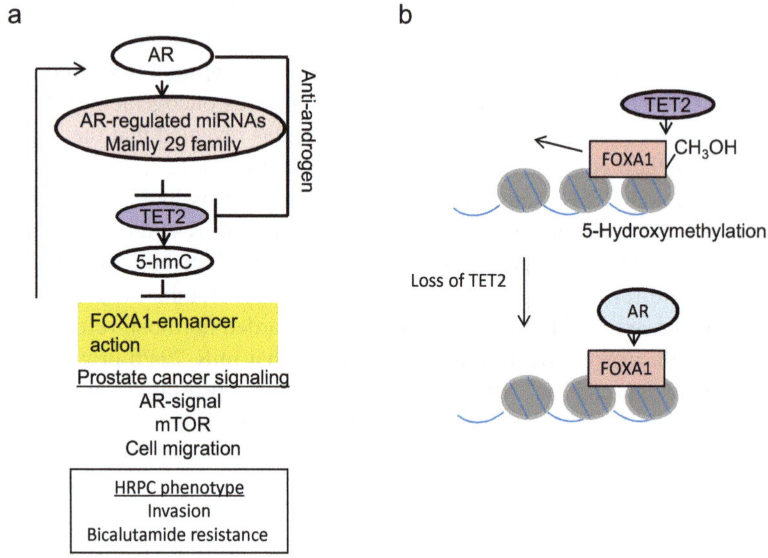

Fig. 2 Androgen induced miRNA-mediated repression of DNA 5-hydroxymethylated cytosine (5-hmC). (**a**) Androgen-induced miRNA mediated TET2 repression inhibits 5-hmC modifications in FOXA1 occupied enhancer regions. (**b**) By removal of 5-hmC, FOXA1 is activated and induce cancer-associated genes such as *mTOR* or androgen-regulated genes

ase (HMTase) complex [70]. MLL complex plays an important role for androgen-mediated gene induction and its activity is regulated finely. After androgen stimulation, protein kinase C-related kinase 1 (PRK1) promotes histone H3 threonine 11 phosphorylation (H3T11P) [71]. Protein kinase C beta 1 (PKCβ1) phosphorylates histone H3T6 prevents lysine specific demethylase including lysine-specific demethylase 1 (LSD1) from histone H3K4 demethylation [72]. Furthermore, PRK1 kinase activity facilitates demethylation of H3K9 by cooperating with LSD1 [71]. WD repeat containing protein 5 (WDR5), a subunit of the SET1/MLL complex, associates with H3T11P and then promotes the recruitment of the MLL complex for H3K4 tri-methylation (H3K4me3) in ARBSs [73]. Thus, WDR5 is a critical epigenetic integrator and is overexpressed in prostate cancers. In addition, menin protein binding to the N-terminus of MLL is important for MLL target gene expressions. Menin directly binds to AR and recruited MLL complex. Menin is highly expressed in CRPC tissues and associated with castration-resistant tumor growth [74]. Importantly, small molecule inhibitors against menin-MLL interaction could be the new useful drug for CRPC.

Histone modification is also important for increased AR expression in CRPC [75]. To introns of the *AR* gene, recruitments of AR and its associated cofactors such as LSD1, which represses transcription by inhibiting histone H3K4 methylation are induced by androgen. This feedback loop mechanism regulates AR expression negatively by androgen. Interestingly, after long-term incubation in castration level of

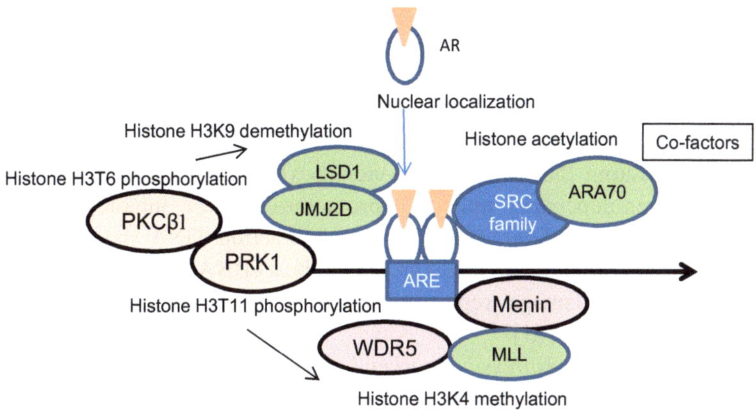

Fig. 3 The mechanisms of AR-dependent histone modification. Upon androgen treatment, several histone modifying enzymes were recruited to AR binding sites. H3T6 phosphorylation directs LSD1 for not H3K4 but H3K9 demethylation, cooperating with JMJ2D. H3T11 phosphorylation also accelerates LSD1 function and WDR5-mediated MLL recruitments. MLL complex associates with AR through menin and promotes histone H3K4 methylation for activating AR dependent gene expression. SRC family or ARA70 are AR interacting cofactors for histone acetylation

androgens, AR expression increases in prostate cancer cells and then low levels of androgens can activate AR regulated genes in CRPC without repressing genes such as the *AR* itself.

LncRNAs Are Regulated by Androgen for Prostate Cancer Progression

Various types of lncRNAs are transcribed widely in the human genome [76]. According to GENCODE v19, there are 13,870 genes which produce 23,898 lncRNAs. LncRNAs have biogenesis and structure similar to mRNAs and are polyadenylated. They function in either nucleus or cytoplasm and their aberrant expressions are associated with many human diseases such as cancer [77–79].

Global nuclear run-on sequencing (GRO-seq) was developed as a new technology to detect androgen-mediated sequential gene expression changes [62, 63]. First, androgen-treated cell nuclei are isolated for nuclear run-on reactions. RNA polymerases run on about 100 bases in the presence of a ribonucleotide analog (5-bromouridine 5′-triphosphate [BrUTP]) in the run-on step. Next, BrU-containing RNA is collected by immunoprecipitation using an antibody recognizing the nucleotide analog. By using the purified RNA, a cDNA library is prepared for sequencing. It was shown that the production of enhancer-templated non-coding RNAs (eRNAs) important for nucleosome remodeling to induce enhancer/promoter interaction by looping and gene activation. It was also observed that androgen promotes both transcriptional initiation and elongation. By combining GRO-seq data with the AR and FOXA1ChIP-seq, a large repository of active enhancers tuned dynamically to alternate gene expression network underlie sequential gene expression changes in prostate cancer. AR is widely recruited to these eRNA-bound enhancer- promoter regions for activating the genes in the vicinity (Fig. 4b). Knockdown of eRNA inhibits androgen-dependent enhancer promoter-enhancer interaction [80]. To explain the mechanism of enhancer promoter interaction, DNA nicking activity of topoisomerase I (TOP1) was found to produce robust eRNA for enhancer activation. Furthermore, DNA damage repair machinery is recruited kinetically to the AR-regulated enhancers [81].

Prostate cancer gene expression marker 1 (PCGEM1) was originally found as an androgen-regulated and prostate tissue-specific lncRNA [82]. Overexpression of *PCGEM1* in prostate tumors were observed and associated with the anti-apoptotic activity by inhibiting p53 and p21 induction [83]. *Prostate cancer noncoding RNA 1 (PRNCR1)* was identified by investigating the surrounding region of SNPs (single nucleotide polymorphisms) correlated with prostate cancer susceptibility. Importantly, both *PCGEM1* and *PRNCR1* cooperatively functions for AR-mediated gene regulation [84]. The associations of PCGEM1 and PRNCR1 with AR were confirmed as the mechanism of AR activation. Moreover, PCGEM1 was found to interact with pygopus homolog2 (Pygo2) and PRNCR1 with DOT1-like histone H3 methyltransferase (DOT1L). By modulating AR proteins with such interacted enzymes, these two lncRNAs were shown to be responsible for AR-associated loop formation between enhancer and promoter (Fig. 4b). Reduction of these lncRNA expressions inhibits CRPC xenograft tumor growth in vivo. However, the roles of these two lncRNAs are still controversial [85].

Steroid receptor RNA activator (SRA) modulate the functions of various nuclear receptors, such as AR, estrogen receptor (ER), progesterone receptor (PR), glucocorticoid receptor (GR) and thyroid hormone receptor (TR). *SRA* associates with a coactivator SRC-1 (steroid receptor coactivator) and six stem-loop motifs in *SRA* are required for co-activation [86, 87]. Interestingly, overexpression of *SRA* was found in various tumors. In various tumors including prostate cancer, *SRA* expression is upregulated compared with normal tissues.

HOX Antisense Intergenic RNA (HOTAIR) is a lncRNA transcribed in the antisense direction from the HOXC gene cluster. *HOTAIR* expression is correlated with the disease progressions of breast and prostate cancer [88, 89]. *HOTAIR* high expressions in these cancers are correlated with poor prognosis. This finding reflects the regulation of steroid hormone function by *HOTAIR*. Although the estrogen-mediated induction of *HOTAIR* is still controversial [90, 91], *HOTAIR* increased ER protein level and promote estrogen-induced signaling [91]. In addition, *HOTAIR* is negatively regulated by androgen treatment and induced by depleting androgen. *HOTAIR* block the association of E3-ubiquitine ligase MDM2 with AR by binding to AR to stabilize AR protein level and activate the androgen receptor mediated transcription for driving CRPC development [89].

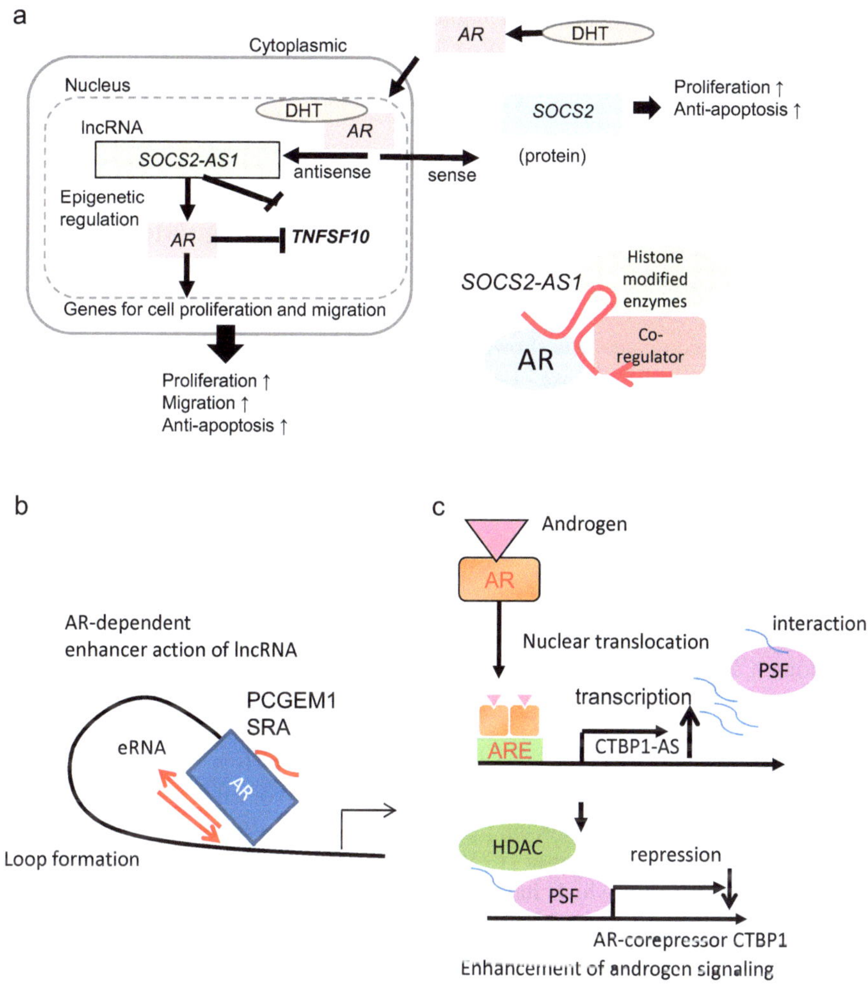

Fig. 4 The role of lncRNA in AR signaling. (**a**) The role of *SOCS2-AS1*, our newly identified androgen-regulated lncRNA, in prostate cancer progression. *SOCS2-AS1* interacts with AR for cofactor recruitments and epigenetic regulation. (**b**) The role of eRNA or other AR interacting lncRNA. These lncRNAs promotes loop formation for promoter/enhancer interaction. (**c**) Epigenetic regulation by androgen-regulated lncRNA, *CTBP1-AS*, which interacts with RNA-binding protein, PSF. This complex binds to and deacetylates specific gene promoters for prostate cancer progression

Suppressor of cytokine signaling 2-antisense transcript 1 (*SOCS2-AS1*) was found in our directional RNA-seq and ChIP-seq analysis (Fig. 4a) [38]. *SOCS2-AS1* is highly expressed in castration-resistant model cells and promotes cell proliferation and inhibits apoptosis induced by docetaxel. *SOCS2-AS1* repressed apoptosis-related genes such as TNFSF10/TRAIL [92], which is an AR target genes. For molecular mechanism in this gene regulation, we found *SOCS2-AS1* is involved with AR activation by promoting coregulatory recruitments to ARBSs. Interaction of AR with *SOCS2-AS1* was observed by our RIP-analysis.

Trans-Regulatory Mechanism for Epigenetic and Transcriptional Regulation by Androgen-Regulated lncRNAs

Global transcriptome analysis showed that most of the genome can be transcribed from both sense and antisense strands. More than 1000 pairs of sense/antisense transcripts were obtained and antisense transcription is involved in such bidirectional gene regulation [93–96]. Sense-transcript is regulated by antisense through several mechanisms. For example, post-transcriptional degradation is caused by antisense transcript. Another mechanism is recruitments of antisense RNA associated transcription factors for epigenetic regulation.

In prostate cancer, lncRNA, Prostate cancer antigen 3 (*PCA3),* was found to be an overexpressed in prostate cancer tissues. In 95% of the prostate tumors, the expression of *PCA3* is upregulated compared with adjacent normal prostate tissues. In addition, *PCA3* RNA levels can also be measured by urinary test more specifically than prostate specific antigen (PSA) measurement [97]. Therefore, it can be a helpful biomarker to diagnose prostate cancer [98]. *PCA3* functions as an oncogenic lncRNA by inhibiting its overlapped gene PRUNE2, which is a tumor suppressor gene. PCA3 represses PRUNE2 expression by formation of a double-stranded RNA with PRUNE2 mRNA for reducing post transcriptionally [99].

The *cyclin dependent kinase (CDKN) 2B antisense RNA1 (CDKN2B-AS1)* is an antisense lncRNA, which harbors the CDK inhibitors, *CDKN2A/CDKN2B.* These CDK inhibitors functions as tumor suppressor genes by regulating cell cycles. Dimethylation of H3K9 and demethylation of H3K4 at the gene promoter are promoted by this lncRNA [96]. Thus, the transcription of CDKN2B is specifically repressed by this antisense RNA forming heterochromatin. *ANRIL (antisense noncoding RNA in the INK4 locus)* and chromobox7 (CBX7), a member of Polycomb repressive complex 1 (PRC1) are upregulated in prostate cancer. Histone H3K27 methylation at the promoter regions of CDKN2A/2B are observed by CBX7/ANRIL complex recruitments to these regions [100]. *HOTAIR* associates with the polycomb repressive complex 2 (PRC2) for acting as a transcriptional regulators *in trans*. PRC2 is recruited to the *HOXD* locus HOTAIR dependently, leading to silenced transcription across a 40-kb region. Moreover, *HOTAIR* associates with LSD1/CoREST/REST complex. This interaction coupled PRC2 and LSD1 to induce histone H3K27 methylation and K4 demethylation for gene silencing [101]. Thus, LncRNAs interacts with chromatin remodeling complexes to promote heterochromatin formation in specific loci, resulting in reduced target gene expression.

By CAGE analysis, we identified a new androgen-responsive lncRNA, *CTBP1-AS* (Fig. 4c) [14]. We found that C-terminal binding protein 1 (CTBP1) [102] functions as a transcriptional repressor for AR and negatively regulates AR downstream signals. *CTBP1-AS* is demonstrated to be induced by AR binding to its promoter region. In addition, *CTBP1-AS* associates with a RNA binding protein, PSF (PTB-associated splicing factor) to transcriptionally repress its target genes via histone deacetylation [103, 104]. We demonstrated that *CTBP1-AS* and PSF repressed cell cycle associated genes such as p53 or SMAD3 and AR-downstream signals. Tumor growth of CRPC models in vivo was inhibited by knocking down *CTBP1-AS*.

These analyses of lncRNA functions revealed a novel transcriptional regulatory mechanism by AR. Several lncRNAs such as *SRA, SOCS2-AS1, PCGEM1 and PRNCR1* associate with AR and promote recruitment of cofactors. Other mechanisms contain loop forming between promoter and enhancer (eRNA, *PCGEM1* and *PRNCR1*) or enhancing AR protein stability (*HOTAIR*) to activate AR action. Regulation of genes related with cancer development or cell cycle controls by interacting with RNA-binding transcriptional repressor (*CTBP1-AS*) would be another mechanism to promote cancer progression. Because only a limited number of lncRNA functions have been demonstrated, we should investigate molecular functions of more lncRNAs in tissue and spatial specific manner in the future.

Summary

Over the recent past years, the massive utilization of biological techniques and functional genomics increased dramatically our knowledge on the regulatory networks of AR and other nuclear receptor signaling, which control disease progression such as prostate cancer. Nonetheless, a better understanding of how cancer cells integrate such multiple signal pathways and transduce them systematically onto chromatin is still needed. In addition, development of new drugs targeting these pathways is the major problem for clinical application.

In this chapter, we provide multiple evidences, demonstrating how AR modulates its target gene expression or epigenetic status. AR downstream signals are associated with prostate cancer progression and AR associated histone modifiers such as LSD1, PKN1, WDR5 and MLL complex are found to be key molecules for activating AR-dependent gene expression. Surprisingly, recent integrative genomic approaches identified novel lncRNAs associated with AR or expressed in AR binding enhancer regions, which are responsible for forming AR complex or chromatin looping formation. In addition, our study of AR downstream signals indicated androgen-regulated miRNAs or lncRNAs functions for epigenetic modifications and gene controls in cancer development or AR activation. Particularly we demonstrated that DNA hydroxymethylation by TET2 and control of RNA binding protein, PSF, may expand the biological mechanism in androgen signaling. Although their role has not been fully addressed, analyses of these signals unravel the complex and multistep process that lead to tumor formation and drug resistance and held promise for novel therapeutic targets.

References

1. Balk SP, Knudsen KE (2008) AR, the cell cycle, and prostate cancer. Nucl Recept Signal 6:e001
2. Debes JD, Tindall DJ (2004) Mechanism of androgen-refractory prostate cancer. N Engl J Med 351:1488–1490
3. Heemers HV, Tindall DJ (2007) Androgen receptor (AR) coregulators: a diversity of functions converging on and regulating the AR transcriptional complex. Endocr Rev 28:778–808
4. Jenster G et al (1991) Domains of the human androgen receptor involved in steroid binding, transcriptional activation, and subcellular localization. Mol Endocrinol 5:1396–1404
5. Jenster G et al (1995) Identification of two transcription activation units in the N-terminal domain of the human androgen receptor. J Biol Chem 270:7341–7346
6. Callewaert L et al (2006) Interplay between two hormone-independent activation domains in the androgen receptor. Cancer Res 66:543–553
7. Chamberlain NL et al (1996) Delineation of two distinct type 1 activation functions in the androgen receptor amino-terminal domain. J Biol Chem 271:26772–26778
8. Dehm SM et al (2007) Selective role of an NH2-terminal WxxLF motif for aberrant androgen receptor activation in androgen depletion-independent prostate cancer cells. Cancer Res 67:10067–10077
9. Schmidt LJ, Tindall DJ (2011) Steroid 5 alpha-reductase inhibitors targeting BPH and prostate cancer. J Steroid Biochem Mol Biol 125:32–38
10. Heery DM et al (1997) A signature motif in transcriptional co-activatorsmediates binding to nuclear receptors. Nature 387:733–736
11. Buchanan G et al (2001) Collocation of androgen receptor gene mutations in prostate cancer. Clin Cancer Res 7:1273–1281
12. Taplin ME et al (1995) Mutation of the androgen-receptor gene in metastatic androgen-independent prostate cancer. N Engl J Med 332:1393–1398
13. Taplin ME et al (2003) Androgen receptor mutations in androgen-independent prostate cancer: cancer and Leukemia Group B Study 9663. J Clin Oncol 21:2673–2678
14. Takayama K et al (2013) Androgen-responsive long noncoding RNA CTBP1-AS promotes prostate cancer. EMBO J 32:1665–1680
15. Shang Y, Myers M, Brown M (2002) Formation of the androgen receptor transcription complex. Mol Cell 9:601–610
16. Chen CD et al (2004) Molecular determinants of resistance to antiandrogen therapy. Nat Med 10:33–39
17. Locke JA et al (2008) Androgen levels increase by intratumoral de novo steroidogenesis during progression of castration-resistant prostate cancer. Cancer Res 68:6407–6415
18. Sun S et al (2010) Castration resistance in human prostate cancer is conferred by a frequently occurring androgen receptor splice variant. J Clin Invest 120:2715–2730
19. Waltering KK et al (2009) Increased expression of androgen receptor sensitizes prostate cancer cells to low levels of androgens. Cancer Res 69:8141–8149
20. Antonarakis ES et al (2014) AR-V7 and resistance to enzalutamide and abiraterone in prostate cancer. N Engl J Med 371:1028–1038
21. Antonarakis ES et al (2016) Androgen receptor variant-driven prostate cancer: clinical implications and therapeutic targeting. Prostate Cancer Prostatic Dis 19:231–241
22. Takayama K, Inoue S (2013) Transcriptional network of androgen receptor in prostate cancer progression. Int J Urol 20(8):756–768
23. Takayama K et al (2007) Identification of novel androgen response genes in prostate cancer cells by coupling chromatin immunoprecipitation and genomic microarray analysis. Oncogene 26:4453–4463
24. Takayama K et al (2009) Amyloid precursor protein is a primary androgen target gene that promotes prostate cancer growth. Cancer Res 69:137–142

25. Wang Q et al (2009) Androgen receptor regulates a distinct transcription program in androgen-independent prostate cancer. Cell 138:245–256
26. Yu J et al (2010) An integrated network of androgen receptor, polycomb, and TMPRSS2-ERG gene fusions in prostate cancer progression. Cancer Cell 17:443–454
27. Urbanucci A et al (2012) Overexpression of androgen receptor enhances the binding of the receptor to the chromatin in prostate cancer. Oncogene 31:2153–2163
28. Tan PY et al (2012) Integration of regulatory networks by NKX3-1 promotes androgen-dependent prostate cancer survival. Mol Cell Biol 32:399–414
29. He B et al (2014) GATA2 facilitates steroid receptor coactivator recruitment to the androgen receptor complex. Proc Natl Acad Sci U S A 111(51):18261–18266
30. Obinata D et al (2016) Targeting Oct1 genomic function inhibits androgen receptor signaling and castration-resistant prostate cancer growth. Oncogene. 35(49):6350–6358
31. Takayama K et al (2015a) RUNX1, an androgen- and EZH2-regulated gene, has differential roles in AR-dependent and -independent prostate cancer. Oncotarget 6:2263–2276
32. Takayama K et al (2015b) TET2 repression by androgen hormone regulates global hydroxymethylation status and prostate cancer progression. Nat Commun 6:8219
33. Shiraki T et al (2003) Cap analysis gene expression for high-throughput analysis of transcriptional starting point and identification of promoter usage. Proc Natl Acad Sci U S A 100:15776–15781
34. Takayama K et al (2011) Integration of cap analysis of gene expression and chromatin immunoprecipitation analysis on array reveals genome-wide androgen receptor signaling in prostate cancer cells. Oncogene 30(5):619–630
35. Gutschner T, Diederichs S (2012) The hallmarks of cancer: a long non-coding RNA point of view. RNA Biol 9:703–719
36. Djebali S, Davis CA, Merkel A et al (2012) Landscape of transcription in human cells. Nature 489:101–108
37. Mercer TR, Mattick JS et al (2013) Structure and function of long noncoding RNAs in epigenetic regulation. Nat Struct Mol Biol 20:300–307
38. Misawa A et al (2016) Androgen-induced lncRNA SOCS2-AS1 promotes cell growth and inhibits apoptosis in prostate cancer cells. J Biol Chem 291(34):17861–17880
39. Feinberg AP (2007) Phenotypic plasticity and the epigenetics of human disease. Nature 447:433–440
40. Gius D et al (2005) The epigenome as a molecular marker and target. Cancer 104:1789–1793
41. Struhl K, Segal E (2013) Determinants of nucleosome positioning. Nat Struct Mol Biol 20:267–273
42. Kimberly PK, Vezina CM (2015) DNA methylation as a dynamic regulator or development and disease process: spotlight on the prostate. Epigenomics 7:413–425
43. Yu M et al (2012) Base-resolution analysis of 5-hydroxymethylcytosine in the mammalian genome. Cell 149:1368–1380
44. Stroud H et al (2011) 5-Hydroxymethylcytosine is associated with enhancers and gene bodies in human embryonic stem cells. Genome Biol 12:R54
45. Bertoli G et al (2016) MicroRNAs as biomarkers for diagnosis, prognosis and theranostics in prostate cancer. Int J Mol Sci 17:421
46. Takayama K, Inoue S (2016) The emerging role of noncoding RNA in prostate cancer progression and its implication on diagnosis and treatment. Brief Funct Genomics 15:257–265
47. Xiao J et al (2012) miR-141 modulates androgen receptor transcriptional activity in human prostate cancer cells through targeting the small heterodimer partner protein. Prostate 72(14):1514–1522
48. Murata T et al (2010) miR-148a is an androgen-responsive microRNA that promotes LNCaP prostate cell growth by repressing its target CAND1 expression. Prostate Cancer Prostatic Dis 13:356–361

49. Shi XB et al (2007) An androgen-regulated miRNA suppresses Bak1 expression and induces androgen-independent growth of prostate cancer cells. Proc Natl Acad Sci U S A 104:19983–19988
50. Sun D et al (2011) miR-99 family of microRNAs suppresses the expression of prostate-specific antigen and prostate cancer cell proliferation. Cancer Res 71(4):1313–1324
51. Li T et al (2009) MicroRNA-21 directly targets MARCKS and promotes apoptosis resistance and invasion in prostate cancer cells. Biochem Biophys Res Commun 383:280–285
52. Liu LZ et al (2011) MiR-21 induced angiogenesis through AKT and ERK activation and HIF-1α expression. PLoS One 6:e19139
53. Lu Z et al (2008) MicroRNA-21 promotes cell transformation by targeting the programmed cell death 4 gene. Oncogene 27(31):4373–4379
54. Sun T et al (2014) MiR-221 promotes the development of androgen independence in prostate cancer cells via downregulation of HECTD2 and RAB1A. Oncogene 33(21):2790–2800
55. Jalava SE et al (2012) Androgen-regulated miR-32 targets BTG2 and is overexpressed in castration-resistant prostate cancer. Oncogene 31:4460–4471
56. Coppola V et al (2013) BTG2 loss and miR-21 upregulation contribute to prostate cell transformation by inducing luminal markers expression and epithelial-mesenchymal transition. Oncogene 32:1843–1853
57. Ribas J et al (2009) miR-21: an androgen receptor-regulated microRNA that promotes hormone-dependent and hormone-independent prostate cancer growth. Cancer Res 69:7165–7169
58. Ambs S et al (2008) Genomic profiling of microRNA and messenger RNA reveals deregulated microRNA expression in prostate cancer. Cancer Res 68:6162–6170
59. Jiang H et al (2014) Diverse roles of miR-29 in cancer. Oncol Rep 31(4):1509–1516
60. Wang Y et al (2013) The role of miRNA-29 family in cancer. Eur J Cell Biol 92(3):123–128
61. Gebeshuber CA et al (2009) miR-29a suppresses tristetraprolin, which is a regulator of epithelial polarity and metastasis. EMBO Rep 10(4):400–405
62. Wang C et al (2011a) miR-29b regulates migration of human breast cancer cells. Mol Cell Biochem 352(1–2):197–207
63. Wang D et al (2011b) Reprogramming transcription by distinct classes of enhancers functionally defined by eRNA. Nature 474:390–394
64. Kong G et al (2011) Upregulated microRNA-29a by hepatitis B virus X protein enhances hepatoma cell migration by targeting PTEN in cell culture model. PLoS One 6(5):e19518
65. Langsch S et al (2016) miR-29b mediates NF-κB signaling in KRAS-induced non-small cell lung cancers. Cancer Res. 76(14):4160–4169
66. Nickerson ML et al (2013) Somatic alterations contributing to metastasis of a castration-resistant prostate cancer. Hum Mutat 34(9):1231–1241
67. Koboldt DC et al (2016) Rare variation in TET2 is associated with clinically relevant prostate carcinoma in African-Americans. Cancer Epidemiol Biomarkers Prev 25(11):1456–1463
68. Chi P et al (2010) Covalent histone modifications-miswritten, misinterpreted and mis-erased in human cancers. Nat Rev Cancer 10:457–469
69. Dasgupta S et al (2014) Nuclear receptor coactivators: master regulators of human health and disease. Annu Rev Med 65:279–292
70. Eissenberg JC, Shilatifard A (2010) Histone H3 lysine 4 (H3K4) methylation in development and differentiation. Dev Biol 339:240–249
71. Metzger E et al (2008) Phosphorylation of histone H3 at threonine 11 establishes a novel chromatin mark for transcriptional regulation. Nat Cell Biol 10:53–60
72. Metzger E et al (2010) Phosphorylation of histone H3T6 by PKCbeta(I) controls demethylation at histone H3K4. Nature 464(7289):792–796
73. Kim JY et al (2014) A role for WDR5 in integrating threonine 11 phosphorylation to lysine 4 methylation on histone H3 during androgen signaling and in prostate cancer. Mol Cell 54(4):613–625
74. Malik R et al (2015) Targeting the MLL complex in castration-resistant prostate cancer. Nat Med 21(4):344–352

75. Cai C et al (2011) Androgen receptor gene expression in prostate cancer is directly suppressed by the androgen receptor through recruitment of lysine-specific demethylase 1. Cancer Cell 20:457–471
76. Derrien T et al (2012) The GENCODE v7 catalog of human long noncoding RNAs: analysis of their gene structure, evolution, and expression. Genome Res 22:1775–1789
77. Kan Z et al (2010) Diverse somatic mutation patterns and pathway alterations in human cancers. Nature 466:869–873
78. Moran VA et al (2012) Emerging functional and mechanistic paradigms of mammalian long non-coding RNAs. Nucleic Acids Res 40:6391–6400
79. Du Z et al (2013) Integrative genomic analyses reveal clinically relevant long noncoding RNAs in human cancer. Nat Struct Mol Biol 20:908–913
80. Hsieh CL et al (2014) Enhancer RNAs participate in androgen receptor-driven looping that selectively enhances gene activation. Proc Natl Acad Sci U S A 111(20):7319–7324
81. Puc J et al (2015) Ligand-dependent enhancer activation regulated by topoisomerase-I activity. Cell 160(3):367–380
82. Srikantan V et al (2000) PCGEM1, a prostate-specific gene, is overexpressed in prostate cancer. Proc Natl Acad Sci U S A 97:12216–12221
83. Petrovics G et al (2004) Elevated expression of PCGEM1, a prostate-specific gene with cell growth-promoting function, is associated with high-risk prostate cancer patients. Oncogene 23:605–611
84. Yang L et al (2013) lncRNA-dependent mechanisms of androgen-receptor regulated gene activation programs. Nature 500:598–602
85. Prensner JR et al (2014) The IncRNAs PCGEM1 and PRNCR1 are not implicated in castration resistant prostate cancer. Oncotarget 5(6):1434–1438
86. Lanz RB et al (1999) steroid receptor coactivator, SRA, functions as an RNA and is present in an SRC-1 complex. Cell 97(1):17–27
87. Lanz RB et al (2002) Distinct RNA motifs are important for coactivation of steroid hormone receptors by steroid receptor RNA activator (SRA). Proc Natl Acad Sci U S A 99(25):16081–16086. Epub 2002 Nov 20
88. Gupta RA et al (2010) Long non-coding RNA HOTAIR reprograms chromatin state to promote cancer metastasis. Nature 464:1071–1076
89. Zhang A et al (2015) LncRNA HOTAIR enhances the androgen-receptor-mediated transcriptional program and drives castration-resistant prostate cancer. Cell Rep 13(1):209–221
90. Bhan A et al (2013) Antisense transcript long noncoding RNA (lncRNA) HOTAIR is transcriptionally induced by estradiol. J Mol Biol 425(19):3707–3722
91. Xue X et al (2016) LncRNA HOTAIR enhances ER signaling and confers tamoxifen resistance in breast cancer. Oncogene 35:2746–2755
92. Farooqi AA, Bhatti S, Ismail M (2012) TRAIL and vitamins: opting for keys to castle of cancer proteome instead of open sesame. Cancer Cell Int 12:22
93. Katayama S et al (2005) Antisense transcription in the mammalian transcriptome. Science 309:1564–1566
94. Ogawa Y et al (2008) Intersect, ion of the RNA interference and X-inactivation pathways. Science 320:1336–1341
95. Rosok O, Sioud M (2004) Systematic identification of sense-antisense transcripts in mammalian cells. Nat Biotechnol 22:104–108
96. Yu W et al (2008) Epigenetic silencing of tumour suppressor gene p15 by its antisense RNA. Nature 451:202–206
97. Hessels D, Schalken JA (2009) The use of PCA3 in the diagnosis of prostate cancer. Nat Rev Urol 6:255–261
98. Bussemakers MJ et al (1999) DD3: a new prostate-specific gene, highly overexpressed in prostate cancer. Cancer Res 59:5975–5979
99. Salameh A et al (2015) PRUNE2 is a human prostate cancer suppressor regulated by the intronic long noncoding RNA PCA3. Proc Natl Acad Sci U S A 112(27):8403–8408

100. Yap KL et al (2010) Molecular interplay of the noncoding RNA ANRIL and methylated histone H3 lysine 27 by polycomb CBX7 in transcriptional silencing of INK4a. Mol Cell 38:662–674
101. Tsai MC et al (2010) Long noncoding RNA as modular scaffold of histone modification complexes. Science 329(5992):689–693
102. Shi Y et al (2003) Coordinated histone modifications mediated by a CtBP co-repressor complex. Nature 422:735–738
103. Shav-Tal Y, Zipori D (2002) PSF and p54(nrb)/NonO--multi-functional nuclear proteins. FEBS Lett 531:109–114
104. Song X et al (2004) Binding of mouse VL30 retrotransposon RNA to PSF protein induces genes repressed by PSF: effects on steroidogenesis and oncogenesis. Proc Natl Acad Sci U S A 101:621–626

Adenoid Cystic Carcinoma of the Lacrimal Gland: Clinical, Genetic and Molecular Characteristics

Steven Pappas, Ke Jin, Brian C. Tse, David T. Tse, Daniel Pelaez, and Wensi Tao

Abstract Lacrimal Gland Adenoid Cystic Carcinoma (LGACC) is a rare but devastating cancer with a high modality rate. In 75% of cases, perineural migration of LGACC can spread intracranially and invade into orbital bone. Currently, patients with LGACC are treated with chemotherapy and exenteration. Despite these interventions, LGACC has a high frequency of local recurrence and distant metastasis. Only 50% of patients survive to 5 years after diagnosis, and just 25% survive to 15 years. To overcome the difficulties in preventing cancer recurrence and metastasis, better treatments for LGACC are urgently needed. To better understand the pathophysiology of LGACC, we have reviewed the recent literature on clinical and research advances in LGACC. In this chapter, we mainly focus on the genetic and

Steven Pappas and Ke Jin contributed equally to this work.

S. Pappas, B.S. • B.C. Tse, M.D. • D.T. Tse, M.D.
Department of Ophthalmology, Bascom Palmer Eye Institute, Dr. Nasser Al-Rashid Orbital Vision Research Center, Miami, FL, USA

K. Jin, B.S.
The Sheila and David Fuente Graduate Program in Cancer Biology, Sylvester Comprehensive Cancer Center, Miami, FL, USA

D. Pelaez, Ph.D. (✉)
Department of Ophthalmology, Bascom Palmer Eye Institute, Dr. Nasser Al-Rashid Orbital Vision Research Center, Miami, FL, USA

Department of Biomedical Engineering, University of Miami Miller School of Medicine, Miami, FL 33136, USA
e-mail: dpelaez@med.miami.edu

W. Tao, Ph.D. (✉)
McKnight Vision Research Center, University of Miami School of Medicine, 1638 NW 10th Ave., Miami, FL 33136, USA

Department of Ophthalmology, Bascom Palmer Eye Institute, Dr. Nasser Al-Rashid Orbital Vision Research Center, Miami, FL, USA
e-mail: WTao@med.miami.edu

A.A. Farooqi, M. Ismail (eds.), *Molecular Oncology: Underlying Mechanisms and Translational Advancements*, DOI 10.1007/978-3-319-53082-6_11

mechanistic studies on important tumorigenic signaling molecules such as MYB, Notch and FGFR. MYB is a proto-oncogene and key regulator of stem cells. In LGACC, MYB-NFIB fusion transcripts are formed by chromatin rearrangements in the MYB locus, leading to the overexpression of MYB. Mutations in the PEST domain and heterodimerization domain of Notch cause accumulation of the Notch intracellular domain (NICD), which is the biologically active form of Notch. The fibroblast growth factor receptor pathway also plays an important role during lacrimal gland development. Growing evidence indicates that FGFR is an effective biological target in other types of ACC. Small molecule inhibitors for FGFR may therefore shed new light on the treatment of LGACC.

Keywords Adenoid cystic carcinoma • Lacrimal gland • Notch • MYB • Fibroblast Growth factor • FGF receptor

Overview

Although lacrimal gland carcinoma is quite rare, it is a devastating disease with a high mortality rate. Lacrimal gland carcinoma accounts for about 9% of all orbital lesions [1–3]. About half of all lacrimal gland tumors are malignant. Of these malignant forms, by far the most common (>60% of cases) is an epithelial neoplasm known as adenoid cystic carcinoma (ACC) [4]. ACC can occur in several other glandular tissues, most commonly in the salivary glands, but also in Bartholin's glands of the vagina, tracheal goblet cells, and mammary gland tissue [5].

Clinicians and surgeons who have dealt with ACC of lacrimal gland (LGACC) know it as a notoriously destructive cancer that often confers a poor prognosis despite aggressive surgical management, chemotherapy, and/or radiation [6]. ACC's viciousness is largely related to its propensity for early perineural spread intracranially (seen in some 75% of cases) and invasion of orbital bone [7, 8]. Its local and regional recurrence and late distant metastasis rates are also disturbingly high, leaving 50% of patients dead within 5 years of being diagnosed. Only 25% of LGACC patients survive to 15 years [9–11].

Normal Physiology of Lacrimal Gland

Human tears are made up of three component layers: aqueous, lipid, and mucous [12]. Meibomian glands located inside the tarsal plates secrete the lipid layer, while conjunctival goblet cells elaborate mucous [13]. The lacrimal gland is responsible for producing the tear film's aqueous layer, a watery secretion rich in soluble proteins (antibodies, lactoferrin, lysozymes, and soluble mucins) that help protect and maintain homeostasis of the corneal surface [14]. In humans, the lacrimal glands are located in the superolateral aspect of each orbit, and are composed of orbital and palpebral portions linked by interlobular ducts. Their secreted aqueous fluid may enter the ocular surface via several excretory ducts [15].

Since the ocular surface is exposed directly to air, tear film plays an essential role in lubricating the corneal epithelium, flushing out foreign particles and protecting the corneal surface from microbial infection. Disruption of tear formation homeostasis can give rise to a litany of clinical problems, including dry eye disease, corneal abrasions and ulcers, keratitis, etc. [14]. LGACC patients with partial or entire lacrimal gland removal almost inevitably develop postoperative dry eye syndrome, which requires lifelong supplementation with artificial tears [16]. So while the lacrimal gland may receive very little press or glamorous limelight, it nevertheless exerts a mightily powerful influence on patients' quality of life.

Clinical Background

Although the odds of developing ACC are less than 1 in 2 million, patients unlucky enough to get the disease are up against a nasty enemy. Missing a diagnosis can lead to critical delays in treatment, augmenting the disease's already formidable mortality [16]. Thus, recognizing the risk factors, patient demographics, and key clinical features of ACC is crucial for prompt initiation of therapy and optimization of outcomes [11]. Moreover, given LGACC's dogged tendency to recur and aggressively metastasize a few years after initial treatment (with surgery, chemotherapy, and radiation), understanding the disease's chemo-resistance mechanisms should be a priority in future collaborations between clinicians and basic scientists.

Demographics

Although children and teens can develop ACC, the disease is vastly more common in young and middle-aged adults. The mean age for diagnosis of lacrimal gland ACC is 40, with females being afflicted slightly more often than males [11]. No evidence published to date has described any clear relationship of ACC to ethnicity, race, or nationality [4].

Clinical Presentation

The lacrimal gland is a bilobed, unencapsulated eccrine gland located in the superotemporal aspect of the orbit. Its two lobes—the orbital lobe and the much smaller palpebral lobe—are divided anatomically by the levator aponeurosis's lateral horn [15]. Importantly, only the palpebral lobe can be visualized in the upon lid eversion during a physical exam. As a result, tumors confined to the orbital lobe may not obviously manifest themselves until late in the course of the disease [16]. As might be expected given the gland's anatomical location, tumors of the lacrimal gland tend to cause subacute proptosis of the eye inferiorly and nasally. Such displacement of the globe is almost always painful (in contrast to most benign tumors), and is frequently compounded by decreased ocular motility. Other common presenting signs of LGACC include diplopia, "S-shaped" blepharoptosis, and/or frontotemporal hypoesthesia secondary to sensory nerve invasion (particularly in the distribution of the lacrimal nerve) [16]. On average, diagnosis is made within six months of the onset of such symptoms.

One important differential diagnosis for LGACC is pleomorphic adenoma, the most common lacrimal gland tumor. Benign and histologically mixed, pleiomorphic adenomas are typically painless, and only rarely harbor the potential for malignant transformation.

Pathophysiology

Histopathologic Presentation

Adenoid cystic carcinomas of the lacrimal gland are composed of mutated ductal and myoepithelial cells. Three histologic growth patterns predominate in ACC: cribriform, solid, and tubular (ductal) [17]. These histological types may be seen individually or together in various combinations, but the cribriform ("Swiss cheese" or sieve-like) pattern is most common and the solid pattern least frequent. Cribriform ACC is characterized by large cyst-like structures that dominate the histological landscape. These cystic architectures contain stroma filled with amorphous, basophilic glycosaminoglycans and hyalinized, eosinophilic basal lamina. By contrast, the tubular and solid patterns of ACC are histologically preponderated by basaloid myoepithelial cells. In these two patterns, little if any glycosaminoglycan deposition can be appreciated, and basal lamina-containing spaces are very scarce. Despite their differences, the three patterns all share a predilection for invasive perineural growth.

The immunohistochemical profile of adenoid cystic carcinoma has only recently begun to be characterized. Ki-67 immunostaining may be helpful in distinguishing adenoid cystic carcinoma from other lacrimal gland malignancies (like polymorphous low-grade adenocarcinoma), but no clear association between Ki-67 and clinical outcome has yet been established. Likewise, the majority of ACC tumors express E-cadherin, CD117, and EGFR, but the correlation of their expression with prognosis remains unknown.

Neoplasms of the lacrimal gland are classified in the same manner (i.e., using the same TNM staging/grading system) as corresponding tumors of the salivary gland.

Genetic and Molecular Profiling

Adenoid cystic carcinomas characteristically overexpress the oncogene MYB, which encodes a transcription factor (TF) normally expressed by undifferentiated, proliferating progenitor cells. Ordinarily, MYB is down-regulated as differentiation proceeds. In the majority of documented cases, excessive or constitutive MYB activation results from a t(6;9)(q22–23;p23–24) chromosomal translocation that fuses the MYB gene with another TF-encoding gene called NFIB. Indeed, the MYB-NFIB fusion oncogene has been identified in more than 85% of adenoid cystic carcinomas of the head, neck, and breast.

Whole exome sequencing has recently shed light on the mutation "signature" of ACC [18]. The most interesting of these mutations belong to two transcription factors, MYB and Notch. Nucleotide sequence analyses and RT-PCR studies have confirmed that aberrant MYB activation is a frequent event in lacrimal gland ACCs [19]. Although no reports about Notch mutation or expression in lacrimal gland ACCs have been published, Notch receptors and ligands are known to have significantly higher expression in embryonic lacrimal glands than in adult lacrimal glands. Since developmental genes are almost always important in cancer, it is not unreasonable to suspect that the Notch signaling pathway may play a role in lacrimal gland ACCs.

MYB Fusion Transcript

The MYB transcription factor is one of the key regulators of stem and progenitor cells [20–22]. MYB binds to DNA at a specific MYB binding site, then recruits several co-activator proteins like CBP and p300 to initiate target gene transcription [23, 24]. Of the more than 80 MYB target genes that have been reported, most are associated with critical processes such as cell growth, apoptosis, and cell cycle transition [25]. MYB can also cooperate with other transcriptional factors, such as CEBP family proteins, resulting in enhanced MYB transcriptional activity [26].

Like many other developmental genes, MYB plays a role in multiple cancer types and is recognized as a canonical oncogene. Although MAP kinase and Wnt signaling pathways have been reported to regulate MYB expression [27],

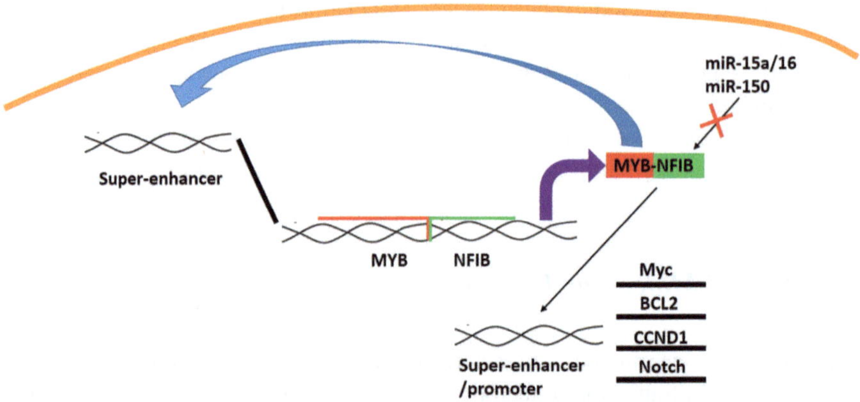

Fig. 1 MYB-NFIB translocation disrupts the 3' UTR, preventing mRNA degradation induced by miR-15a/16 and miR-150. Then, the MYB-NFIB fusion protein binds to the super-enhancers that translocate either upstream or downstream of the MYB gene, enhancing MYB expression. At the same time, MYB binds to the super-enhancers and promoters of its own target genes to upregulate their expression

overexpression of MYB is more commonly related to the attenuation sequences that reside in the first intron of the MYB gene. Mutations in this region that overcome the blockade of transcription elongation result in high levels of MYB expression, and have been demonstrated as critical mutations in most colorectal cancers [28]. The mechanism is slightly different in breast cancer—in that tissue, estrogen receptor-α (ERα) blocks unmutated attenuation sequences in the first MYB intron. Such dysinhibition powerfully elevates MYB expression without the requirement for first intron mutations [29].

Whole-genome sequencing has revealed chromatin rearrangements in the MYB locus that drive the overexpression of MYB, including MYB-NFIB gene fusion and the translocation of super-enhancers to the MYB locus. The MYB-NFIB fusion oncogene was identified in the majority (>85%) of adenoid cystic carcinomas (in all tissues) [30] and in 50% of lacrimal gland ACCs [19]. The *MYB-NFIB* translocation disrupts the *MYB* 3′ untranslated region (UTR), which is targeted by miR-15a/16 and miR-150, two microRNAs that down-regulate MYB expression [31]. Thus, the MYB-NFIB fusion drives the overexpression of MYB and its downstream target genes. Recently, the juxtaposition of super-enhancer regions to the *MYB* locus was identified as a common feature of ACCs. The MYB protein can bind to these super-enhancer regions, forming a positive feedback loop that exacerbates overexpression of MYB and its target genes [32] (Fig. 1).

Although no small molecular compounds directly targeting MYB have yet been developed, several potential therapeutic approaches may be considered based on our significant knowledge of the MYB protein and its gene network. One strategy involves targeting MYB's transcriptional co-factors, proteins that facilitate the stability of the multi-protein MYB transcriptional complex. Two such co-factors, p300 and CBP, have been shown to be critical for the activity of MYB. Thus, individually inhibiting these cofactors or blocking their interaction could represent two effective anti-MYB approaches. A second strategy involves targeting estrogen receptor-α (ERα). As described above, the attenuation sequence in the first intron of MYB is critical for the down-regulation of MYB expression. Since ERα is known to block this attenuation sequence in breast cancers, inhibition of ERα may be a valid approach to manipulating MYB levels in mammary gland tissue. A third tactic involves targeting MYB's downstream target genes. Like all transcription factors, MYB regulates normal cells and cancer cells by modulating the expression levels of its target genes. Thus, inhibiting important MYB target genes such as BCL2 and COX2 could help suppress the effects of excess MYB activity. Finally, pharmacologic control of MYB might be achieved through targeting of the BET bromodomain. As previously mentioned, the translocation of super-enhancers to the MYB locus to form a positive feedback loop has been identified as a common feature of ACCs. Thus, breaking this feedback loop by inhibiting super-enhancers could provide an efficacious therapeutic approach. BRD4 occupancy is critical for the function of super-enhancers, so BET Bromodomain inhibitors could theoretically serve as tools to disrupt the super-enhancers' function [25, 32].

Notch Signaling

The Notch pathway is involved in myriad cell processes. It is particularly important for normal development, exerting influence on cell differentiation, survival, proliferation, etc. [33]. Abnormal Notch signaling plays an indispensable role in T cell acute lymphoblastic leukemia (T-ALL) [34], as well as in solid tissue carcinomas of the breast [35], pancreas [36], and esophagus [37]. The Notch receptor family is comprised of four type I transmembrane receptors (NOTCH1–4) which are canonically activated by Notch ligands expressed on the surface of neighboring cells. Notch receptors are composed of an extracellular domain (ECD), a transmembrane domain, and an intracellular domain (ICD). Upon ligand binding, the Notch intracellular domain (NICD) is released from the cell membrane after two proteolytic cleavages (S2 cleavage by TACE and S3 cleavage by gamma secretase). The liberated NICD then translocates to cell nucleus, where it releases the CSL repression complex and forms an activation complex with CSL, Maml, and other co-activators like p300 (Fig. 2). Formation of this activation complex then leads to the transcription of Notch target genes. Several target genes, such as cyclin D1 and c-Myc have been well-defined, and are known to be involved in tumorigenesis [38]. We also know that the Notch transcriptional complex is subject to multiple modifications that can modulate the activity of the Notch signaling pathway. For example, CK2 phosphorylates N1ICD, resulting in decreased binding of the Notch1 ternary complex to DNA [39]; and CDK8 phosphorylates N1ICD, resulting in PEST-dependent degradation [40].

Like all transcriptional factors, Notch regulates cell processes by controlling the expression of downstream target genes. In most cases, Notch is considered to be an oncogene. Notch directly induces the expression of well-known oncogenes like c-Myc and CCND1, and the cooperation between Notch and RAS has been shown

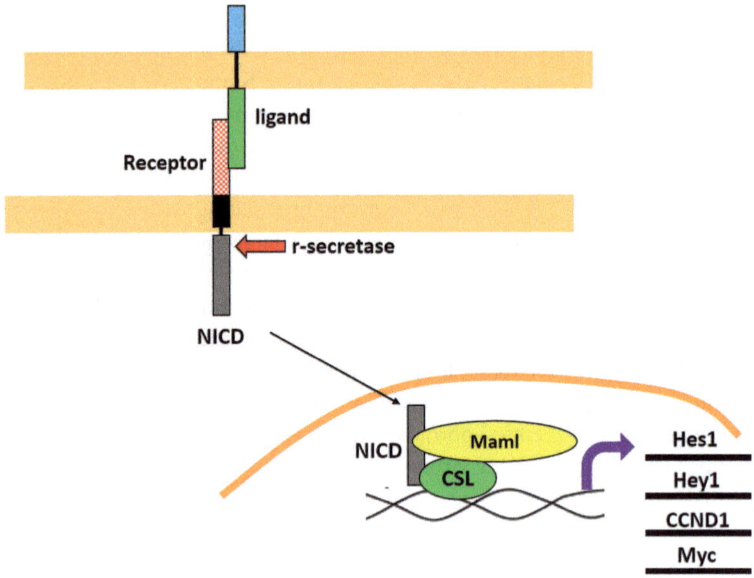

Fig. 2 Canonical Notch signaling. Notch signaling is canonically initiated by Notch ligands on adjacent cells. Notch receptors are composed of an extracellular domain (ECD), a transmembrane domain, and an intracellular domain (ICD). Upon ligand binding, Notch intracellular domain (NICD) is released from the cell membrane after two proteolytic cleavages (S2 cleavage by TACE and S3 cleavage by gamma secretase) and translocates to the nucleus. In the nucleus, NICD releases the CSL repression complex and forms an activation complex with CSL, Maml, and other coactivators like p300, leading to the transcription of target genes

to facilitate malignant transformation of cells in breast tissue [41]. Notch signaling also contributes to cell proliferation, invasion, and epithelial to mesenchymal transition in ACC of the salivary gland [44]. Additionally, Notch has been reported to inhibit tumor suppressor genes such as p53 [42]. However, in other cases, Notch can paradoxically function as a tumor suppressor. In prostate cancer cells with low levels of the tumor suppressor PTEN, ectopic activation of Notch increases levels of PTEN and inhibits cell proliferation [43]. Thus, the function of Notch signaling is highly context-dependent.

Because of the importance of Notch signaling in different malignancies, Notch is a remarkably attractive therapeutic target in cancer treatment. However, clinical methods to target Notch pathway remain limited. To date, no Notch inhibitors have been approved for clinical use, and the only Notch inhibitors currently being investigated clinical trials are gamma secretase inhibitors (GSIs). Gamma secretase is critical for the cleavage of Notch receptors after the binding of Notch ligands to Notch receptors on the cell surface [45]. However, gamma secretase also cleaves other substrates in addition to Notch, imbuing it with a problematic lack of specificity. A novel Notch inhibitor, IMR-1, has been developed to target the assembly of the Notch transcriptional complex. It has been shown to disrupt the recruitment of Maml1 to the Notch transcriptional complex on chromatin, thereby attenuating

Notch target gene transcription [46]. IMR-1 may therefore represent a promising alternative treatment strategy for Notch-dependent cancer by overcoming the specificity limitation of GSIs.

FGF-FGFR Signaling

During embryonic development, FGF-FGFR signaling is required for the branching morphogenesis of lacrimal gland [47]. Fibroblast growth factor (FGF) initiates this signaling pathway by binding to the FGF receptor. The FGF receptor in turn activates several downstream signaling pathways: RAS/Mitogen-Activating Protein (MAP) Kinase, phosphoinositide 3 kinase (PI3K)/AKT, and Phospholipase C [48]. Of these three pathways, the RAS/MAP kinase pathway is the most highly activated by the FGF receptor signal [49]. Upon binding FGF10, FGFR is dimerized and trans-activated by phosphorylation of specific residues. The SH2 domain of Grb2 binds to SH2 and to phosphorylated tyrosine residues of FGFR, allowing recruitment of the nucleotide exchange factor SOS. SOS is a guanine nucleotide exchange factor that can active Ras by exchanging GDP for GTP. SOS's activation of Ras causes activation of more downstream signaling pathways, such as Raf, MEK, and MAP kinase (Erk1,2).

Two SOX family genes (Sox9 and Sox10) downstream of FGFR2 also play important roles during lacrimal gland development. Together with FGF signaling, Sox9 regulates Sox10 expression, which controls the lacrimal gland's acinar structure formation and extracellular matrix (ECM) production [50]. Since FGF10 is a paracrine signaling molecule, its diffusion is tightly regulated by affinity for the ECM proteoglycan heparan sulfate [51, 52]. In sum, FGF10 controls Sox9, which controls Sox10 signaling, which modulates expression of ECM components to control FGF10 (Fig. 3).

Given the FGF-FGFR signaling pathway's central role in lacrimal gland development, it is not unreasonable to suspect that it may also play a role in lacrimal gland ACCs. Indeed, therapies targeting FGFR are currently being investigated in a clinical trial for progressive metastatic adenoid cystic carcinoma (not of lacrimal gland origin). Dovitinib is a small molecule inhibitor of FGFR 1, 2, and 3. The drug can reduce tumor cell proliferation and angiogenesis, both in cell culture and in the ACC xenograft model [53, 54]. From the current research on other types of ACC, we can anticipate that new drugs targeting FGFR will soon become relevant to the treatment of LGACC.

Disease Management

Management of ACC varies by institution, but most cases are treated with multidisciplinary modalities, using combinations of surgery, radiation therapy, and/or chemotherapy (neoadjuvant and/or adjuvant, intravenous and/or intra-arterial).

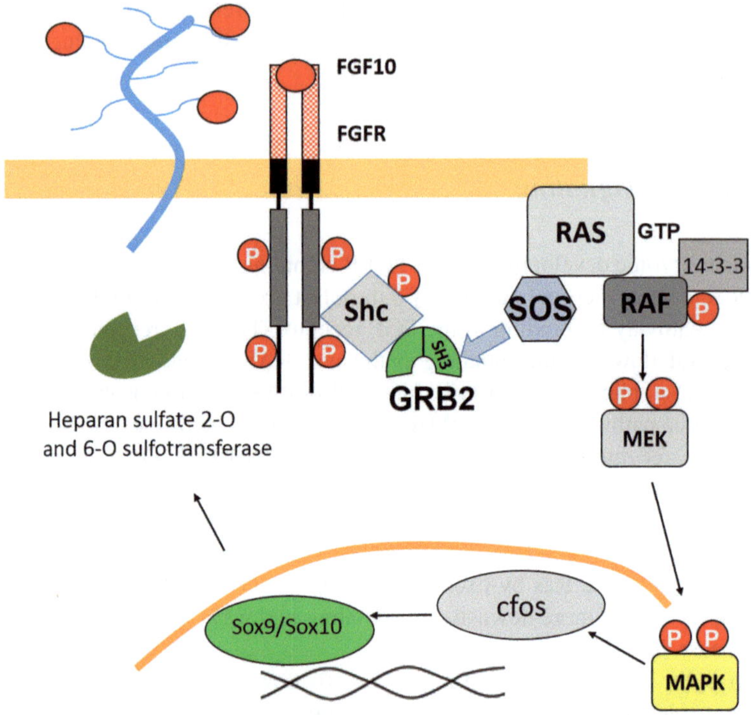

Fig. 3 FGF10-FGFR signaling: a feedback loop. FGFR is dimerized and transactivated by phosphorylation upon the binding of FGF10. Ras is recruited by the interaction between Grb2 and SOS, leading to the activation of the downstream signaling pathways Raf, MEK, and MAP kinase (Erk1,2). Two SOX family genes (Sox9 and Sox10) downstream of the MAP kinase pathway control the modification of heparan sulfate proteoglycan, which binds to FGF10

Historically, the standard of care has been orbital exenteration (often with removal of the bony walls of the lacrimal gland fossa) and adjuvant radiation therapy [55]. But paralleling the non-inferiority of lumpectomy compared to radical mastectomy in certain breast cancers, orbital exenteration has not demonstrated a survival benefit over globe-sparing tumor excision. Thus, it is sensible to consider globe-preserving surgery with adjuvant radiation or concurrent chemoradiation in certain patients with ACC, as the cosmetic consequences of exenteration are profound.

Recently, Tse et al. introduced the neoadjuvant intraarterial cytoreductive chemotherapy (IACC) protocol [56]. During treatment, a catheter is introduced into an artery that supplies the lacrimal gland [56]. It delivers a powerful, concentrated dose of chemotherapy directly to the tumor. This novel approach has so far conferred a 100% survival rate at 10 years (compared to <50% at 10 years with conventional therapy) [57]. However, the IACC protocol can only be applied in patients with an "intact lacrimal artery.

Microdissection genotyping analyses of LGACC tumor samples indicate that allelic loss of microsatellite markers at 1p36, followed by loss of heterozygosity involving 9p21, 22q12, 10q23, and 9q22 in temporal sequence, may be an early indication of LGACC [58, 59]. Such genomic analyses could thus be useful in surveillance and screening for LGACC.

In sum, preliminary data and observations suggest that multidisciplinary eye-sparing strategies provide reasonable local control rates and ocular toxicity profiles. Neoadjuvant intra-arterial or IV chemotherapy appears useful for reducing the size of lacrimal gland tumors, and could in theory be the ideal combination with eye-sparing surgery. Modern radiation delivery techniques (i.e., proton therapy) may enhance outcomes by lessening toxic side effects to nearby brain and ocular parenchyma, but also remain to be studied under the rigorous purview of well-powered randomized trials. Finally, supplementation of pharmacological therapies with metabolic techniques such as glucose and glutamine restriction, ketogenic diet, and hyperbaric oxygen therapy—all of which seek to undermine cancer cells by attacking their unique metabolic traits, known since Warburg's experiments in the 1930s—merits further exploration.

References

1. Alkatan HM, Al-Harkan DH, Al-Mutlaq M, Maktabi A, Elkhamary SM (2014) Epithelial lacrimal gland tumors: a comprehensive clinicopathologic review of 26 lesions with radiologic correlation. Saudi J Ophthalmol 28:49–57. doi:10.1016/j.sjopt.2013.12.007
2. Zeng J et al Epithelial tumors of the lacrimal gland in the Chinese: a clinicopathologic study of 298 patients. Graefes Arch Clin Exp Ophthalmol 248:1345–1349. doi:10.1007/s00417-010-1349-2 (2010)
3. Lee DA, Campbell RJ, Waller RR, Ilstrup DM (1985) A clinicopathologic study of primary adenoid cystic carcinoma of the lacrimal gland. Ophthalmology 92:128–134
4. Chawla B et al (2013) Clinicopathologic review of epithelial tumors of the lacrimal gland. Ophthal Plast Reconstr Surg 29:440–445. doi:10.1097/IOP.0b013e31829f3a0c
5. Khan AJ et al (2001) Adenoid cystic carcinoma: a retrospective clinical review. Int J Cancer 96:149–158
6. Brada M, Henk JM (1987) Radiotherapy for lacrimal gland tumours. Radiother Oncol 9:175–183
7. Mardi K, Kaushal V, Uppal H (2011) Cytodiagnosis of intracranial metastatic adenoid cystic carcinoma: spread from a primary tumor in the lacrimal gland. J Cytol 28:200–202. doi:10.4103/0970-9371.86348
8. Reese AB, Jones IS (1964) Bone resection in the excision of epithelial tumors of the lacrimal gland. Arch Ophthalmol 71:382–385
9. Zeidan BA et al (2006) Adenoid Cystic Carcinoma of the lacrimal gland metastasising to the liver: report of a case. World J Surg Oncol 4:66. doi:10.1186/1477-7819-4-66
10. Bacalja J et al (2014) Adenoid cystic carcinoma of the lacrimal gland metastatic to the kidney: case report and review of the literature. Scott Med J 59:e14–e17. doi:10.1177/0036933014530836
11. Esmaeli B et al (2004) Outcomes in patients with adenoid cystic carcinoma of the lacrimal gland. Ophthal Plast Reconstr Surg 20:22–26. doi:10.1097/01.IOP.0000105518.72611.4F
12. Galicia-Carreon J, Santacruz C, Hong E, Jimenez-Martinez MC (2013) The ocular surface: from physiology to the ocular allergic diseases. Rev Alerg Mex 60:172–183
13. Knop, E., Knop, N. & Schirra, F. [Meibomian glands. Part II: physiology, characteristics, distribution and function of meibomian oil]. Ophthalmologe 106, 884–892, doi:10.1007/s00347-009-2019-9 (2009).

14. Conrady CD, Joos ZP, Patel BC (2016) Review: the lacrimal gland and its role in dry eye. Aust J Ophthalmol 2016:7542929. doi:10.1155/2016/7542929
15. Kels BD, Grzybowski A, Grant-Kels JM (2015) Human ocular anatomy. Clin Dermatol 33:140–146. doi:10.1016/j.clindermatol.2014.10.006
16. Mendoza-Santiesteban E et al (2010) Diagnosis and surgical treatment of orbital tumors. Semin Ophthalmol 25:123–129. doi:10.3109/08820538.2010.500188
17. Weis E et al (2009) Epithelial lacrimal gland tumors: pathologic classification and current understanding. Arch Ophthalmol 127:1016–1028. doi:10.1001/archophthalmol.2009.209
18. Stephens PJ et al (2013) Whole exome sequencing of adenoid cystic carcinoma. J Clin Invest 123:2965–2968. doi:10.1172/JCI67201
19. von Holstein SL et al (2013) Adenoid cystic carcinoma of the lacrimal gland: MYB gene activation, genomic imbalances, and clinical characteristics. Ophthalmology 120:2130–2138. doi:10.1016/j.ophtha.2013.03.030
20. Carpinelli MR et al (2004) Suppressor screen in Mpl−/− mice: c-Myb mutation causes supraphysiological production of platelets in the absence of thrombopoietin signaling. Proc Natl Acad Sci U S A 101:6553–6558. doi:10.1073/pnas.0401496101
21. Emambokus N et al (2003) Progression through key stages of haemopoiesis is dependent on distinct threshold levels of c-Myb. EMBO J 22:4478–4488. doi:10.1093/emboj/cdg434
22. Malaterre J et al (2007) c-Myb is required for progenitor cell homeostasis in colonic crypts. Proc Natl Acad Sci U S A 104:3829–3834. doi:10.1073/pnas.0610055104
23. Dai P et al (1996) CBP as a transcriptional coactivator of c-Myb. Genes Dev 10:528–540
24. Oelgeschlager M, Janknecht R, Krieg J, Schreek S, Luscher B (1996) Interaction of the coactivator CBP with Myb proteins: effects on Myb-specific transactivation and on the cooperativity with NF-M. EMBO J 15:2771–2780
25. Ramsay RG, Gonda TJ (2008) MYB function in normal and cancer cells. Nat Rev Cancer 8:523–534. doi:10.1038/nrc2439
26. Oelgeschlager M, Nuchprayoon I, Luscher B, Friedman AD (1996) C/EBP, c-Myb, and PU.1 cooperate to regulate the neutrophil elastase promoter. Mol Cell Biol 16:4717–4725
27. van de Wetering M et al (2002) The beta-catenin/TCF-4 complex imposes a crypt progenitor phenotype on colorectal cancer cells. Cell 111:241–250
28. Hugo H et al (2006) Mutations in the MYB intron I regulatory sequence increase transcription in colon cancers. Genes Chromosomes Cancer 45:1143–1154. doi:10.1002/gcc.20378
29. Drabsch Y et al (2007) Mechanism of and requirement for estrogen-regulated MYB expression in estrogen-receptor-positive breast cancer cells. Proc Natl Acad Sci U S A 104:13762–13767. doi:10.1073/pnas.0700104104
30. Ho AS et al (2013) The mutational landscape of adenoid cystic carcinoma. Nat Genet 45:791–798. doi:10.1038/ng.2643
31. Persson M et al (2009) Recurrent fusion of MYB and NFIB transcription factor genes in carcinomas of the breast and head and neck. Proc Natl Acad Sci U S A 106:18740–18744. doi:10.1073/pnas.0909114106
32. Drier Y et al (2016) An oncogenic MYB feedback loop drives alternate cell fates in adenoid cystic carcinoma. Nat Genet 48:265–272. doi:10.1038/ng.3502
33. Allenspach EJ, Maillard I, Aster JC, Pear WS (2002) Notch signaling in cancer. Cancer Biol Ther 1:466–476
34. Rakowski LA et al (2013) Convergence of the ZMIZ1 and NOTCH1 pathways at C-MYC in acute T lymphoblastic leukemias. Cancer Res 73:930–941. doi:10.1158/0008-5472.CAN-12-1389
35. Reedijk M (2012) Notch signaling and breast cancer. Adv Exp Med Biol 727:241–257. doi:10.1007/978-1-4614-0899-4_18
36. Ristorcelli E, Lombardo D (2010) Targeting Notch signaling in pancreatic cancer. Expert Opin Ther Targets 14:541–552. doi:10.1517/14728221003769895
37. Wang Z et al (2014) Notch signaling drives stemness and tumorigenicity of esophageal adenocarcinoma. Cancer Res 74:6364–6374. doi:10.1158/0008-5472.CAN-14-2051

38. Ranganathan P, Weaver KL, Capobianco AJ (2011) Notch signalling in solid tumours: a little bit of everything but not all the time. Nat Rev Cancer 11:338–351. doi:10.1038/nrc3035
39. Ranganathan P et al (2011) Hierarchical phosphorylation within the ankyrin repeat domain defines a phosphoregulatory loop that regulates Notch transcriptional activity. J Biol Chem 286:28844–28857. doi:10.1074/jbc.M111.243600
40. Fryer CJ, White JB, Jones KA (2004) Mastermind recruits CycC:CDK8 to phosphorylate the Notch ICD and coordinate activation with turnover. Mol Cell 16:509–520. doi:10.1016/j.molcel.2004.10.014
41. Mittal S, Subramanyam D, Dey D, Kumar RV, Rangarajan A (2009) Cooperation of Notch and Ras/MAPK signaling pathways in human breast carcinogenesis. Mol Cancer 8:128. doi:10.1186/1476-4598-8-128
42. Beverly LJ, Felsher DW, Capobianco AJ (2005) Suppression of p53 by Notch in lymphomagenesis: implications for initiation and regression. Cancer Res 65:7159–7168. doi:10.1158/0008-5472.CAN-05-1664
43. Whelan JT, Kellogg A, Shewchuk BM, Hewan-Lowe K, Bertrand FE (2009) Notch-1 signaling is lost in prostate adenocarcinoma and promotes PTEN gene expression. J Cell Biochem 107:992–1001. doi:10.1002/jcb.22199
44. Bell D et al (2014) Expression and significance of notch signaling pathway in salivary adenoid cystic carcinoma. Ann Diagn Pathol 18:10–13. doi:10.1016/j.anndiagpath.2013.10.001
45. Takebe N, Nguyen D, Yang SX (2014) Targeting notch signaling pathway in cancer: clinical development advances and challenges. Pharmacol Ther 141:140–149. doi:10.1016/j.pharmthera.2013.09.005
46. Astudillo L et al (2016) The small molecule IMR-1 inhibits the notch transcriptional activation complex to suppress tumorigenesis. Cancer Res 76:3593–3603. doi:10.1158/0008-5472.CAN-16-0061
47. Makarenkova HP et al (2000) FGF10 is an inducer and Pax6 a competence factor for lacrimal gland development. Development 127:2563–2572
48. Turner N, Grose R (2010) Fibroblast growth factor signalling: from development to cancer. Nat Rev Cancer 10:116–129. doi:10.1038/nrc2780
49. Corson LB, Yamanaka Y, Lai KM, Rossant J (2003) Spatial and temporal patterns of ERK signaling during mouse embryogenesis. Development 130:4527–4537. doi:10.1242/dev.00669
50. Chen Z et al (2014) FGF signaling activates a Sox9-Sox10 pathway for the formation and branching morphogenesis of mouse ocular glands. Development 141:2691–2701. doi:10.1242/dev.108944
51. Qu X et al (2011) Lacrimal gland development and Fgf10-Fgfr2b signaling are controlled by 2-O- and 6-O-sulfated heparan sulfate. J Biol Chem 286:14435–14444. doi:10.1074/jbc.M111.225003
52. Qu X et al (2012) Glycosaminoglycan-dependent restriction of FGF diffusion is necessary for lacrimal gland development. Development 139:2730–2739. doi:10.1242/dev.079236
53. Kim KB et al (2011) Phase I/II and pharmacodynamic study of dovitinib (TKI258), an inhibitor of fibroblast growth factor receptors and VEGF receptors, in patients with advanced melanoma. Clin Cancer Res 17:7451–7461. doi:10.1158/1078-0432.CCR-11-1747
54. Kang YK et al (2013) Phase II study of dovitinib in patients with metastatic and/or unresectable gastrointestinal stromal tumours after failure of imatinib and sunitinib. Br J Cancer 109:2309–2315. doi:10.1038/bjc.2013.594
55. Alabiad CR et al (2014) En bloc resection of lacrimal sac tumors and simultaneous orbital reconstruction: surgical and functional outcomes. Ophthalmic plastic and reconstructive surgery 30:459–467. doi:10.1097/IOP.0000000000000134
56. Meldrum ML, Tse DT, Benedetto P (1998) Neoadjuvant intracarotid chemotherapy for treatment of advanced adenocystic carcinoma of the lacrimal gland. Arch Ophthalmol 116:315–321
57. Tse DT, Benedetto P, Dubovy S, Schiffman JC, Feuer WJ (2006) Clinical analysis of the effect of intraarterial cytoreductive chemotherapy in the treatment of lacrimal gland adenoid cystic carcinoma. Am J Ophthalmol 141:44–53. doi:10.1016/j.ajo.2005.08.068

58. Tse DT et al (2006) Microdissection genotyping analysis of the effect of intraarterial cytoreductive chemotherapy in the treatment of lacrimal gland adenoid cystic carcinoma. Am J Ophthalmol 141:54–61. doi:10.1016/j.ajo.2005.09.002
59. Tse DT (2005) Clinical and microdissection genotyping analyses of the effect of intra-arterial cytoreductive chemotherapy in the treatment of lacrimal gland adenoid cystic carcinoma. Trans Am Ophthalmol Soc 103:337–367

Role of TRAIL and miR-34a as Therapeutic Agents in Prostate Cancer: Increasing the Armory of Micro-Musketeers

Agnieszka Sobczak-Kupiec, Muhammad Javed Iqbal, Muhammad Zahid Qureshi, Qaisar Mansoor, Seyed Mohammad Nabavi, Jelena Purenovic, Ilhan Yaylim, Ammad Ahmad Farooqi, and Muhammad Ismail

Abstract Prostate cancer is a genomically complex disease and data obtained through in-vitro, preclinical and clinical researches has significantly improved our understanding of the dysregulations of spatio-temporally controlled signaling cascades. Using high-throughput technologies, it has been shown that signaling cascades are re-wired in androgen dependent and androgen independent prostate cancer. Inactivation of tumor suppressor genes, overexpression of oncogenes, genetic/epigenetic mutations, tumor heterogeneity and loss of apoptosis are some of the most extensively studied molecular mechanisms. TRAIL has emerged as one amongst the most deeply studied protein reportedly involved in killing of cancer cells while leaving normal cells intact. In this chapter we set spotlight on most recent breakthroughs made in our understanding of prostate cancer biology and how oncogenic and tumor suppressor proteins stoichiometrically control TRAIL induced

A. Sobczak-Kupiec
Institute of Inorganic Chemistry and Technology, Cracow University of Technology, Cracow, Poland

M.J. Iqbal
Department of Biotechnology, University of Gujrat, Sialkot Sub-campus, Sialkot, Pakistan

M.Z. Qureshi (✉)
Department of Chemistry, GCU, Lahore, Pakistan
e-mail: qureshicnv@yahoo.com

Q. Mansoor • A.A. Farooqi • M. Ismail
Institute of Biomedical and Genetic Engineering (IBGE), Islamabad, Pakistan

S.M. Nabavi
Applied Biotechnology Research Center, Baqiyatallah University of Medical Sciences, Tehran, Iran

J. Purenovic
Faculty of Technical Sciences, Cacak University of Kragujevac, Cacak, Serbia

I. Yaylim
Department of Molecular Medicine, Institute of Experimental Medicine, Istanbul Medical Faculty, Istanbul University, Istanbul, Turkey

A.A. Farooqi, M. Ismail (eds.), *Molecular Oncology: Underlying Mechanisms and Translational Advancements*, DOI 10.1007/978-3-319-53082-6_12

apoptosis in prostate cancer cells. The chapter is partitioned into different sections which sequentially discuss tumor suppressing roles of TRAIL and miR-34a in prostate cancer. We also provide an overview of the nanotechnological approaches currently being used to effectively deliver TRAIL and miR-34a to the target site.

Keywords TRAIL • DR4 • DR5 • Apoptosis • Intracellular signaling • miRNA • Therapeutics

Introduction

Researches over the years have gradually and systematically unveiled many underlying mechanisms of prostate cancer development and progression [1]. Increasingly it is being realized that prostate cancer cells are inter-tumorally and intra-tumorally heterogeneous which are contributory in prostate carcinogenesis and resistance against wide ranging therapeutics [2]. Rapidly accumulating knowledge related to identification of molecular alterations, cancer subtypes, deregulated signaling cascades, Darwinian evolution in response to therapeutic pressures and the complicated multidirectional trajectories of tumor spread between primary and metastatic sites has helped us to understand multifaceted nature of cancer and identify different strategies to improve clinical outcomes. Recent advancements in high-throughput, genome-wide profiling technologies, such as next-generation sequencing (NGS) and RNA interference strategies, have provided near complete resolution of signaling landscape of prostate cancer [1, 2]. Major breakthrough in analysis of transcriptomic and genomic profile of prostate cancer was made in 2010 which involved the investigation of more than 200 tumors [3]. Team of researchers used arrays for mapping of the prostate cancer onco-genome to measure copy number and gene expression. Complete exon re-sequencing was also carried out for identification of specific mutations [3].

It is clear that prostate cancer cells rewire intracellular signaling cascades upon exposure to conventionally used, and next-generation hormonal therapeutics. Presence of androgen receptor splice variants (AR-Vs) has added another layer of complexity to the standardization of therapy [4]. Androgen receptor amplifications, presence of AR-Vs, mutations and persistent signaling are some of the mechanisms which are instrumental in development of castration resistant prostate cancer (CRPC) [5].

Loss of apoptosis is also a well-studied mechanism in prostate cancer. Researchers have identified different apoptosis inducing molecules (TRAIL, FasL, TNFα) which induced apoptosis in cancer cells. However these molecules and their receptors are frequently downregulated in prostate cancer. TNF-related apoptosis-inducing ligand (TRAIL) has gained considerable appreciation as one amongst the most deeply studied molecule noted to selectively target cancer cells while sparing normal cells.

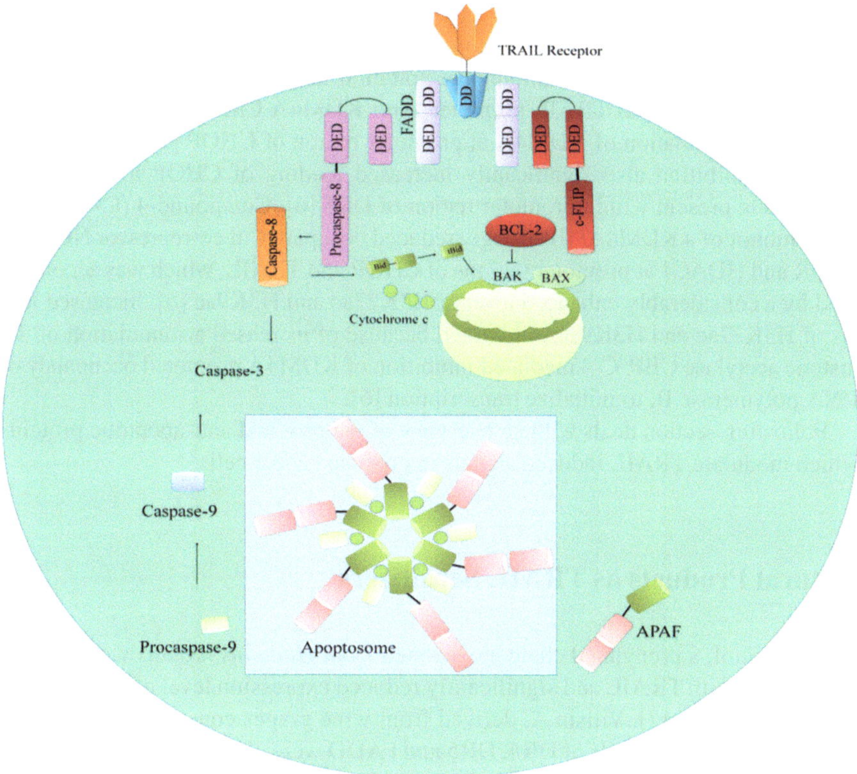

Fig. 1 TRAIL mediated intracellular signaling. Signals are transduced through extrinsic pathway and intrinsic pathway

TRAIL induced apoptosis in cancer cells through its receptors (DR4 and DR5). Binding of TRAIL with its receptor induced trimerization of death receptor that promoted recruitment of signaling machinery at death receptor that consisted of FAS-associated death domain (FADD), an adaptor molecule and pro-caspase-8. This multi-protein machinery is known as DISC (Death Inducing Signaling Complex) and active caspase 8 generated from an efficient DISC, is frequently inhibited by higher levels of c-FLIP in cancer cells. Pro-caspase 8 was converted into functionally active caspase-8 that further activated caspase-3. Intrinsically controlled pathway is triggered via entry of truncated Bid (tBid) into mitochondrion. Bid is proteolytically processed by caspase-8 to form tBid and triggers release of second mitochondria-derived activator of caspase (SMAC) and cytochrome c from mitochondrion. Cytochrome c interacted with Apaf-1 (apoptotic protease activating factor 1) and activated initiator caspase-9. Shown in Fig. 1.

Histone lysine demethylase 4A (KDM4A; JMJD2A), belongs to Jumonji C (JmjC) domain-containing KDM4 subfamily of histone demethylases. KDM4A epigenetically silenced TRAIL and DR5 in prostate cancer cells. mRNA and protein levels of DR5 and TRAIL were found to be notably enhanced in KDM4A silenced cancer cells [6]. Chromatin Immunoprecipitation analysis revealed that KDM4A directly interacted with TRAIL promoter. Anti-KDM4A ChIP assay provided evidence of accumulation of KDM4A at promoter region of CHOP gene. Essentially, KDM4A inhibition also significantly increased loading of CHOP to the CHOP binding site present within promoter region of DR5 [6]. Compound-4 (C-4), selective inhibitor of a KDM4A/4B strongly reduced occupancy of co-repressor NCOR1/ NCoR and HDAC1 at promoter regions of CHOP and TRAIL, which was accompanied by a considerably enhanced level of H3K27ac and H3K9ac [6]. Increased levels of H3K27ac and H3K9ac were noted because of increased accumulation of the histone acetylase CBP. C-4 mediated inhibition of KDM4A promoted occupancy of RNA polymerase II, to initialize transcription [6].

Following section deals with an overview of the pro- and anti-apoptotic proteins which modulate TRAIL induced signals in prostate cancer cells.

Natural Products as TRAIL Sensitizers

Xanthohumol, a prenylated chalcone isolated from *Humulus lupulus* worked synergistically with TRAIL and significantly reduced expression level of Bcl-xL after 8 h of incubation [7]. Vitisin A, derived from wine grapes considerably inhibited Bcl-2 and Bcl-XL. Levels of DR4, DR5 and FADD were also noted to be enhanced in Vitisin A treated PC-3 cells [8]. Delphinidin, a polyphenol dose dependently enhanced protein level of DR5 in LNCaP and DU145 cells. Furthermore, expression levels of negative regulators of apoptosis including cIAP-2, XIAP, Bcl-2, MCL-1 and survivin were reduced in Delphinidin treated prostate cancer cells [9]. Isoegomaketone isolated from *Perilla frutescens* efficiently induced extrinsic and intrinsic pathway in prostate cancer cells [10]. Levels of Bax and AIF were notably enhanced in treated cancer cells. Isoegomaketone enhanced DR5 expression in a ROS-independent manner, mainly through CHOP and p53 dependent pathway [10].

It is understandable that phytochemicals have shown efficacy in improving the TRAIL mediated apoptosis in cancer cells mainly through modulation of pro- and anti-apoptotic proteins and increasing the cell surface expression of death receptors. Therefore, combining different pre-clinically tested phytochemicals with TRAIL based therapeutics may further be tested in Clinical trials.

Increasingly it is being realized that targeted nanoparticles notably reduce off-target effects, mainly because of targeted localization in tumors and active cellular uptake. In the upcoming sections we set spotlight on the advancements made in improving the delivery of well appreciated anticancer agents including TRAIL and miR-34a.

Nanotechnologically Assisted TRAIL Delivery in Different Cancers

Myristic acid (MC) modified Low molecular weight polyethylenimine was complexed with DNA, to yield transfectionally effective MC-PEI(10 K)/DNA NPs [11]. Tumor-necrosis–factor-related apoptosis-inducing ligand (TRAIL) is a protein with reported efficacy against different cancers. TRAIL loaded MC-PEI(10 K)/DNA NPs considerably enhanced survival time of intracranial U87 glioblastoma-bearing mice [11].

Poly(amine-co-esters) have been studied extensively because of their ability to readily condense DNA and form nanosized polyplexes. Poly(N-methyldiethyleneamine sebacate) (PMSC), has previously been used for efficient delivery of genes [12]. In aqueous medium, sebacate units of PMSC interacted strongly, which resulted in formation of hydrophobic domains that induced non-covalent crosslinkage of PMSC-DNA polyplex and increased their stability. PolyE–mRGD contained tumor-targeting and tissue-penetrating ability, and intravenously administered coated III-20% PDL/pLucDNA polyplexes allowed significantly enhanced cargo delivery to the tumor site [12]. After preparation, PDL/pEGFP-TRAIL were coated with polyE-mRGD. To evaluate efficacy, polyE-mRGD coated material was administered in tumor bearing mice via tail vein [12].

TRAIL Delivery in Prostate Cancer

Delivery of TRAIL to the prostate cancer cells using different nanotechnological approaches is currently being tested for efficacy [13]. In accordance with this approach, a novel targeted delivery system particularly, nano-ghosts (NGs) has shown potential. Mesenchymal stem cells (MSCs) are used as a source and NGs are reconstructed from the whole cell membrane. Process of MSC-NGs generation is reproducible and carried out by isolation of intact MSC cell membranes (ghost cells), homogenization of nano-sized vesicles (nano-ghosts) and entrapment of TRAIL [13]. Over the time, MSC-NGs accumulated inside nucleolus and cytoplasm of PC3 prostate cancer cells. Incubation of PC3 cells with NGs for more than 12 h induced clustering of NGs around PC3 cancer cells [13]. Transferrin conjugated, generation 3 diaminobutyric polypropylenimine (DAB) dendrimer loaded with TRAIL plasmid showed activity against DU145, PC-3 and LNCaP prostate cancer cells. However, intravenously administered TRAIL plasmid loaded dendriplex inhibited tumor growth in 10% of PC-3 tumors [14].

There is a recently published report suggesting that delivery of therapeutic drugs through different delivery systems may also prove to be effective. Piperlongumine, a phytochemical was encapsulated in polymer-based NPs comprised of PLGA and coated with a polyvinyl alcohol surfactant layer [15]. Chemical conjugation of TRAIL to the liposomal surface, helped in free interaction of TRAIL with its receptors [15]. Use of different NPs, each with different cargos, helped in maximizing the effects of each therapeutic agent.

Nanoparticle assisted delivery of TRAIL has also shown potential in xenografted mice as evidenced by markedly enhanced bioavailability to the target site. Better understanding of the structure of nanoparticles will prove to be helpful in designing of efficient delivery systems for therapeutic agents.

miR-34a

miR-34a, miR-34b and miR-34c are members of miR-34 family. miR-34a was encoded by its own transcript, however miR-34b and miR-34c had a common primary transcript. Epigenetic downregulation of miR-34a has previously been reported in prostate cancer tissues [16]. miR-34a expression was also found to be notably reduced in PC-3 and DU145 cancer cells. Autophagy, a highly organized catabolic process is also noted be activated in prostate cancer cells having lower expression of miR-34a. Autophagy-related proteins (ATG4B, Beclin-1 and LC3B II/I) were remarkably reduced in miR-34a expressing prostate cancer cells through inhibition of AMPK/mTOR pathway [16].

Target Genes of miR-34a

Persistently active Ras triggered induction of the WNT mediated transduction cascade by increasing expression of WNT-related genes in advanced prostate cancer cells. Lower levels of miR-34a were detected in WNT ligand treated RasB1 and PC3 cells [17]. miR-34a negatively regulated TCF7 (WNT signaling-related gene) and BIRC5 (anti-apoptotic gene). Tumor growth was markedly reduce in mice xenografted with miR-34a overexpressing RasB1 cells [17].

LEF1, a member of LEF1/T-cell factor (TCF) family is reportedly involved in modulation of nuclear response to the canonical WNT induced transduction cascade by interacting with β-catenin [18]. In the nucleus, LEF1/TCF protein directly interacted with β-catenin to trigger target genes. There was a twofold decrease in expression LEF1 in miR-34a transfected LNCaP-AI cancer cells [18].

Increasing the Expression of miR-34a in Prostate Cancer Cells

BioResponse 3,3″-diindolylmethane (BR-DIM) has been shown to upregulate expression of miR-34a in prostate cancer cells [19]. 5-aza-dC, a demethylating agent has also been shown to transcriptionally upregulate miR-34a by promoter demethylation in C4-2B and LNCaP prostate cancer cells [20].

Nanotechnological Delivery of miR-34a

Chitosan nanoparticles are naturally occurring polysaccharides having lower toxicity and immunogenicity. Systemically administered miR-34a using Chitosan nanoparticles remarkably reduced tumor volume of established prostate tumors in the bone in nude mice injected with PC3MM2-LG (transfected to express luciferase and GFP) cells [21]. miR-34a and doxorubicin have recently been investigated to be effective against DU145 and PC3 prostate cancer cells when delivered simultaneously by a self-assembled, reducible, disulfide cross-linked stearyl-peptide-based micellar system (SHRss) using a copolymer building unit [22].

Disialoganglioside GD2 (GD2)-antibody conjugated to the surface of porous silica NPs have been shown to effectively deliver miR-34a. Systemic administration of anti-GD2-miR34a-NP in tumor bearing mice considerably reduced tumor growth [23]. Polyamidoamine (PAMAM) are cations with dendritic structure and electrostatically interact with negatively charged pDNA to form nanocomplexes. PAMAM-PEG-aptamer was developed to efficiently deliver miR-34a to non-small cell lung cancer cells [24].

Better, deeper and sharper understanding of the route of administration, molecular characteristics and temporally controlled delivery of NPs are very essential design variables that must be considered for improving efficacy of therapeutics. Together with the targeting capacity of site-specific peptides and antibodies, these approaches will prove to be helpful in maximizing selective accumulation of therapeutic agents and integration of nanomedicines into clinical practice.

Crosslinkers

There is an exciting piece of evidence suggesting that self-assembled block copolymers were considerably lower toxicity in 2D prostate tumor cell culture than free chemotherapeutic drug, however, surprisingly, micelles were cytotoxic in the 3D prostate MCTS. Paclitaxel has reportedly enhanced killing activity when conjugated with poly(ethylene glycol methyl ether acrylate)-b-poly(carboxyethyl acrylate) block copolymer and self-assembled to generate micelle based delivery systems [25]. For a comparative analysis of effects of micelle stability on the results, micelle core was attached with diamino nondegradable cross-linker. DAO-cross-linked POEGMEA-b-PCEA-PTX conjugate micelles demonstrated an improved drug delivery system [25].

Conclusion

Preclinical and clinical studies have substantially enhanced our knowledge related to genetic, genomic and proteomic landscape of prostate cancer. Reconstituting cancer cells with tumor suppressor genes is an important area of research and different anticancer molecules are being transfected into cancer cells to see how cells respond to therapeutic drugs. Both TRAIL and miR-34a have entered into clinical trials and it will be interesting to see clinical outcomes of these agents in different populations. Restoration of expression of TRAIL receptors and miR-34a is also an area of intense research and different phytochemicals and synthetic agents have shown potential in significantly upregulating the expression of these molecules. It will be also very exciting to witness therapeutic efficacy of co-delivery of TRAIL and miR-34a using different efficient delivery systems. We have to further refine our knowledge related to context dependent behavior of protein network in androgen dependent and androgen independent prostate cancer.

References

1. Spratt DE, Zumsteg ZS, Feng FY, Tomlins SA (2016) Translational and clinical implications of the genetic landscape of prostate cancer. Nat Rev Clin Oncol. doi:10.1038/nrclinonc.2016.76
2. Yap TA, Smith AD, Ferraldeschi R, Al-Lazikani B, Workman P, de Bono JS (2016) Drug discovery in advanced prostate cancer: translating biology into therapy. Nat Rev Drug Discov. doi:10.1038/nrd.2016.120
3. Taylor BS, Schultz N, Hieronymus H, Gopalan A, Xiao Y, Carver BS, Arora VK, Kaushik P, Cerami E, Reva B, Antipin Y, Mitsiades N, Landers T, Dolgalev I, Major JE, Wilson M, Socci ND, Lash AE, Heguy A, Eastham JA, Scher HI, Reuter VE, Scardino PT, Sander C, Sawyers CL, Gerald WL (2010) Integrative genomic profiling of human prostate cancer. Cancer Cell 18(1):11–22. doi:10.1016/j.ccr.2010.05.026
4. Antonarakis ES, Armstrong AJ, Dehm SM, Luo J (2016) Androgen receptor variant-driven prostate cancer: clinical implications and therapeutic targeting. Prostate Cancer Prostatic Dis 19(3):231–241. doi:10.1038/pcan.2016.17
5. Antonarakis ES, Armstrong AJ (2011) Evolving standards in the treatment of docetaxel-refractory castration-resistant prostate cancer. Prostate Cancer Prostatic Dis 14(3):192–205. doi:10.1038/pcan.2011.23
6. Wang J, Wang H, Wang LY, Cai D, Duan Z, Zhang Y, Chen P, Zou JX, Xu J, Chen X, Kung HJ, Chen HW (2016) Silencing the epigenetic silencer KDM4A for TRAIL and DR5 simultaneous induction and antitumor therapy. Cell Death Differ 23(11):1886–1896
7. Kłósek M, Mertas A, Król W, Jaworska D, Szymszal J, Szliszka E (2016) Tumor necrosis factor-related apoptosis-inducing ligand-induced apoptosis in prostate cancer cells after treatment with xanthohumol-a natural compound present in *Humulus lupulus* L. Int J Mol Sci 17(6). doi:10.3390/ijms17060837. pii: E837
8. Shin D, Kwon HY, Sohn EJ, Nam MS, Kim JH, Lee JC, Ryu SY, Park B, Kim SH (2015) Upregulation of death receptor 5 and production of reactive oxygen species mediate sensitization of PC-3 prostate cancer cells to TRAIL induced apoptosis by vitisin A. Cell Physiol Biochem 36(3):1151–1162. doi:10.1159/000430286
9. Ko H, Jeong MH, Jeon H, Sung GJ, So Y, Kim I, Son J, Lee SW, Yoon HG, Choi KC (2015) Delphinidin sensitizes prostate cancer cells to TRAIL-induced apoptosis, by inducing DR5 and causing caspase-mediated HDAC3 cleavage. Oncotarget. 6(12):9970–9984

10. Lee JH, Cho HD, Jeong IY, Lee MK, Seo KI (2014) Sensitization of tumor necrosis factor-related apoptosis-inducing ligand (TRAIL)-resistant primary prostate cancer cells by isoegomaketone from *Perilla frutescens*. J Nat Prod 77(11):2438–2443. doi:10.1021/np500452e
11. Li J, Gu B, Meng Q, Yan Z, Gao H, Chen X, Yang X, Lu W (2011) The use of myristic acid as a ligand of polyethylenimine/DNA nanoparticles for targeted gene therapy of glioblastoma. Nanotechnology 22(43):435101. doi:10.1088/0957-4484/22/43/435101
12. Zhou J, Liu J, Cheng CJ, Patel TR, Weller CE, Piepmeier JM, Jiang Z, Saltzman WM (2011) Biodegradable poly(amine-co-ester) terpolymers for targeted gene delivery. Nat Mater 11(1):82–90
13. Toledano Furman NE, Lupu-Haber Y, Bronshtein T, Kaneti L, Letko N, Weinstein E, Baruch L, Machluf M (2013) Reconstructed stem cell nanoghosts: a natural tumor targeting platform. Nano Lett 13(7):3248–3255. doi:10.1021/nl401376w
14. Al Robaian M, Chiam KY, Blatchford DR, Dufès C (2014) Therapeutic efficacy of intravenously administered transferrin-conjugated dendriplexes on prostate carcinomas. Nanomedicine (Lond) 9(4):421–434. doi:10.2217/NNM.13.25
15. Sharkey CC, Li J, Roy S, Wu Q, King MR (2016) Two-stage nanoparticle delivery of piperlongumine and tumor necrosis factor-related apoptosis-inducing ligand (TRAIL) anti-cancer therapy. Technology (Singap World Sci) 4(1):60–69
16. Liao H, Xiao Y, Hu Y, Xiao Y, Yin Z, Liu L, Kang X, Chen Y (2016) Methylation-induced silencing of miR-34a enhances chemoresistance by directly upregulating ATG4B-induced autophagy through AMPK/mTOR pathway in prostate cancer. Oncol Rep 35(1):64–72. doi:10.3892/or.2015.4331
17. Chen WY, Liu SY, Chang YS, Yin JJ, Yeh HL, Mouhieddine TH, Hadadeh O, Abou-Kheir W, Liu YN (2015) MicroRNA-34a regulates WNT/TCF7 signaling and inhibits bone metastasis in Ras-activated prostate cancer. Oncotarget 6(1):441–457
18. Liang J, Li Y, Daniels G, Sfanos K, De Marzo A, Wei J, Li X, Chen W, Wang J, Zhong X, Melamed J, Zhao J, Lee P (2015) LEF1 targeting EMT in prostate cancer invasion is regulated by miR-34a. Mol Cancer Res 13(4):681–688. doi:10.1158/1541-7786.MCR-14-0503
19. Li Y, Sarkar FH (2016) Role of BioResponse 3,3'-diindolylmethane in the treatment of human prostate cancer: clinical experience. Med Princ Pract 25(Suppl2):11–17. doi:10.1159/000439307
20. Kong D, Heath E, Chen W, Cher M, Powell I, Heilbrun L, Li Y, Ali S, Sethi S, Hassan O, Hwang C, Gupta N, Chitale D, Sakr WA, Menon M, Sarkar FH (2012) Epigenetic silencing of miR-34a in human prostate cancer cells and tumor tissue specimens can be reversed by BR-DIM treatment. Am J Transl Res 4(1):14–23
21. Gaur S, Wen Y, Song JH, Parikh NU, Mangala LS, Blessing AM, Ivan C, Wu SY, Varkaris A, Shi Y, Lopez-Berestein G, Frigo DE, Sood AK, Gallick GE (2015) Chitosan nanoparticle-mediated delivery of miRNA-34a decreases prostate tumor growth in the bone and its expression induces non-canonical autophagy. Oncotarget 6(30):29161–29177. doi:10.18632/oncotarget.4971
22. Yao C, Liu J, Wu X, Tai Z, Gao Y, Zhu Q, Li J, Zhang L, Hu C, Gu F, Gao J, Gao S (2016) Reducible self-assembling cationic polypeptide-based micelles mediate co-delivery of doxorubicin and microRNA-34a for androgen-independent prostate cancer therapy. J Control Release 232:203–214. doi:10.1016/j.jconrel.2016.04.034
23. Tivnan A, Orr WS, Gubala V, Nooney R, Williams DE, McDonagh C, Prenter S, Harvey H, Domingo-Fernández R, Bray IM, Piskareva O, Ng CY, Lode HN, Davidoff AM, Stallings RL (2012) Inhibition of neuroblastoma tumor growth by targeted delivery of microRNA-34a using anti-disialoganglioside GD2 coated nanoparticles. PLoS One 7(5):e38129
24. Wang H, Zhao X, Guo C, Ren D, Zhao Y, Xiao W, Jiao W (2015) Aptamer-dendrimer bioconjugates for targeted delivery of miR-34a expressing plasmid and antitumor effects in non-small cell lung cancer cells. PLoS One 10(9):e0139136
25. Du AW, Lu H, Stenzel MH (2015) Core-cross-linking accelerates antitumor activities of paclitaxel–conjugate micelles to prostate multicellular tumor spheroids: a comparison of 2D and 3D models. Biomacromolecules 16(5):1470–1479

Components from the Traditional Chinese Medicine Acts as Protein Kinase Inhibitors

Minghua Liu, Ge Zhao, Shousong Cao, Yangyang Zhang, Xiaofang Li, and Xiukun Lin

Abstract Protein kinases play critical roles in control of cell growth, proliferation, migration, survival and angiogenesis and the enzymes mediate biological effects through their catalytic activity. In recent years, numerous protein kinase inhibitors have been developed and, some of them have been used clinically. Traditional Chinese Medicine (TCM) has been used in China for thousands of years, and components isolated from TCM represent a large class of bioactive substances, and some of them display anticancer activity via inhibiting protein kinases signaling pathway. In the present article, we comprehensively reviewed several components isolated from anticancer TCMs that exhibited significantly inhibitory activity towards a range of protein kinases. These components, which belong to diverse structural classes, are reviewed herein, based upon the kinases that they inhibit. The prospects and problems in development of the anticancer TCMs are also discussed.

Keywords Traditional Chinese Medicine • Protein kinase inhibitors • Anticancer activity

Introduction

The protein kinase family catalyze the transfer of a phosphate group from a high energy molecule such as adenine triphosphate (ATP) to a specific amino acid in a protein [1]. Protein kinases play important roles in regulating cellular functions, including proliferation, survival, apoptosis, motility as well as metabolism and DNA damage repair, etc. Protein kinases such as cellular Src (c-Src), c-Abl, mitogen activated protein kinase (MAPK), phosphotidylinositol-3-kinase (PI3K), serine/threonine-specific protein kinase (AKT) and the epidermal growth factor receptor (EGFR), are commonly activated in cancer cells and known to play roles in tumorigenesis. Many of these occur in the same signaling pathway; EGFR kinase family members (HER1 [EGFR], HER2, HER3, and HER4) transmit signals through

---

M. Liu • G. Zhao • S. Cao • Y. Zhang • X. Li • X. Lin (✉)
Department of Pharmacology, School of Pharmacy, Southwest Medical University,
No. 319, Zhongshan Road, Jiangyang District, Luzhou, Sichuan 646000, China
e-mail: linxiukun@yahoo.com

A.A. Farooqi, M. Ismail (eds.), *Molecular Oncology: Underlying Mechanisms and Translational Advancements*, DOI 10.1007/978-3-319-53082-6_13

MAPK and PI3K to promote cell proliferation [2]. The central role of kinases in virtually all networks of signal transduction is the driving motivation useful for the development of compounds modulating their activities [3].

In recent years, an increasing number of novel compounds have been isolated from Traditional Chinese Medicines (TCMs), and many of them have been reported to possess potent anticancer activity via inhibition of protein kinase mediated signaling pathways, including PI3K/AKT/mTOR, P38 MAPK and ERK. In this review, we focus on those compounds isolated from TCMs with inhibitory effects on protein kinases and present an overview of their anticancer effects and potentials in pharmaceutics for cancer therapy. The problem and prospect for developing protein kinase inhibitors from TCS are also presented.

Mark Family and Components Isolated from TCMs

MAPK, a serine/threonine specific protein kinase, regulates a variety of biological processes including cell survival, proliferation, differentiation, and apoptosis through downstream signal transduction cascades [4]. The classical MAPK family consists of three subfamilies, i.e. the ERKs, the c-Jun N-terminal kinases (JNKs)/stress-activated protein kinases (SAPKs), and the p38 MAPKs [5, 6]. JNKs and p38 MAPKs play critical roles in the signaling mechanisms that orchestrate cellular response to various types of cellular stress [7, 8]. It has been acknowledged that the ERK signaling pathway is also very important in carcinogenesis. Selective inhibitors of these kinases are likely to affect cellular events with high specificities and are therefore the molecules of significant interest for discovery and development of anticancer pharmaceuticals [9].

Curcuma longa L. is an important herb used in TCM to treat various types of pain and inflammation. Curcumin (Fig. 1), an apolyphenolic compound, is isolated from the rhizomes of *Curcuma longa L.* Recent studies have shown that curcumin has anti-tumor effect to inhibit cell proliferation and promote cell apoptosis in several types of cancer including hepatocellular carcinoma, lung cancer, breast cancer, colorectal cancer, etc. [10–13]. Curcumin significantly activates the JNK and p38 MAPK, but not the ERK, signaling pathways via phosphorylation, thus down-regulating anti-apoptotic proteins Bcl-2, Bcl-XL, Mcl-1, and survivin in human HCT-116 colon cancer cells during apoptosis process [14]. Curcumin induces apoptosis of THP-1 human monocytic leukemia cells by activation of the JNK/ERK signaling pathway [15]. Curcumin can also block cell cycle progression at the G_2/M phase and induce apoptosis by regulation of ERK1/2 phosphorylation in nasopharyngeal carcinoma cells [16]. Curcumin halts the growth of human HepG2 liver xenograft tumors in nude mice. Curcumin down-regulates the expression of p-ERK1/2 and p-AKT in tumor tissues by immunohistochemical analyses [17]. Furthermore, curcumin inhibits proliferation of colorectal carcinoma cells by modulating the Akt/mTOR signaling pathway [13]. Curcumin as an antitumoral agent is currently under phase II clinical development for prevention of colorectal cancer.

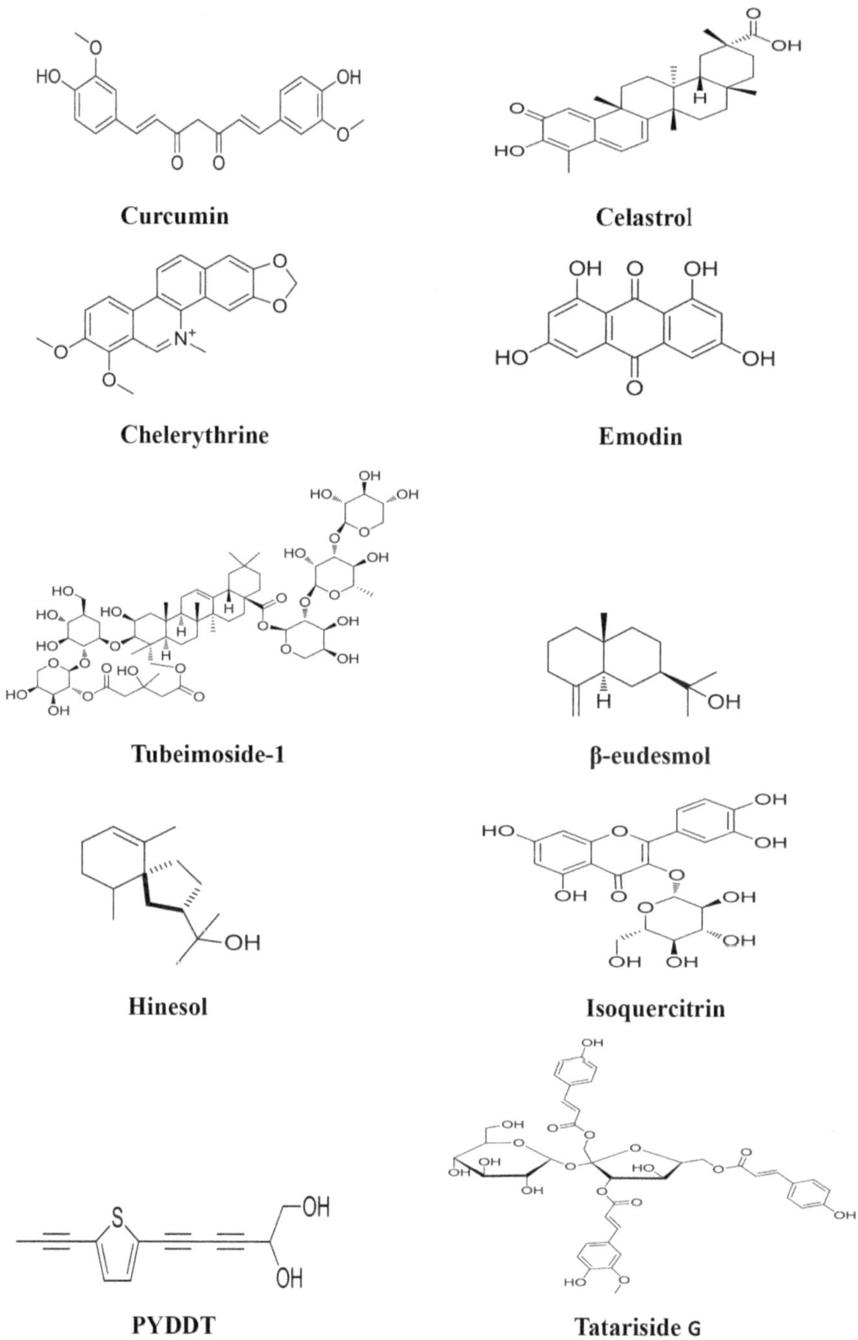

Fig. 1 Chemical structures of components isolated from TCMs with inhibitory effects via MAPK pathway

Pharmacokinetic studies show that the absorbed curcumin conjugates with glucuronic acid and sulphate, and metabolized to glucuronic acid and sulphate conjugates in the intestine and liver [18]. Excretion of curcumin glucuronides from intestinal cells occurs predominantly at the apex and to a lesser extent at the basolateral side, thus limiting its absorption [19]. In cancer patients, the serum concentration peaks at 1–2 h after intake and does not exceed 0.60 μg/mL (0.16 μmol/L) even at a dose of 8 g curcumin per day for 3 months [20]. In a dose-escalation study, curcumin was not detected in the serum for up to 4 h after administration of single doses of 0.5–8.0 g curcuminoids, and only low concentrations between 0.03 and 0.06 μg/mL were detected after single oral dose of 10 or 12 g [21]. The low bioavailability of curcumin is attributed to its limited absorption, efficient re-secretion from intestinal cells and rapid intestinal and hepatic conversion to its metabolites dihydro-, tetrahydro- and hexahydrocurcumin and their respective conjugates with glucuronic acid and sulphate, which considerable hampers its therapeutic efficacy and clinical application [22]. Recently, the nanoparticle of curcumin was developed, and the bioavailability of the compound was greatly improved [23].

Tripterygium wilfordii Hook. f., distributed in Asia, is another herb used in TCM to treat autoimmune and inflammatory diseases such as rheumatoid arthritis and tuberculosis. Celastrol (Fig. 1), a triterpenoid isolated from the plant has attracted great attention due to its potent anticancer effects and its diverse molecular targets involved in tumorigenesis [24–30]. The anticancer mechanisms of the compound include inducing apoptosis in tumor cells, affecting angiogenesis, regulating the related proteins of tumor and so on. Recent studies have shown that Reactive oxygen species (ROS)/c-Jun NH2-terminal kinase (JNK) signal pathway plays a critical role in celastrol induced cell apoptosis; treatment of cancer cells with celastrol activates caspase-3, -8, -9, DR5 and cleavage of PARP, Bid, upregulates the expression of LC3B-II. The augmentation of JNK phosphorylation and ROS generation is another important event in celastrol induced cell apoptosis [31]. In addition, celastrol is able to suppress the expression of vascular endothelial growth factor receptor (VEGFR), and inhibits the growth of human glioma xenografts in nude mice [29]. Additionally, treatment with celastrol resulted in significant inhibition of the tumor growth without host toxicity in nude mice bearing prostate tumors [27]. These studies suggest that celastrol is a promising candidate for development as an anticancer agent. A sensitive and precise LC–MS/MS assay was developed to determine the pharmacokinetic profiles of celastrol in rats [32]. The results showed that oral administration of pure celastrol leads only to an bioavailability of 17.06%, whereas after oral administration of TGV tablets, the absolute bioavailability of celastrol in female rats increased up to 94.19%, demonstrating improved absorption properties of celastrol [32].

Chelidonium majus L. is used in TCM to treat ulcer and gastrointestinal pain. Chelerythrine (Fig. 1) is a benzene alkaloid isolated from the herb. Chelerythrine has been proved to possess potent antitumor effect on various cancers, in particular breast, colon and prostate cancers [33]. The mechanism of action of chelerythrine involves several pathways, including cell cycle arrest and inhibition of protein synthesis. Chelerythrine activated JNK/p38 MAPK pathways in a concentration and time-dependent manners in HeLa cervical cancer cells [34]. Treatment of chelerythrine resulted in activation of MEK/ERK1/2 signaling pathway, up-regulation of downstream kinases (p90RSK), and finally induction of apoptosis in human osteosarcoma cells [35]. Chelerythrine can also induce G1 phase arrest and bimodal cell death in human leukemia HL-60 cells [36]. In addition, chelerythrine is a specific inhibitor of protein kinase C (PKC), blocking PKC translocation from cytosol to membrane, contributed to the progression of apoptotic tumor cell death [37]. Recent study also demonstrated that chelerythrine possesses the activity of inhibiting the telomerase activity and promoting cancer cell death via binding with human telomeric DNA to form the four-stranded G-quadruplex [38].

Emodin (Fig. 1) is an active ingredient derived from the rhizome of *Rheum palmatum L.*, which is widely used in TCM as a laxative over thousands years [39, 40]. In the last decades, increased attention is focused on the anticancer activities of emodin since studies have shown that the compound exhibited the effects of antiproliferation and apoptosis-induction in a number of human cancers such as colon, cervical and gastric cancer [41, 42]. Emodin inhibited proliferation and induced apoptosis of hepatocellular carcinoma cells both in vitro and in vivo through MAPK and PI3K/AKT signaling pathways in a dose-dependent manner [43]. Emodin significantly activates the phosphorylation of ERK and p38, which associated with apoptosis of hepatocellular carcinoma (HCC) cells. Moreover, emodin can induce apoptosis of colorectal cancer cells through activating p53/p38/Puma pathway by triggering ROS production [44]. Pharmacokinetic study revealed that emodin was predominantly found in liver and brain after oral intake of *Polygonum cuspidatum*, which is a widely used in TCM [45]. After intragastric administration at doses of 20 and 40 mg/kg, emodin rapidly underwent phase II metabolism to form its glucuronide derivative, and the parent form of emodin was almost undetectable in vivo [46]. Glucuronidation metabolism appeared to be one of the main reasons for the very poor oral bioavailability of emodin as found in a cultured Caco-2 cell model [47].

Bolbostemma paniculatum (Maxim.) Franquet is used in TCM to treat swollen skin, tuberculosis and abscess of the lung. Tubeimoside-1 (Fig. 1) as a novel compound with potent anticancer activity is isolated from the plant [48, 49]. Tubeimoside-1 inhibited the growth of several cancer cells including gliomas, lung cancer and liver cancer [50–52]. Tubeimoside-1 induced phosphorylation of apoptosis signal-regulating kinase 1 (ASK-1) and its downstream target proteins JNK and p38 in a dose-dependent manner, leading to mitochondrial apoptosis in DU145 human prostate cancer cells [53]. Activation of MAPK-JNK signaling pathway plays an important role in tubeimoside-1 induced cell cycle arrest in lung cancer cells [54]. Tubeimoside-1 can also sensitize cell response to cisplatin in cisplatin-resistant human ovarian cancer cells (A2780/DDP) through down-regulation of ERK and up-regulation of p38 [55]. Tubeimoside-1 increased the expression of CHOP and phosphorylated p38, resulting in G_2/M phase arrest and apoptosis in SKOV-3 human ovarian carcinoma cells [56]. In addition, tubeimoside-1 can induce oxidative stress-mediated apoptosis and G_2/M phase arrest in HepG2 liver cancer cells via NF-kappaB, JNK and p53 pathways [48]. LC/MS analysis was performed to check the pharmacokinetics of tubeimoside-1 after intravenous and oral administration in rats [57]. Tubeimoside-1 was found with very slow clearance via hepatic tissues. The absolute oral bioavailability of tubeimoside-1 was only 0.23%, suggesting that tubeimoside-1 has poor absorption or undergoes acid-induced degradation.

Atractylodes lancea rhizome is recognized to possess the diuretic and stomachic effects in TCM, and used to treat abdominal distention and dismembered sores in China. Two oil products, β-eudesmol (Fig. 1) and hinesol (Fig. 1) are isolated from the plant. Recent study showed that β-eudesmol is able to activate JNK/MAPK signaling pathway, and induce cell death through mitochondria-mediated intrinsic apoptosis modulated by JNK-dependent downregulation of Bcl-2 in HL60 leukemia cells [58]. β-eudesmol induced the decrease of matrix metalloproteinases (MMP) and the release of cytochrome C from mitochondria in HL60 leukemia cells accompanied with the activation of caspase-9, caspase-3, and cleavage of PARP. β-eudesmol exhibited the inhibitory effect on the growth of various cancer cells including HeLa cervical cancer, SGC-7901 gastric cancer, and liver cancer BEL-7402 cells in vitro [59]. Hinesol, a sesquiterpenoid component isolated from the herb, also induced apoptosis via JNK signaling pathway. Hinesol treatment significantly activated JNK and ERK, but did not alter the activation of p38; thus hinesol may represent a novel anticancer agent in the treatment of leukemia [60].

Bidens bipinnata L. has been used in TCM as a basic drug historically in the local area of Guangxi, China, to treat many kinds of diseases such as malaria, diarrhoea, dysentery, hepatitis, acute nephritis, hypertension, hyperlipidaemia, and diabetes. Isoquercitrin (Fig. 1) is a flavonoid compound with anticancer activity isolated from *Bidens bipinnata L* [61, 62]. Isoquercitrin strongly inhibited the phosphorylation of ERK and p38MAPK proteins while promoting the phosphorylation of JNK, thus inducing apoptosis in HepG2 liver cancer cells in a caspase-dependent manner [63]. Isoquercitrin can also block the liver cancer cells at the G_1 phase and exhibited inhibitory effect on transplanted tumor growth in vivo [63].

The roots of *Echinops grijsii*, is believed to possess the effects of antiinflammation, detoxicating and expelling miasma in TCM, and used to relieve the distention of the breast and stimulating milk secretion [64, 65]. A thiophene derivative, 2-(Pro-1-ynyl)-5- (5,6-dihydroxypenta-1,3-diynyl) thiophene (PYDDT) (Fig. 1) is isolated from the herb. PYDDT induces the production of ROS, and the activation of JNK but not p38 and ERK1/2, leading to induction of mitochondrial-mediated apoptosis in human colon cancer SW620 cells [66]. PYDDT-induced apoptosis was characterized by the cleavage of PARP, activation of caspase 9 and caspase 3, release of cytochrome C from mitochondria, loss of mitochondrial membrane potential, down-regulation of Bcl-2, and mitochondrial translocation of Bax.

Fagopyrum tataricum (L.) Gaertn (tartary buckwheat) has been widely used as an important folk medicine in China as a nutritional food. Studies have shown that the herb has multiple benefits including antioxidant, antitumor, antihypotensive, hypoglycemic, and hypolipidaemic effects [67, 68]. Tatariside G (Fig. 1), a novel phenylpropanoid glycosides compound, was isolated from the roots of *Fagopyrum tataricum (L.) Gaertn*. Recent study revealed that tatariside G notably inhibited cell viability and induced apoptosis in human cervical cancer HeLa cells through both activation of p38/JNK phosphorylation and inhibition of Akt phosphorylation [69]. Tatariside G could elevate the cleaved protein expression of caspase-3 and caspase-9 in a dose-dependent manner, and decreased mitochondrial membrane potential (MMP) in HeLa cells [69].

Targeting PI3K/AKT

The PI3K signaling pathway contributes to tumor development and progression in many types of human malignancies. It is well acknowledged that activation of AKT, the major downstream effecter of PI3K, is frequently observed in human tumors [70, 71], and the activation of AKT promotes the development of cancer as well as resistance to chemotherapy and radiation therapy. Additionally, immunohistochemical analysis has shown that AKT activation is a poor prognostic factor in various cancers [72]. Therefore, PI3K/AKT signaling pathway is an attractive target for cancer therapy [73, 74]. Several components isolated from TCMs were found to induce cell death via inhibiting PI3K/AKT pathway.

Alkannin (Fig. 2) is the major active ingredient isolated from *Arnebia euchroma roots*, which has long been used as anti-inflammation and anti-tumor herb in Chinese folk medicine [75]. Studies have shown that alkannin exerted antitumor effects by inhibiting cancer cell proliferation and inducing apoptosis via inhibiting DNA topoisomerase I/II activity, anti-telomerase activity and anti-angiogenesis [76–78]. SYUNZ-16, a synthesized alkannin derivative, is one of the compounds with potent antitumor activities [79–82]. SYUNZ-16 displayed potent cytotoxicity in diversified cancer cell lines including nasopharyngeal carcinoma, hepatocellular cancer, leukemia, cervical cancer, gastric cancer and breast cancer. SYUNZ-16 inhibits AKT signaling pathway, and down-regulates the phosphorylation of AKT in a dose and time-dependent manner , subsequently initiating apoptotic events in Hep3B liver cancer and GLC-82 lung cancer cells [83]. SYUNZ-16 can obviously inhibit the proliferation of these cancer cells via induction of apoptosis with the activation of caspase-3 and PARP cleavage [83]. SYUNZ-16 can also partially attenuate the phosphorylation levels of forkhead transcription factors (FKHR and FKHRL1), which are important substrates of AKT [84]. SYUNZ-16 exhibits inhibitory effects on murine S-180 sarcoma allografts and GLC-82 lung cancer xenografts in vivo [83].

Toad venom (venenum bufonis, also called Chan'su) is derived from the dried skin secretions of giant toads (*Bufo gargarizans Cantor or Bufo melanostictus Schneider*) and has been widely used alone or in combination with other herbal ingredients for cancer treatment over centuries in China. An injectable formulation of toad venom called cinobufacin (Huchansu) was developed to treat various solid tumors in China in 1990s. Clinical studies have shown that cinobufacin significantly increased the antitumor efficacy of docetaxol or cisplatin in the combination therapy. Decreased toxicity and improved life quality were also observed in the clinical trial with cancer patients [85]. Arenobufagin (Fig. 1), one of the components of toad venom, was reported to have a broad spectrum of antitumor activity in cancer cells,

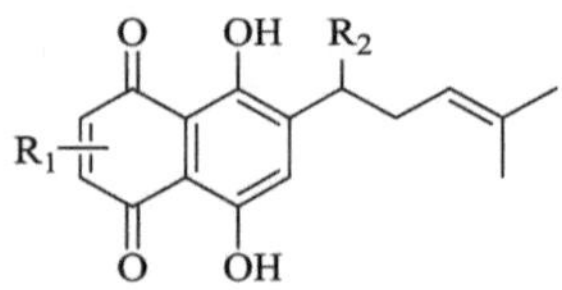

$R_1=R_2=N(CH_2CH_2)_2O$

SYUNZ-16

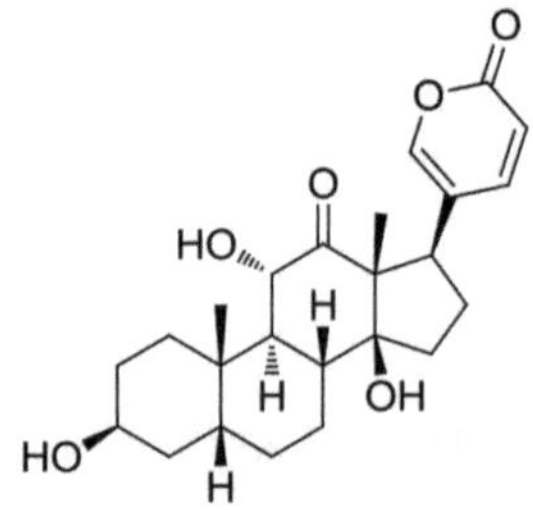

Arenobufagin

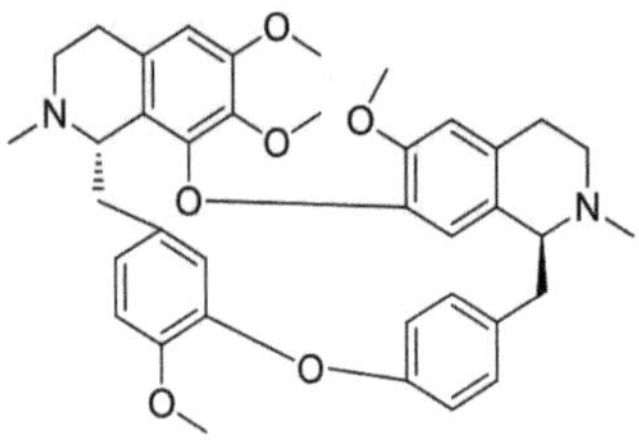

Tetrandrine

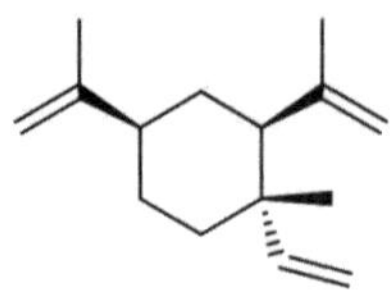

β-Elemen

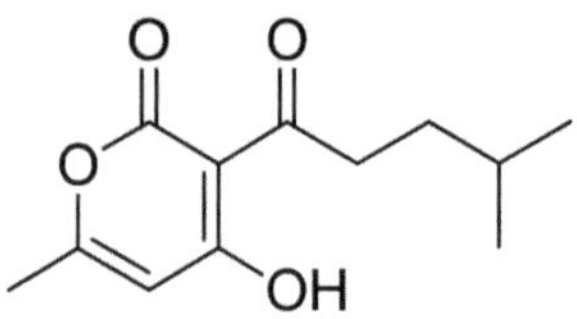

Pogostemon

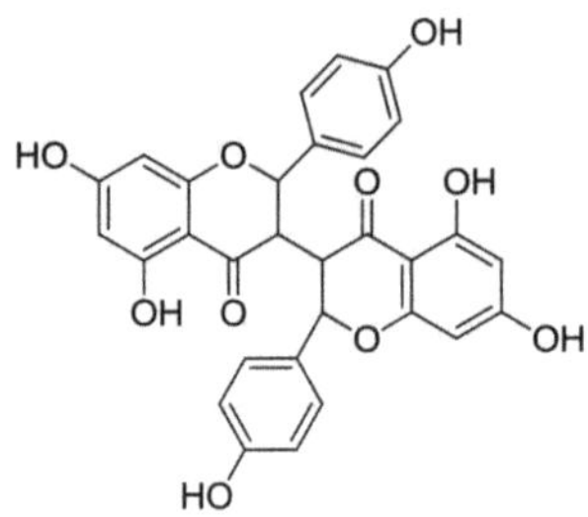

Chamaejasmine

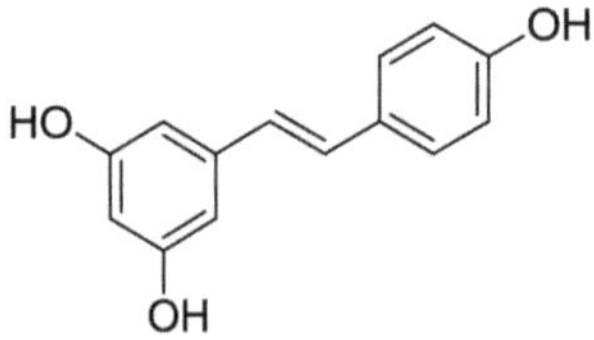

Resveratrol

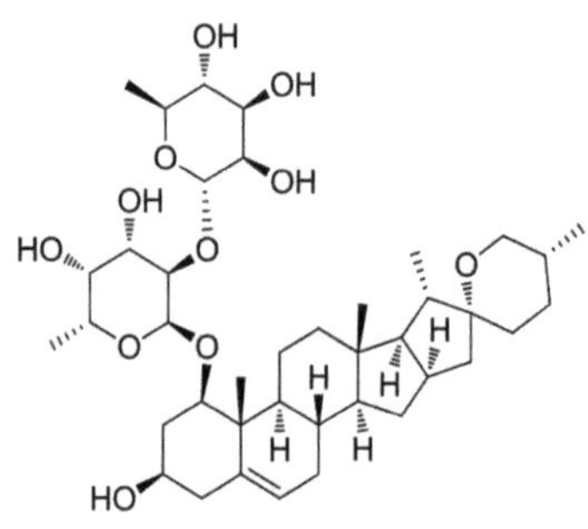

Ophiopogonin B

Fig. 2 Chemical structures of components isolated from TCMs with inhibitory effects on PI3K/AKT pathway

including MCF-7, MCF-7/ADR, HepG2, and some other carcinoma cell lines [86–88]. PI3K/AKT signaling pathway plays a central role in arenobufagin-mediated cell death. Arenobufagin can inhibit AKT with involvement of Phosphatase and tensin homolog (PTEN) activation as well as PDK1 and PI3K inhibition, and induces apoptosis in HCC cells. Arenobufagin treatment leads to marked decrease in the expression of mTOR. Inhibition of PI3K/AKT/mTOR pathway can promote the development of both autophagy and apoptosis induced by arenobufagin [89–91]. Arenobufagin induces mitochondria-mediated apoptosis in HepG2 and HepG2/ADM cells, accompanied with a decrease of mitochondrial potential, and an increase of Bax/Bcl-2 expression ratio. Activation of caspase-3 and caspase-9 as well as cleavage of PARP was also found in arenobufagin induced cell apoptosis [92]. In addition, arenobufagin is able to block VEGF-mediated angiogenesis [93]. Therefore, arenobufagin as the main active ingredients of toad venom has the potential to be developed as a novel anticancer agent [94, 95]. The pharmacokinetic characteristics of arenobufagin has been studied in six Sprague-Dawley rats by ultra fast liquid chromatography–tandem mass spectrometry [96]. Arenobufagin can be detected in plasma within 5 min to a peak concentration of 1.98 ng/mL after intraperitoneal administration 4.0 mg/kg, which indicates that arenobufagin can be absorbed quickly [96].

Radix Stephaniae tetrandrae is used to treat the syndrome of dampness-heat related diseases in TCM over thousands of years and it is widely used to treat cystitis, prostatitis, urethritis, pyelonephritis, vaginitis as well as rheumatism in China. A bisbenzylisoquinoline alkaloid, tetrandrine (Fig. 2) is isolated from the roots of *Radix Stephaniae tetrandrae* [97, 98]. Studies have shown that tetrandrine is able to inhibit cell proliferation and induces apoptosis of cancer cells [99, 100]. ERK and PI3K-AKT signaling pathways play a critical role in tetrandrine induced cell apoptosis [101]. Treatment of cancer cells with tetrandrine leads to the suppression of AKT activation, which in turn regulated the function of Bcl-2 family proteins and activated caspase cascades [102]. Tetrandrine also has the potential of immunomodulation and anti-inflammatory activity, which plays a positive role in HCC therapy [103]. Based on a long history of clinical application in TCM, tetrandrine is considered to be a safe agent, and may be an attractive candidate compound for liver cancer therapy. The Pharmacokinetic properties of tetrandrine were studied with a simple HPLC method in rabbits. The concentration-time data of tetrandrine fitted the classical two-compartment model, whether the drug was administered intravenously or orally [104]. The ratio of tetrandrine AUC (10 mg/kg by gavage) to AUC (5 mg/kg by intravenous injection) was about 30% and ratio of their Cmax was less than 20%, suggesting that tetrandrine is less absorbed from digestive tract or has a strong first pass effect as the gavage dose is double that of intravenous dose [104].

Rhizoma zedoariae possesses the effects of subsiding swelling, relieving pain in TCM and used to tread rheumatalgia, headache and chest pain. Elemene (1-methyl-1-vin-yl-2,4-diiso-propenyl-cyclohex-ane, Fig. 2), a noval lipid-soluble component, is extracted from the rhizoma of zedoariae [105]. β-Elemene, the most active component of elemene, has been shown to be effective against various cancers in vitro and in vivo, such as lung cancer, colorectal cancer and glioblastoma [105–108].

Recently, β-Elemene has been approved by the State Food and Drug Administration of China for the treatment of some solid tumors [109]. β-Elemene induces apoptosis and autophagy through inhibition of the PI3K/Akt/ mTOR/p70S6K1 signaling pathway in human gastric cancer cells [110]. Following treatment with β-Elemene, the level of phospho-AKT was obviously downregulated, leading to the down-regulation of downstream phosphor-mTOR as well as phospho-p70S6K1. The cleavage of PARP and conversion of LC3 I to LC3 II is consistent with the change of PI3K/Akt/mTOR/p70S6K1 activity. β-Elemen can induce G2/M phase arrest and apoptotic cell death in non-small lung cancer cells with activation of caspases-9, -3 and 7 [109]. β-Elemen promotes apoptosis through inhibiting the expression of Bcl-2 and survivin in MCF-7 human breast cancer cells [111]. In addition, β-Elemen can suppress the expressions of VEGF, basic fibroblast growth factor (bFGF), and epidermal growth factor (EGF), and exhibit anti-cancer ability on laryngeal cancer cells both in vitro and in vivo [112, 113]. β-Elemenal was a primary metabolite in bile of rat after β-Elemen intravenous administration. A sensitive gas chromatographic–mass spectrometric assay was developed to determine the level of β-Elemen and β-Elemenal in human plasma [114]. The peak plasma concentration (Cmax) and area under curve (AUC) of β-Elemen were prone to increase in proportion to the dose, but there were no significant differences among Cl values in the range of dosages. Moreover, no β-Elemenal was detected in plasma, and there was no other obvious homologous fragment elsewhere, which indicated that β-Elemen may be mainly decomposed into some small hydrophilic metabolites. Further investigations are needed to determine the biological process of β-Elemen in vivo [114].

Pogostemon cablin (Blanco) Benth, commonly known as "Guang-huoxiang" in China, is a TCM herb widely used to treat gastrointestinal diseases in many Asian countries [115]. Pogostone (Fig. 2) is one of the major constituent of *Pogostemon cablin*, and possesses various bioactivities, such as anti-fungal [116], anti-bacterial [117], pesticidal [118], and anti-inflammatory activities [119]. Recent studies have revealed that pogostone exhibited potent anti-proliferative activities against multiple human cancer cell lines, especially on human colorectal cancer cells HCT116 (IC50: 18.7 ± 1.93 μg/mL) [120]. Pogostone significantly inhibited AKT and mTOR phosphorylation in a dose-dependent manner, which contributed to the initiation of autophagy and apoptosis in HCT116 cells [120]. After treatment of pogostone, a dose-dependent increase in the levels of LC3 -II, cleaved caspase-3 and caspase-7, and a significant decrease in pro-caspase-3 levels were observed in HCT116 cells. Pogostone also inhibited the growth of HCT116 tumor, and reduced the tumor volume significantly with well tolerated by the host in vivo. Pogostone may be developed as a promising drug in the treatment of human colorectal cancer. The preclinical pharmacokinetic investigation of pogostone has been performed in rats after intravenous and oral administration [121]. The results showed that the blood concentration of pogostone appeared to increase nonproportionally between 5 and 20 mg/kg under the intravenous route [121].

Stellera chamaejasme L. is used to treat skin ulcer and abdominal distension in TCM. Chamaejasmine (Fig. 2), a flavone compound isolated from *Stellera chamaejasme L,* displays potent cytotoxicity in multiple cancer cell lines, including human lung cancer A549 cells, and human breast cancer MDA-MB-231 cells [122–124]. Recent study showed that chamaejasmine could induce apoptosis in HeLa cervical cancer cells, mediated through PI3K/Akt signaling cascades [125]. Treatment of chamaejasmine inactivates AKT to trigger apoptosis in human hep-2 larynx carcinoma cells [126].

Polygonum cuspidatum is believed to possess the effects of dissipating blood stasis and pain relief. Resveratrol 3,4,5-trihydroxystilbene, (Fig. 2), a polyphenol compound, is isolated and extracted from *Polygonum cuspidatum* with broad bioactivity including anti-bacterial, anti-inflammatory, anticancer, anti-hyperlipidemia anti-lipid peroxidation and pro-apoptotic effects [127, 128]. Resveratrol inhibited PI3K and Akt phosphorylations, and subsequently triggered the dephosphorylation of glycogen synthase kinase 3 beta (GSK3β), which resulted in cyclin D1 degradation and eventually cell cycle arrest and apoptosis in MGC803 human gastric cancer cells [129]. Furthermore, resveratrol can inhibit the invasion and metastasis of colorectal cancer cells through metastasis associated lung adenocarcinoma transcript 1 (MALAT1) mediated Wnt/β-catenin signal pathway [130]. However, the water solubility of resveratrol was very poor with approximately 0.03 mg/mL [131]. In vivo pharmacokinetic study confirmed that the oral bioavailability of resveratrol approaches zero, although administrated with relatively high concentrations of the compounds [132]. Therefore, it is important to enhance the bioavailability of resveratrol, which is considered as the main challenge in successfully applying resveratrol in clinical and health-promoting interventions [133].

Ophiopogonin B (OP-B, Fig. 2) is a bioactive component of *Radix Ophiopogon japonicus,* which is often used in TCM to treat pulmonary disease [134]. OP-B can significantly decrease cell viability in a panel of NSCLC cell lines. OP-B inhibited the PI3K/Akt/mTOR/p70S6K signaling pathway, suppressed p-AKT at both Ser308 and Thr473 and induced autophagy in NCI-H157 and H460 human lung cancer cells [135]. As a prospective inhibitor of AKT/mTOR, OP-B can also exhibit autophagy-dependent antitumor effects via repression AKT/mTOR signaling pathway in human cervical cancer HeLa cells [136]. OP-B can induce autophagy and apoptosis in A549 human lung cancer cells both in vitro and in vivo [137]. Moreover, OP-B significantly decreases cell proliferation and induces apoptosis in SGC-7901 human gastric cancer cells via triggering the JNK1/2 and ERK1/2 signaling pathways [138].

Epidermal Growth Factor Receptor (EGFR) as Targets

EGFR (also known as erbB1 or HER1) belongs to the family of tyrosine kinase receptors that include erbB2 (Neu, HER2), erbB3 (HER3), and erbB4 (HER4). EGFR once combined with EGF can promote the related genes in the cell nucleus, leading to cell proliferation. EGFR is commonly highly expressed in a variety of malignant tumors [9], and the abnormal activation of EGFR is closely correlated with tumor cell biology, acting as an indicator of poor prognosis for the patients with cancer.

The root of *Panax ginseng C. A. Mey (Ginsheng)* is believed to possess the activity of nourishing vitality and is widely used in China for patients with poor health condition. Ginsenoside Rg3 (GS-Rg3, Fig. 3) is one of the active ingredients in Ginsheng with significant antitumor activity. It is also the main component of Shenyi capsule, the first drug used for controlling the metastasis and recurrence of cancer patients in China. GS-Rg3 shows antitumor effects in a variety of cancers such as gastric, lung, colon, breast, and liver cancers etc. [139, 140]. GS-Rg3 displays various anticancer activities including inhibiting tumor growth, invasion and metastasis, and suppressing angiogenesis in tumor tissues and improving immunity. Synergistic anticancer effects are found when it combined with chemotherapeutic agents [141]. GS-Rg3 inhibited epithelial-mesenchymal transition (EMT) and invasion of lung cancer by down-regulating fucosyltransferase 4 (FUT4) mediated EGFR inactivation and blocking MAPK and NF-κB signal pathways [142]. GS-Rg3 reduced the expressions of EGFR and pEGFR in MCF-7 breast cancer cells in a dose-dependent manner, suggesting that GS-Rg3 inhibits the tumor growth by targeting EGFR and its down-stream signal transduction pathways [143]. GS-Rg3 is also an inhibitor of VEGF and bFGF; significantly decreasing the expression of these angiogenesis factors in human A549 lung cancer and human umbilical vein endothelial cells (HUVEC) [144]. In vitro as well as in vivo study have been carried out to determine the blood level of GS-Rg3 in rat plasma and its major metabolites using an HPLC/Q/TOF analytical approach. GS-Rg3 has an average half-life of 18.5 min after intravenous administration dosed at 5 mg/kg, whereas it was not detected in rat plasma after oral administration at 100 mg/kg [145]. GS-Rg3 was metabolized to ginsenoside Rh2 and protopanaxadiols (PPD) when anaerobically incubated with human fecal microflora, and the deglycosylated metabolites display activities comparable to or higher than that of GS-Rg3 [146]. However, GS-Rg3 has poor solubility and oral bioavailability, which limits its clinical application. Recently, a derivative of the compound, 20(S)-ginsenoside Rg3, was designed and developed as a new drug. Pharmacokinetics has been studied in healthy volunteers in China [147]. 20(S)-ginsenoside Rg3 was generally well tolerated, and exhibited a pharmacokinetic profile suitable for once-every-2-days dosing regimen [147].

Epimedium koreanum Nakai is believed to possess the effects of nourishing Yin and strengthening Yang, promoting blood circulation. Icariside II (Fig. 3), a flavonoidglycoside compound, is isolated from the stems and leaves of epimedium koreanum Nakai [148]. Studies have shown that icariside II exhibited potent cytotoxicity against a broad spectrum of human cancer cells through various pathways [149, 150]. Icariside II displays significant antitumor activity against A431 human epidermoid carcinoma cells in vitro and in mice bearing osteosarcoma sarcoma-180 in vivo by suppressing the phosphorylation of EGFR, down-regulating EGFR downstream signal PI3K/AKT and Raf/MEK/ERK as well as mTOR pathways in these cancer cells [151, 152]. Icariside II metabolites in rats were analyzed using an ultra-performance liquid chromatography/quadrupole-time-of-flight mass spectrometry method. The results showed that the metabolized mainly via desugarisation,

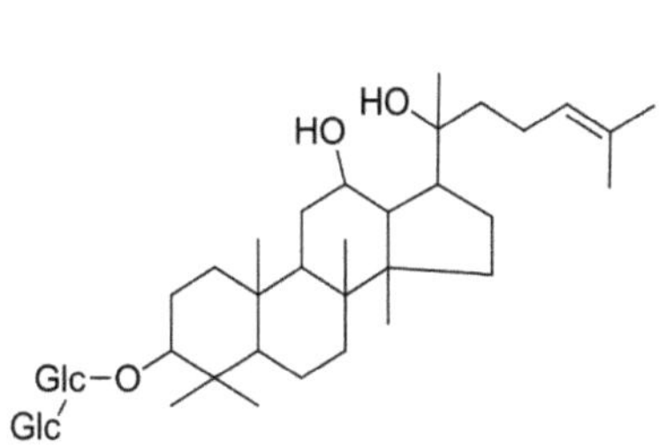

GS-Rg3

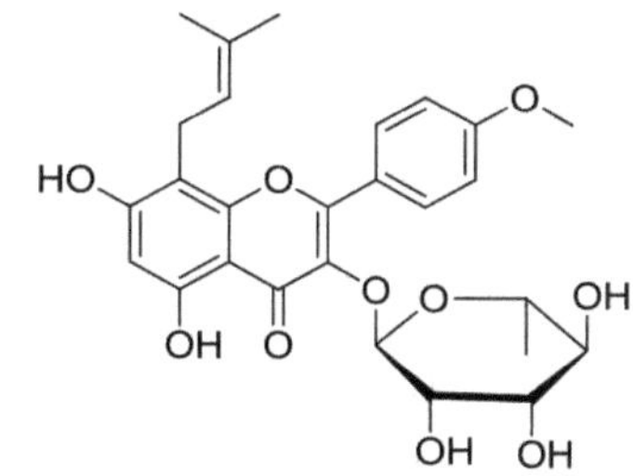

Icariside II

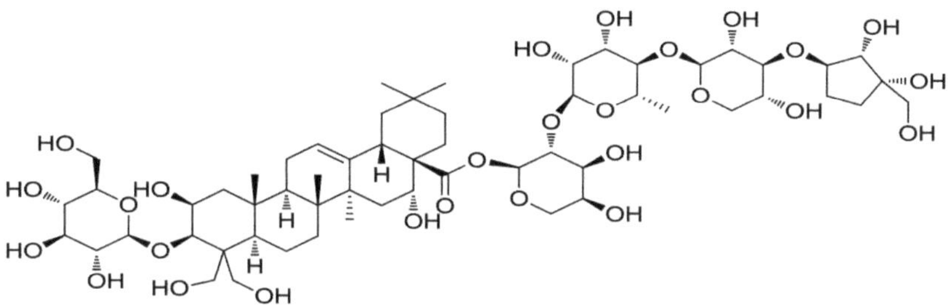

Platycodin D

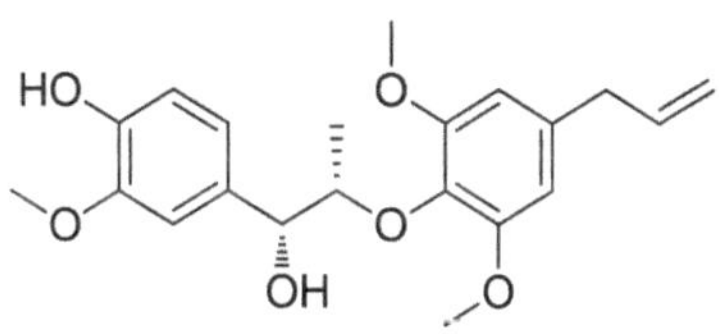

myrislignan

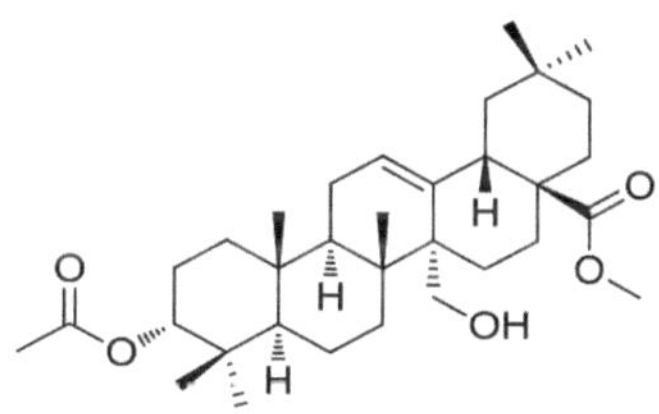

OA

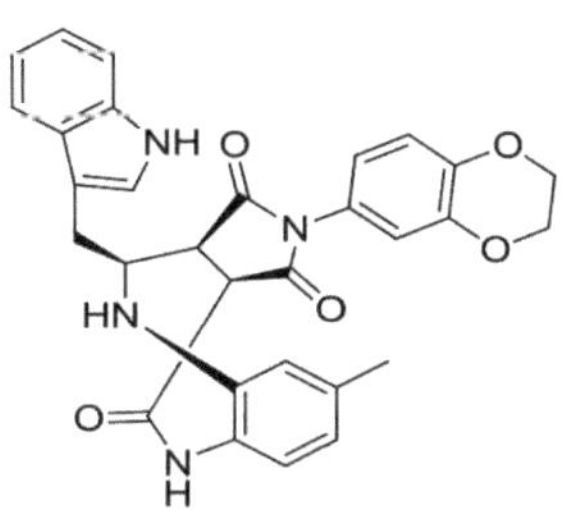

VS1

Fig. 3 Chemical structures of components isolated from TCM that target epidermal growth factor receptor (EGFR)

dehydrogenation, hydrogenation, hydroxylation, demethylation, glucuronidation, dehydration and glycosylation pathways in vivo. Specific hydrolysis of 7-O glucoside in the gut lumen and glucuronic acid conjugation in the liver was considered as the main physiologic processes of icariside II [153].

The root of *Platycodon grandiflorum (Companulaceae)* has been extensively used to treat several types of chronic inflammatory diseases in TCM [154]. Platycodin D (PD, Fig. 3), one of the major saponin components contained in the herb is reported to display antitumor effect on several cancer cell lines [155]. EGFR/PI3K/AKT pathway plays a critical role in PD induced cell apoptosis and PD downregulates the expression of EGFR in MDA-MB-231 breast cancer cells subsequently leading to the inhibition of the PI3K/AKT and MAPK pathways [156]. Additionally, PD could induce apoptosis and trigger ERK- and JNK-mediated autophagy in human hepatocellular carcinoma BEL-7402 cells [157].

The seed of *Myristica fragrans Houtt (Nutmeg)* is used to treat diarrhea and epigastric pain in TCM. Recent study showed that one of the components myrislignan (Fig. 3) isolated from nutmeg, displayed potent anticancer activity against A549 lung cancer cells both in vitro and in vivo [158]. The effects of myrislignan on apoptosis and cell proliferation are mediated by activation of MAPK and inhibition of EGFR signal pathway.

Peganum harmala L. is used to treat cancer in TCMs and Uygur medicine. A novel compound called 3α-acetoxy-27-hydroxyolean-12-en-28-oic acid methyl ester (OA, Fig. 3) was isolated from the herb [159]. OA possesses potent anticancer activity against NSCLC via inhibiting the activation of EGFR and its downstream signals. Guo et al. developed a model to identify the ERBB3 inhibitors from natural products and TCMs. Several compounds with anticancer activity were identified; among them, VS1 (Fig. 3) is the most promising component with IC_{50} value of 269 μM against A549 lung cancer cells [160].

Conclusions

TCM is widely used in China to reduce the side effects of chemotherapeutic drugs and improve the outcome of conventional treatment. The discussed components here are isolated from TCMs and their modes of actions are summarized in Table 1. However, it should be kept in mind that numerous components from TCMs display antitumor activity via multiple targets. Most components discussed above show pro-apoptotic activity mediated by activation of caspases and downregulation of mitochondrial antiapoptotic proteins. One point should be emphasized that in some cases, the mixed extracts of TCM display more potent antitumor effects than the single individual component and exhibited synergistic effects with most TCM preparation. Our recent study revealed that the crude extract of clove bud can induce cell death via apoptotic pathway and inhibit the growth of cancer cells both in vitro and in vivo. However, the isolated bioactive component, Oleanolic acid, displays much weaker antitumor activity compared to the crude extract in the nude mouse models

Table 1 Components from the Traditional Chinese Medicine Acts as Protein Kinase Inhibitors

Name of anti-tumor TCMs	Sources	Classification	Kinase inhibitors and cell lines	References
Curcuma	*Curcuma longa L.*	Polyphenols	JNK/p38 MAPK/ERK HCT-116, THP-1, CNE1, CNE2 and HepG2 cells	[14–17]
Celastrol	*Tripterygium wilfordii Hook. f.*	Triterpene	JNK	[31]
			HOS, MG-63, U-2OS and Saos-2 cells	
Chelerythrine	*Chelidonium majus L.*	Benzophenanthridine alkaloid	JNK/p38 MAPK/ERK	[34, 35]
			HeLa, HOS and U-2OS cells	
Emodin	*Rheum palmatum L.*	Anthraquinone	ERK/p38 MAPK	[43, 44]
			SMMC-7721, SW480 and SW620 cells	
Tubeimoside-1	*Bolbostemma paniculatum Franquet*	Triterpenoid saponin	JNK/p38 MAPK/ERK	[48, 53–56]
			DU145, A549, PC9 A2780/DDP, SKOV-3 and HepG2 cells	
β-eudesmol	*Atractylodes lancea rhizome*	Sesquiterpenol	JNK	[58]
			HL60 cell	
Hinesol	*Atractylodes lancea rhizome*	Sesquiterpenol	JNK/ERK	[60]
			HL60 cell	
Isoquercitrin	*Bidens bipinnata L.*	Flavonoid	JNK/p38 MAPK/ERK	[63]
			HepG2 cell	
PYDDT	*Echinops grijsii*	Alkynol group-substituted thiophene	JNK	[66]
			SW620 cell	
Tatariside G	*Fagopyrum tataricum (L.) Gaertn*	Phenylpropanoid glycosides	JNK/p38 MAPK	[69]
			HeLa cell	

(continued)

Table 1 (continued)

Name of anti-tumor TCMs	Sources	Classification	Kinase inhibitors and cell lines	References
SYUNZ-16	*Arnebia euchroma roots*	b,b-Dimethylacrylalkannin	AKT	[83]
			Hep3B and GLC-82 cells	
Arenobufagin	*Bufo gargarizans Cantor or Bufo melanostictus Suhneider*	C24 steroids	PI3K/Akt/mTOR	[92]
			HepG2 and HepG2/	
			ADM cells	
Tetrandrine	*Radix Stephaniae tetrandrae*	Bisbenzylisoquinoline alkaloid	ERK and PI3K/AKT	[99, 102]
			HT-29, Huh7, HepG2 and BEL7402 cells	
β-Elemene	*Rhizomazedoariae*	Terpene	PI3K/Akt/mTOR	[110]
			MGC803 and SGC7–901 cells	
Pogostone	*Pogostemon cablin (Blanco) Benth*	Ketone	PI3K/Akt/mTOR	[120]
			HCT116 cell	
Chamaejasmine	*Stellera chamaejasme L.*	Flavonoid	PI3K/Akt	[125, 126]
			HeLa and Hep-2 cells.	
Resveratrol	*Polygonum cuspidatum*	Polyphenol	PI3K/Akt	[129]
			MGC803 cell	
Ophiopogonin-B	*Radix Ophiopogon japonicus*	Saponin	PI3K/Akt/mTOR	[135, 136]
			NCI-H157, H460 and HeLa cells	
Ginsenoside Rg3	*Ginsheng*	Saponin	EGFR and VEGF	[142–144]
			A549, H1299, H358, MCF-7 and HUVEC304 cells	
Icariside II	*Yin Yanghuo*	Flavonoid	EGFR	[151, 152]
	Horny Goat Weed		A431 cell	

Name of anti-tumor TCMs	Sources	Classification	Kinase inhibitors and cell lines	References
Platycodin D	*Platycodon grandiflorum*	Saponin	EGFR	[156]
			MDA-MB-231 cell	
Myrislignan	*Myristica fragrans Houtt*	Lignans	EGFR	[158]
			A549 cell	
OA	*Peganum harmala L.*	Triterpene	EGFR	[159]
			A549 cell	
VS1		Heterocycle	ERBB3	[160]
			A549 cell	

of xenografted human tumors, suggesting synergistic antitumor effects exist among the components in the extract of clove bud [161].

In most cases, TCMs are used with combinational preparation; certain kinds of herbs are combined to treat cancer. There are challenges to dissect the mechanisms of the interactions of too many components in the combinational preparation. However, TCM provide a novel strategy for cancer therapy due to its multiple targets and low side effects. However, the underlying mechanisms of most TCM have not been elucidated yet. On the other hands, numerous components isolated from TCMs possess poor bioavailability; novel approaches, including chemical modification, nanotechnology etc. should be employed to improve their efficacy in vivo. It is likely that the efficacy of TCM in cancer treatment may lead to novel strategies in fight against various cancers.

Acknowledgments This work was supported by National Innovative Drug Development Project of China (No. #: 2014ZX-09102043-001) and the 863 High Technology Project of China (No#: 2014AA093503). The study was also supported in part by the Natural Science Foundation of China (No#81302906, 81273550, 81573457, and 41306157), the Shandong Provincial Natural Science Foundation in China (No #: ZR2014HQ031, ZR2011HQ027 and 2016GGD03015) and Zibo Development Program of Sci. & Tech, in Shandong, China (No#2016KJ100048).

Conflict of Interest The authors declare no conflict of interest.

References

1. Sharma PS, Sharma R, Tyagi R (2008) Inhibitors of cyclin dependent kinases: useful targets for cancer treatment. Curr Cancer Drug Targets 8(1):53–75
2. Goldstein DM, Gray NS, Zarrinkar PP (2008) High-throughput kinase profiling as a platform for drug discovery. Nat Rev Drug Discov 7(5):391–397
3. Ferre F, Palmeri A, Helmer-Citterich M (2014) Computational methods for analysis and inference of kinase/inhibitor relationships. Front Genet 5:196
4. Sun ZJ, Chen G, Hu X, Zhang W, Liu Y, Zhu LX, Zhou Q, Zhao YF (2010) Activation of PI3K/Akt/IKK-alpha/NF-kappaB signaling pathway is required for the apoptosis evasion in human salivary adenoid cystic carcinoma: its inhibition by quercetin. Apoptosis 15:850–863
5. Kannan-Thulasiraman P, Katsoulidis E, Tallman MS, Arthur JS, Platanias LC (2006) Activation of the mitogen- and stress-activated kinase 1 by arsenic trioxide. J Biol Chem 281(32):22446–22452
6. Chang L, Karin M, Mammalian MA (2001) Kinase signalling cascades. Nature 410(6824):37–40
7. Dhanasekaran DN, Reddy EP (2008) JNK signaling in apoptosis. Oncogene 27(48):6245–6251
8. Wagner EF, Nebreda AR (2009) Signal integration by JNK and p38 MAPK pathways in cancer development. Nat Rev Cancer 9(8):537–549
9. Nakao Y, Fusetani N (2007) Enzyme inhibitors from marine invertebrates. J Nat Prod 70(4):689–710
10. Cheng CY, Lin YH, Su CC (2010) Curcumin inhibits the proliferation of human hepatocellular carcinoma J5 cells by inducing endoplasmic reticulum stress and mitochondrial dysfunction. Int J Mol Med 26(5):637–638

11. Saha A, Kuzuhara T, Echigo N, Fujii A, Suganuma M, Fujiki H (2010) Apoptosis of human lung cancer cells by curcumin mediated through up-regulation of "growth arrest and DNA damage inducible genes 45 and 153". Biol Pharm Bull 33(8):1291–1299
12. Banerjee M, Singh P, Panda D (2010) Curcumin suppresses the dynamic instability of microtubules, activates the mitotic checkpoint and induces apoptosis in MCF-7 cells. FEBS J 277(16):3437–3448
13. Johnson SM, Gulhati P, Arrieta I (2009) Curcumin inhibits proliferation of colorectal carcinoma by modulating Akt/mTOR signaling. Anticancer Res 29(8):3185–3190
14. Collett GP, Campbell FC (2004) Curcumin induces c-jun N-terminal kinase-dependent apoptosis in HCT116 human colon cancer cells. Carcinogenesis 25(11):2183–2189
15. Yang CW, Chang CL, Lee HC, Chi CW, Pan JP, Yang WC (2012) Curcumin induce the apoptosis of human monocytic leukemia THP-1 cells via the activation of JNK/ERK pathways. BMC Complement Altern Med 12(1):22
16. Wang D, Hu J, Lv L, Xia X, Liu J, Li X (2013) Enhanced inhibitory effect of curcumin via reactive oxygen species generation in human nasopharyngeal carcinoma cells following purple-light irradiation. Oncol Lett 6(1):81–85
17. Chintana PY, Wirachwong P, Suksamrarn A et al (2011) Down regulation of p-ERK1/2 and p-AKT expression by curcumin and tetrahydrocurcumin in hepatocellular carcinoma-induced tumors in nude mice. Asian Biomed 5(3):345–352
18. Ireson CR, Jones DJ, Orr S, Coughtrie MW et al (2002) Metabolism of the cancer chemopreventive agent curcumin in human and rat intestine. Cancer Epidemiol Biomarkers Prev 11:105–111
19. Usta M, Wortelboer HM, Vervoort J, Boersma MG, Rietjens IM, van Bladeren PJ, Cnubben NH (2007) Human glutathione S-transferase-mediated glutathione conjugation of curcumin and efflux of these conjugates in Caco-2 cells. Chem Res Toxicol 20:1895–1902
20. Cheng AL, Hsu CH, Lin JK, Hsu MM et al (2001) Phase I clinical trial of curcumin, a chemopreventive agent, in patients with high-risk or pre-malignant lesions. Anticancer Res 21:2895–2900
21. Lao CD, Ruffin MT, Normolle D et al (2006) Dose escalation of a curcuminoid formulation. BMC Complement Altern Med 6:10
22. Schiborr C, Eckert GP, Rimbach G, Frank J (2010) A validated method for the quantification of curcumin in plasma and brain tissue by fast narrow-bore high-performance liquid chromatography with fluorescence detection. Anal Bioanal Chem 397:1917–1925
23. Zhang CY, Yi JM, Yuan HL et al (2014) Progress in pharmacokinetics of curcumin and its dosage forms. Anhui Med Pharm J 18:1
24. Peng B, Xu L, Cao F, Wei T, Yang C, Uzan G et al (2010) HSP90 inhibitor, celastrol, arrests human monocytic leukemia cell U937 at G0/G1 in thiol-containing agents reversible way. Mol Cancer 9:79
25. Kannaiyan R, Manu KA, Chen L, Li F, Rajendran P, Subramaniam A et al (2011) Celastrol inhibits tumor cell proliferation and promotes apoptosis through the activation of c-Jun N-terminal kinase and suppression of PI3 K/Akt signaling pathways. Apoptosis 16:1028–1041
26. Sethi G, Ahn KS, Pandey MK, Aggarwal BB (2007) Celastrol, a novel triterpene, potentiates TNF-induced apoptosis and suppresses invasion of tumor cells by inhibiting NF-kappaB regulated gene products and TAK1-mediated NF-kappaB activation. Blood 109:2727–2735
27. Yang H, Chen D, Cui QC, Yuan X, Dou QP (2006) Celastrol, a triterpene extracted from the Chinese "Thunder of God Vine," is a potent proteasome inhibitor and suppresses human prostate cancer growth in nude mice. Cancer Res 66:4758–4765
28. Rajendran P, Li F, Shanmugam MK, Kannaiyan R, Goh JN, Wong KF et al (2012) Celastrol suppresses growth and induces apoptosis of human hepatocellular carcinoma through the modulation of STAT3/JAK2 signaling cascade in vitro and in vivo. Cancer Prev Res (Phila) 5:631–643

29. Huang Y, Zhou Y, Fan Y, Zhou D (2008) Celastrol inhibits the growth of human glioma xenografts in nude mice through suppressing VEGFR expression. Cancer Lett 264:101–106
30. Lee JH, Won YS, Park KH, Lee MK, Tachibana H, Yamada K et al (2012) Celastrol inhibits growth and induces apoptotic cell death in melanoma cells via the activation ROS-dependent mitochondrial pathway and the suppression of PI3K/AKT signaling. Apoptosis 17:1275–1286
31. Li HY, Zhang J, Sun LL, Li BH, Gao HL, Xie T, Zhang N, Ye ZM (2015) Celastrol induces apoptosis and autophagy via the ROS/JNK signaling pathway in human osteosarcoma cells: an in vitro and in vivo study. Cell Death Dis 6:e1604
32. Zhang J, Li C-Y, Xu M-J, Wu T et al (2012) Oral bioavailability and gender-related pharmacokinetics of celastrol following administration of pure celastrol and its related tablets in rats. J Ethnopharmacol 144:195–120
33. Chmura SJ, Dolan ME, Cha A, Mauceri HJ, Kufe DW, Weichselbaum RR (2000) In vitro and in vivo activity of protein kinase C inhibitor chelerythrine chloride induces tumor cell toxicity and growth delay in vivo. Clin Cancer Res 6(2):737–742
34. Yu R, Mandlekar S, Tan TH, Kong AN (2000) Activation of p38 and c-Jun N-terminal kinase pathways and induction of apoptosis by chelerythrine do not require inhibition of protein kinase C. J Biol Chem 275(13):9612–9619
35. Yang R, Piperdi S, Gorlick R (2008) Activation of the RAF/mitogen-activated protein/extracellular signal-regulated kinase/extracellular signal-regulated kinase pathway mediates apoptosis induced by chelerythrine in osteosarcoma. Clin Cancer Res 14(20):6396–6404
36. Vrba J, Dolezel P, Vicar J, Modrianský M, Ulrichová J (2008) Chelerythrine and dihydrochelerythrine induce G1 phase arrest and bimodal cell death in human leukemia HL-60 cells. Toxicol In Vitro 22(4):1008–1017
37. Siomboing X, Gressier B, Dine T et al (2001) Investigation of the inhibitory effects of chelerythrine chloride on the translocation of the protein kinase C βI,βII,zeta in human neutrophils. Farmaco 56(11):859–865
38. Yang S, Liu Y, Yang QF et al (2011) The antitumor effect of *Macleaya cordata* and its molecular mechanism research of inducting human telomere DNA to form the Four-stranded G-quadruplex. Chin Herb Med 42(4):738–742
39. Qu W, Wang Y, Wu Q, Liu J, Hao D (2015) Emodin inhibits HMGB1-induced tumor angiogenesis in human osteosarcoma by regulating SIRT1. Int J Clin Exp Med 8:15054–15064
40. Ma L, Li W (2014) Emodin inhibits LOVO colorectal cancer cell proliferation via the regulation of the Bcl-2/Bax ratio and cytochrome c. Exp Ther Med 8:1225–1228
41. Xie MJ, Ma YH, Miao L, Wang Y, Wang HZ, Xing YY, Xi T, Lu YY (2014) Emodin-provoked oxidative stress induces apoptosis in human colon cancer HCT116 cells through a p53-mitochondrial apoptotic pathway. Asian Pac J Cancer Prev 15:5201–5205
42. Yaoxian W, Hui Y, Yunyan Z, Yanqin L, Xin G, Xiaoke W (2013) Emodin induces apoptosis of human cervical cancer HeLa cells via intrinsic mitochondrial and extrinsic death receptor pathway. Cancer Cell Int 13:71
43. Lin W, Zhong M, Yin H, Chen Y, Cao Q, Wang C, Ling C (2016) Emodin induces carcinoma cell apoptosis through MAPK and PI3K/AKT signaling pathways in vitro and in vivo. Oncol Rep 36:961–967
44. Liu B, Yuan B, Zhang L, Mu W, Wang C (2015) ROS/p38/p53/Puma signaling pathway is involved in emodin-induced apoptosis of human colorectal cancer cells. Int J Clin Exp Med 8:15413–15422
45. Lin SP, Chu PM, Tsai SY et al (2012) Pharmacokinetics and tissue distribution of resveratrol, emodin and their metabolites after intake of Polygonum cuspidatum in rats. J Ethnopharmacol 144:671–676
46. Shia CS, Hou YC, Tsai SY et al (2010) Differences in pharmacokinetics and ex vivo antioxidant activity following intravenous and oral administrations of emodin to rats. J Pharm Sci 99:2185–2195

47. Liu W, Feng Q, Li Y et al (2012) Coupling of UDP-glucuronosyltransferases and multidrug resistance-associated proteins is responsible for the intestinal disposition and poor bioavailability of emodin. Toxicol Appl Pharmacol 265:316–324
48. Yin Y, Chen W, Tang C, Ding H, Jang J, Weng M, Cai Y, Zou G (2011) NF-κB, JNK and p53 pathways are involved in tubeimoside-1-induced apoptosis in HepG2 cells with oxidative stress and G2/M cell cycle arrest. Food Chem Toxicol 49:3046–3054
49. Yu TX, Ma RD, Yu LJ (2001) Structure-activity relationship of tubeimosides in anti-inflammatory, antitumor, and antitumor-promoting effects. Acta Pharmacol Sin 22:463–468
50. Jia G, Wang Q, Wang R, Deng D, Xue L, Shao N, Zhang Y, Xia X, Zhi F, Yang Y (2015) Tubeimoside-1induces glioma apoptosis through regulation of Bax/Bcl-2 and the ROS/Cytochrome C/Caspase-3 pathway. Onco Targets Ther 8:303–311
51. Zhang Y, Xu X, He P (2011) Tubeimoside-1 inhibits proliferation and induces apoptosis by increasing the Bax to Bcl-2 ratio and decreasing COX-2 expression in lung cancer A549 cells. Mol Med Rep 4:25–29
52. Wang Y, Deng L, Zhong H, Jiang X, Chen J (2011) Natural plant extract tubeimoside I promotes apoptosis-mediated cell death in cultured human hepatoma (HepG2) cells. Biol Pharm Bull 34:831–838
53. Yang JB, Khan M, He YY, Yao M et al (2016) Tubeimoside-1 induces oxidative stress-mediated apoptosis and G0/G1phase arrest in human prostate carcinoma cells in vitro. Acta Pharmacol Sin 37(7):950–962
54. Hao W, Wang S, Zhou Z (2015) Tubeimoside-1 (TBMS1) inhibits lung cancer cell growth and induces cells apoptosis through activation of MAPK-JNK pathway. Int J Clin Exp Pathol 8(10):12075–12083
55. Liu HZ, Yu C, Yang Z, He JL, Chen WJ, Yin J, Li WM, Liu HT, Wang YX (2011) Tubeimoside I sensitizes cisplatin in cisplatin-resistant human ovarian cancer cells (A2780/DDP) through down-regulation of ERK and up-regulation of p38 signaling pathways. Mol Med Rep 4(5):985–992
56. Chen WJ, Yu C, Yang Z, He JL, Yin J, Liu HZ et al (2012) Tubeimoside-1 induces G2/M phase arrest and apoptosis in SKOV-3 cells through increase of intracellular Ca^{2+} and caspase-dependent signaling pathways. Int J Oncol 40:535–543
57. Liang JM, Zhang WD, Zhang C, Liu RH et al (2007) Quantitative determination of the anti-cancer agent tubeimoside I in rat plasma by liquid chromatography coupled with mass spectrometry. J Chromatogr B 845:84–89
58. Li Y, Li T, Miao C, Li J, Xiao W, Ma E (2013) β-Eudesmol induces JNK-dependent apoptosis through the mitochondrial pathway in HL60 cells. Phytother Res 27(3):338–343
59. Tsuneki H, Ma E, Kobayashi S et al (2005) Antiangiogenic activity of β-eudesmol in vitro and in vivo. Eur J Pharmacol 512:105–115
60. Masuda Y, Kadokura T, Lshii M, Takada K, Kitajima J (2015) Hinesol, a compound isolated from the essential oils of Atractylodes lancea rhizome, inhibits cell growth and induces apoptosis in human leukemia HL-60 cells. J Nat Med 69(3):332–339
61. Yang QH, Yang J, Liu GZ, Wang L, Zhu TC, Gao HL, Kou XG (2013) Study on in vitro anti-tumor activity of *Bidens bipinnata* L. extract. Afr J Tradit Complement Altern Med 10:543–549
62. Wu J, Wan Z, Yi J, Wu Y, Peng W, Wu J (2013) Investigation of the extracts from *Bidens pilosa* Linn. var. radiata Sch. Bip. for antioxidant activities and cytotoxicity against human tumor cells. J Nat Med 67:17–26
63. Huang G, Tang B, Tang K, Dong X et al (2014) Isoquercitrin inhibits the progression of liver cancer in vivo and in vitro via the MAPK signalling pathway. Oncol Rep 31(5):2377–2384
64. Jin W, Shi Q, Hong C, Cheng Y, Ma Z, Qu H (2008) Cytotoxic properties of thiophenes from Echinops grijissi Hance. Phytomedicine 15:768–774
65. Zhang P, Jin WR, Shi Q, He H, Ma ZJ, Qu HB (2008) Two novel thiophenes from Echinops grijissi Hance. J Asian Nat Prod Res 10:977–981

66. Xu DG, Lv W, Dai CY, Zhu FF, Xu GH, Ma ZJ, Chen Z (2015) 2-(Pro-1-ynyl)-5-(5,6-dihydrox-ypenta-1,3-diynyl) Thiophene induces apoptosis through reactive oxygen species-mediated JNK activation in human colon cancer SW620 cells. Anat Rec (Hoboken) 298(2):376–385
67. Lin B, Hu CL, Huang F, Han T (2011) Research progress on chemical constituents and pharmacological effect of Fagopyrum tataricum. Drugs Clinic 26:29–32
68. Karki R, Park CH, Kim DW (2013) Extract of buckwheat sprouts scavenges oxidation and inhibits pro-inflammatory mediators in lipopolysaccharide–stimulated macrophages (RAW264.7). J Integr Med 11:246–252
69. Li Y, Wang SJ, Xia W, Rahman K, Zhang Y, Peng H et al (2014) Effects of tatariside G isolated from fagopyrum tataricum roots on apoptosis in human cervical cancer HeLa cells. Molecules 19(8):11145–11159
70. Brugge J, Hung MC, Mills GB (2007) A new mutational AKTivation in the PI3K pathway. Cancer Cell 12(2):104–107
71. Yu L, Wang LT, Chen SW (2012) Dual character of Toll-like receptor signaling: pro-tumorigenic effects and anti-tumor functions. Biochim Biophys Acta 1835(2):144–154
72. LoPiccolo J, Granville CA, Gills JJ, Dennis PA (2007) Targeting Akt in cancer therapy. Anticancer Drugs 18:861–874
73. Crowell JA, Steele VE, Fay JR (2007) Targeting the AKT protein kinase for cancer chemoprevention. Mol Cancer Ther 6:2139–2148
74. Hennessy BT, Smith DL, Ram PT, Lu Y, Mills GB (2005) Exploiting the PI3K/AKT pathway for cancer drug discovery. Nat Rev Drug Discov 4:988–1004
75. Feng GE, Wang XD, Wang YC (2003) Advances in studies on medicinal Radix Arnebiae Seu Lithospermi. Chin Tradit Herb Drug 9:6–10
76. Yang F, Chen Y, Duan W, Zhang C, Zhu H, Ding J (2006) SH-7, a new synthesized shikonin derivative, exerting its potent antitumor activities as a topoisomerase inhibitor. Int J Cancer 119:1184–1193
77. Lu Q, Liu W, Ding J, Cai J, Duan W (2002) Shikonin derivatives: synthesis and inhibition of human telomerase. Bioorg Med Chem Lett 12:1375–1378
78. Lim ES, Rhee YH, Park MK, Shim BS, Ahn KS, Kang H, Yoo HS, Kim SH (2007) DMNQ S-64 induces apoptosis via caspase activation and cyclooxygenase-2 inhibition in human nonsmall lung cancer cells. Ann N Y Acad Sci 1095:7–18
79. Wang Y, Xie BF, Zhu XF, Feng GK, Deng R, Liu JN et al (2006) The mechanism for SYUNZ-4 inducing apoptosis of U937 cells. Chin J Hematol 27:762–765
80. Xie BF, Feng GK, Huang H, Zhu XF, Wang Y, Deng R et al (2007) Antitumor effect of alkannin derivative, SYUNZ-4. Chin Pharm J 42:1384–1388
81. Xie BF, Feng GK, Huang H, Liu ZC, Wu HQ, Huang ZS, Gu LQ (2006) Apoptosis induct ion of new naphthoquinone-like derivative TEISHNZ on human nasopharyngeal cancer cell. Chin Tradit Herb Drug 37:234–238
82. Xie BF, Feng GK, Huang H, Zhu XF, Zhou JM, Wang Y et al (2006) Investigation of antitumor effect of natural radixarnebiae seu Lithospermi naphthoquinone compounds and its derivatives. Chin Pharmacol Bull 22:505–507
83. Deng R, Tang J, Xie BF, Feng GK, Huang YH, Liu ZC, Zhu XF (2010) SYUNZ-16, a newly synthesized alkannin derivative, induces tumor cells apoptosis and suppresses tumor growth through inhibition of PKB/AKT kinase activity and blockade of AKT/FOXO signal pathway. Int J Cancer 127:220–229
84. Tokunaga E, Oki E, Egashira A, Sadanaga N, Morita M, Kakeji Y, Maehara Y (2008) Deregulation of the Akt pathway in human cancer. Curr Cancer Drug Targets 8:27–36
85. Gong ZP, Chn T, Deng LR, Hu YQ (2010) Research progress on the antitumor clinical application of cinobufacin injection combined with chemotherapy. Anhui Med Pharm J 14:12–14
86. Zhang L, Nakaya K, Yoshida T, Kuroiwa Y (1992) Induction by bufalin of differentiation of human leukemia cells HL60, U937, and ML1 toward macrophage/monocyte-like cells and its

potent synergistic effect on the differentiation of human leukemia cells in combination with other inducers. Cancer Res 52:4634–4641
87. Masuda Y, Kawazoe N, Nakajo S, Yoshida T, Kuroiwa Y, Nakaya K (1995) Bufalin induces apoptosis and influences the expression of apoptosis-related genes in human leukemia cells. Leuk Res 19:549–556
88. Yu CH, Kan SF, Pu HF, Jea Chien E, Wang PS (2010) Apoptotic signaling in bufalin- and cinobufagin-treated androgen-dependent and -independent human prostate cancer cells. Cancer Sci 99:2467–2476
89. Brown VI, Fang J, Alcorn K, Barr R, Kim JM, Wasserman R, Grupp SA (2003) Rapamycin is active against B-precursor leukemia in vitro and in vivo, an effect that is modulated by IL-7-mediated signaling. Proc Natl Acad Sci U S A 100:15113–15118
90. Teachey DT, Obzut DA, Cooperman J et al (2006) The mTOR inhibitor CCI-779 induces apoptosis and inhibits growth in preclinical models of primary adult human ALL. Blood 107:1149–1155
91. Chen G, Hu X, Zhang W et al (2012) Mammalian target of rapamycin regulates isoliquiritigenin-induced autophagic and apoptotic cell death in adenoid cystic carcinoma cells. Apoptosis 17:90–101
92. Zhang DM, Liu JS, Deng LJ et al (2013) Arenobufagin, a natural bufadienolide from toad venom, induces apoptosis and autophagy in human hepatocellular carcinoma cells through inhibition of PI3K/Akt/mTOR pathway. Carcinogenesis 34(6):1331–1342
93. Li M, Wu S, Liu Z et al (2013) Arenobufagin, a bufadienolide compound from toad venom, inhibits VEGF-mediated angiogenesis through suppression of VEGFR-2 signaling pathway. Biochem Pharmacol 83:1251–1260
94. Liu JS, Zhang DM, Kurihara H, Ye WC (2009) Antitumor effects of toad venom and its active components. J Int Pharm Res 4:115–120
95. Hu Y, Yu Z, Yang ZJ, Zhu G, Fong W (2011) Comprehensive chemical analysis of Toad venom by using liquid chromatography/electrospray ionization tandem mass spectrometry. J Pharm Biomed Anal 56:210–220
96. Li G, Han W, Jiang W, Zhang D et al (2013) Quantitative determination of arenobufagin in rat plasma by ultra fast liquid chromatography-tandem mass spectrometry and its application in a pharmacokinetic study. J Chromatogr B 939:86–91
97. Bosch FX, Ribes J, Diaz M, Cleries R (2004) Primary liver cancer: worldwide incidence and trends. Gastroenterology 127:S5–S16
98. Liu L, Cao Y, Chen C, Zhang X, McNabola A, Wilkie D, Wilhelm S, Lynch M, Carter C (2006) Sorafenib blocks the RAF/MEK/ERK pathway, inhibits tumor angiogenesis, and induces tumor cell apoptosis in hepatocellular carcinoma model PLC/PRF/5. Cancer Res 66:11851–11858
99. Chen XL, Ren KH, He HW, Shao RG (2008) Involvement of PI3K/AKT/GSK3 beta pathway in tetrandrine-induced G1 arrest and apoptosis. Cancer Biol Ther 7:1073–1078
100. Yan C, Xin-Ming Q, Li-Kun G, Lin-Lin L, Fang-Ping C, Ying X, Xiong-Fei W, Xiang-Hong L, Jin R (2006) Tetrandrine-induced apoptosis in rat primary hepatocytes is initiated from mitochondria: caspases and endonuclease G (Endo G) pathway. Toxicology 218:1–12
101. Lin ST, Wang Y, Xue Y, Feng DC, Xu Y, Xu LY (2008) Tetrandrine suppresses LPS-induced astrocyte activation via modulating IKKs-IkappaBalpha NF-kappaB signaling pathway. Mol Cell Biochem 315:41–49
102. Liu CY, Gong K, Mao X, Li WH (2011) Tetrandrine induces apoptosis by activating reactive oxygen species and repressing Akt activity in human hepatocellular carcinoma. Int J Cancer 129:1519–1531
103. Shen YC, Chou CJ, Chiou WF, Chen CF (2001) Anti-inflammatory effects of the partially purified extract of radix Stephaniae tetrandrae: comparative studies of its active principles tetrandrine and fangchinoline on human polymorphonuclear leukocyte functions. Mol Pharmacol 60:1083–1090

104. Jiang XH, Yang JQ, Li N, Wang H, Zhou QX (2011) The pharmacokinetical study of plant alkaloid tetrandrine with a simple HPLC method in rabbits. Fitoterapia 82:878–882
105. Li QQ, Wang G, Zhang M, Cuff CF, Huang L, Reed E (2009) beta-Elemene, a novel plant-derived antineoplastic agent, increases cisplatin chemosensitivity of lung tumor cells by triggering apoptosis. Oncol Rep 22:161–170
106. Wang G, Li X, Huang F, Zhao J, Ding H, Cunningham C, Coad JE, Flynn DC, Reed E, Li QQ (2005) Antitumor effect of beta-elemene in non-small-cell lung cancer cells is mediated via induction of cell cycle arrest and apoptotic cell death. Cell Mol Life Sci 62:881–893
107. Xie CY, Yang W, Li M, Ying J, Tao SJ, Li K, Dong JH, Wang XS (2009) Cell apoptosis induced by delta-elemene in colorectal adenocarcinoma cells via a mitochondrial-mediated pathway. Yakugaku Zasshi 129:1403–1413
108. Yao YQ, Ding X, Jia YC, Huang CX, Wang YZ, Xu YH (2008) Anti-tumor effect of beta-elemene in glioblastoma cells depends on p38 MAPK activation. Cancer Lett 264:127–134
109. Tan P, Zhong W, Cai W (2000) Clinical study on treatment of 40 cases of malignant brain tumor by elemene emulsion injection. Zhongguo Zhong Xi Yi Jie He Za Zhi 20:645–648
110. Liu J, Zhang Y, Qu JL et al (2011) b-Elemene-induced autophagy protects human gastric cancer cells from undergoing apoptosis. BMC Cancer 11:183
111. Hu J, Jin W, Yang PM (2004) Reversal of resistance to adriamycin in human breast cancer cell line MCF-7/ADM by beta-elemene. Chin J Oncol 26(5):268–270
112. Tao L, Zhou L, Zheng LY (2006) Elemene displays anti-cancer ability on laryngeal cancer cells in vitro and in vivo. Cancer Chemother Pharmacol 58(7):24–34
113. Tao L, Zhou L, Zheng LY et al (2005) Inhibition of eIF families expression and angiogenesis for human laryngeal carcinoma by elemene administration. Chin J Otorhinolaryngol Head Neck Surg 40(11):840–845
114. Chen ZH, Song YX, Che JJ, Liu XL et al (2009) Validation of a sensitive gas chromatographic–mass spectrometric method for the simultaneous determination of β-elemene and β-elemenal in human plasma. J Chromatogr B 877:408–414
115. Chen H, Liao H, Liu Y, Zheng Y, Wu X, Su Z et al (2015) Protective effects of pogostone from Pogostemonis Herba against ethanol-induced gastric ulcer in rats. Fitoterapia 100:110–117
116. Li YC, Liang HC, Chen HM, Tan LR, Yi YY, Qin Z et al (2012) Anti-Candida albicans activity and pharmacokinetics of pogostone isolated from Pogostemonis Herba. Phytomedicine 20:77–83
117. Peng F, Wan F, Xiong L, Peng C, Dai M, Chen J (2014) In vitro and in vivo antibacterial activity of Pogostone. Chin Med J (Engl) 127:4001–4005
118. Huang SH, Xian JD, Kong SZ, Li YC, Xie JH et al (2013) Insecticidal activity of pogostone against Spodoptera litura and *Spodoptera exigua* (Lepidoptera: Noctuidae). Pest Manag Sci 70:510–516
119. Su JY, Luo X, Zhang XJ, Deng XL et al (2015) Immuno-suppressive activity of pogostone on T cells: blocking proliferation via S phase arrest. Int Immunopharmacol 26:328–337
120. Cao ZX, Yang YT, Yu S, Li YZ et al (2016) Pogostone induces autophagy and apoptosis involving PI3K/Akt/mTOR axis in human colorectal carcinoma HCT116 cells. J Ethnopharmacol 8741(16):30453–30456
121. Chen HM, Li YC, Wu XL, Li CW et al (2013) LC-MS/MS determination of pogostone in rat plasma and its application in pharmacokinetic studies. Biomed Chromatogr 27(9):1092–1099
122. Yu H, Zhang T, Cai L, Qu Y, Hu S, Dong G et al (2011) Chamaejasmine induces apoptosis in human lung adenocarcinoma A549 cells through a ROS-mediated mitochondrial pathway. Molecules 16:8165–8180
123. Zhang T, Yu H, Dong G, Cai L, Bai Y (2013) Chamaejasmine arrests cell cycle, induces apoptosis and inhibits nuclear NF-κβ translocation in the human breast cancer cell line MDA-MB-231. Molecules 18:845–858
124. Yang D, Wang P, Ren X (2015) Apoptosis induced by chamaejasmine in human osteosarcoma cells through p53 pathway. Tumour Biol 36:5433–5439

125. Qiang S, Li M (2017) Chamaejasmine induces apoptosis in HeLa cells through the PI3K/Akt signaling pathway. Anticancer Drugs 28(1):40–50
126. Wang Y, Zhao Y, Liu Y, Tian L, Jin D (2011) Chamaejasmine inactivates Akt to trigger apoptosis in human hep-2 larynx carcinoma cells. Molecules 16:8152–8164
127. Piotrowska H, Kucinska M, Murias M (2012) Biological activity of piceatannol: leaving the shadow of resveratrol. Mutat Res 750:60–82
128. Kucinska M, Piotrowska H, Luczak MW, Mikula-Pietrasik J et al (2014) Effects of hydroxylated resveratrol analogs on oxidative stress and cancer cells death in human acute T cell leukemia cell line: prooxidative potential of hydroxylated resveratrol analogs. Chem Biol Interact 209:96–110
129. Jing X, Cheng W, Wang S, Li P, He L (2016) Resveratrol induces cell c cycle arrest in human gastric cancer MGC803 cells via the PTEN-regulated PI3K/Akt signaling pathway. Oncol Rep 35(1):472–478
130. Ji Q, Liu X, Fu X, Zhang L, Sui H, Zhou L, Sun J, Cai J, Qin J, Ren J, Li Q (2013) Resveratrol inhibits invasion and metastasis of colorectal cancer cells via MALAT1 mediated Wnt/β-catenin signal pathway. PLoS One 8:e78700
131. Vian MA, Tomao V, Gallet S, Coulomb PO, Lacombe JM (2005) Simple and rapid method for cis- and trans-resveratrol and piceid isomers determination in wine by high-performance liquid chromatography using Chromolith columns. J Chromatogr A 1085(2):224–229
132. Wenzel E, Somoza V (2005) Metabolism and bioavailability of trans-resveratrol. Mol Nutr Food Res 49(5):472–481
133. Chang CW, Wong CY, Wu YT, Hsu MC (2016) Development of a solid dispersion system for improving the oral bioavailability of resveratrol in rats. Eur J Drug Metab Pharmacokinet [Epub ahead of print]
134. Wang YH, Qiu C, Wang DW, Hu ZF, Yu BY, Zhu DN (2011) Identification of multiple constituents in the traditional Chinese medicine formula Sheng-Mai San and rat plasma after oral administration by HPLC-DAD-MS/MS. J Pharm Biomed Anal 54:1110–1127
135. Chen M, Du Y, Qui M, Wang M, Chen K, Huang Z et al (2013) Ophiopogonin B-induced autophagy in non-small cell lung cancer cells via inhibition of the PI3K/Akt signaling pathway. Oncol Rep 29(2):430–436
136. Xu QJ, Hou LL, Hu GQ, Xie SQ (2013) Molecular mechanism of ophiopogonin B induced cellular autophagy of human cervical cancer HeLa cells. Yao Xue Xue Bao 48(6):855–859
137. Chen M, Guo Y, Zhao R, Wang X, Jiang M, Fu H, Zhang X (2016) Ophiopogonin B induces apoptosis, mitotic catastrophe and autophagy in A549 cells. Int J Oncol 49(1):316–324
138. Zhang W, Zhang Q, Jiang Y, Li F, Xin H (2016) Effects of ophiopogonin B on the proliferation and apoptosis of SGC-7901 human gastric cancer cells. Mol Med Rep 13(6):4981–4986
139. He BC, Gao JL, Luo X et al (2011) Ginsenoside Rg3 inhibits colorectal tumor growth through the down-regulation of Wnt/β-catenin signaling. Int J Oncol 38(2):437–445
140. Lu P, Su W, Miao ZH et al (2008) Effect and mechanism of ginsenoside Rg3 on postoperative life span of patients with non-small cell lung cancer. Chin J Integr Med 14(1):33–36
141. Keum YS, Han SS, Chun KS et al (2003) Inhibitory effects of the ginsenoside Rg3 on phorbol ester-induced cyclooxygenase-2 expression, NF-kappaB activation and tumor promotion. Mutat Res 523–524:75–85
142. Tian L, Shen D, Li X et al (2016) Ginsenoside Rg3 inhibits epithelial-mesenchymal transition (EMT) and invasion of lung cancer by down-regulating FUT4. Oncotarget 7(2):1619–1632
143. Wang JN, Liu JW (2008) Effect of ginsenoside Rg3 on the epidermal growth factor receptor signaling pathways in human breast cancer cell line MCF-7. Dalian Medical University
144. Chen MW, Ni L, Zhao XG et al (2005) The inhibition of 20 (R)-ginsenoside Rg3 on the expressions of angiogenesis factors proteins in human lung adenocarcinoma cell line A549 and HUVEC304 cell. Zhongguo Zhong Yao Za Zhi 30(5):357–360

145. Qian T, Cai Z, Wong RN, Mak NK, Jiang ZH (2005) In vivo rat metabolism and pharmacokinetic studies of ginsenoside Rg3. J Chromatogr B Analyt Technol Biomed Life Sci 816:223–232
146. Xie HT, Wang GJ, Sun JG, Tucker I et al (2005) High performance liquid chromate-graphic-mass spectrometric determination of ginsenoside Rg3 and its metabolites in rat plasma using solid-phase extraction for pharmacokinetic studies. J Chromatogr B Analyt Technol Biomed Life Sci 818(2):167–173
147. Zhao Q, Li P, Jiang J, Hu P (2016) Pharmacokinetics of single ascending doses and multiple doses of 20(S)-ginsenoside Rg3 in Chinese healthy volunteers. Eur J Drug Metab Pharmacokinet 41(6):845–853
148. Aramwit P, Wirotsaengthong S (2012) Overview of commonly used Chinese herbs. J Med Plants Res 6(29):4505–4521
149. Kang SH, Jeong SJ, Kim SH et al (2012) Icariside II Induces apoptosis in U937 acute myeloid leukemia cells: role of inactivation of STAT3-related signaling. PLoS One 7(4):e28706
150. Wu JF, Guan M, Wong PF, Yu H, Dong JC, Xu JH (2012) Icariside II potentiates paclitaxel-induced apoptosis in human melanoma A375 cells by inhibiting TLR4 signaling pathway. Food Chem Toxicol 50:3019–3024
151. Geng YD, Yang L, Zhang C, Kong LY (2014) Blockade of epidermal growth factor receptor/mammalian target of rapamycin pathway by Icariside II results in reduced cell proliferation of osteosarcoma cells. Food Chem Toxicol 73:7–16
152. Wu J, Zuo F, Du J, Wong PF, Qin H, Xu J (2013) Icariside II induces apoptosis via inhibition of the EGFR pathways in A431 human epidermoid carcinoma cells. Mol Med Rep 8(2):597–602
153. Sun E, Xu F, Qian Q, Cui L, Tan X, Jia X (2014) Ultra-performance liquid chromatography/quadrupole-time-of-flight mass spectrometry analysis of icariside II metabolites in rats. Nat Prod Res 28(19):1525–1529
154. Shin CY, Lee WJ, Lee EB, Choi EY, Ko KH (2002) Platycodin D and D3 increase airway mucin release in vivo and in vitro in rats and hamsters. Planta Med 68:221–225
155. Chun J, Ha IJ, Kim YS (2013) Antiproliferative and apoptotic activities of triterpenoid saponins from the roots of Platycodon grandiflorum and their structure-activity relationships. Planta Med 79:639–645
156. Chun J, Kim YS (2013) Platycodin D inhibits migration, invasion, and growth of MDA-MB-231 human breast cancer cells via suppression of EGFR-mediated Akt and MAPK pathways. Chem Biol Interact 205(3):212–221
157. Li T, Xu XH, Tang ZH, Wang YF, Leung CH, Ma DL et al (2015) Platycodin D induces apoptosis and triggers ERK- and JNK-mediated autophagy in human hepatocellular carcinoma BEL-7402 cells. Acta Pharmacol Sin 36(12):1503–1513
158. Lu X, Yang L, Chen J et al (2016) The action and mechanism of myrisligna on A549 cells in vitro and in vivo. J Nat Med [Epub ahead of print]
159. Wang C, Zhang Z, Wang Y, He X (2016) Cytotoxic constituents and mechanism from Peganum harmala. Chem Biodivers 13(7):961–968
160. Guo R, Zhang Y, Li X, Song X, Li D, Zhao Y (2016) Discovery of ERBB3 inhibitors for non-small cell lung cancer (NSCLC) via virtual screening. J Mol Model 22(6):135
161. Liu H, Schmitz JC, Wei J et al (2014) Clove extract inhibits tumor growth and promotes cell cycle arrest and apoptosis. Oncol Res 21(5):247–259

Impact and Application of Nutraceuticals on Inflammation-Induced Colorectal Cancer Development

Yi Liu

Abstract Chronic inflammation has been shown to contribute to several diseases including colorectal cancer, which is the third leading death cancer in the world. During the past several decades, scientific research on biology of inflammation-induced colorectal cancer has been raised to become a mainstream of biomedical investigation and pharmaceutical development. Due to the important role played by inflammation in common diseases, attempting to prevent or treat them by suppressing the cellular and chemical mediators is an active area of medical research. Most of the prevailing approaches include steroids, non-steroidal anti-inflammatory drugs and immune selective anti-inflammatory derivatives are fraught with side effects. There is an urgent need for an alternative, effective, and well-tolerated treatment with negative side effects, such as the natural compound therapy. Healthy diet includes low intake of carbohydrates and fats (high percentage of unsaturated fat), high intake of fruits and vegetables, and more physical excises. Moreover, bioactive compounds in food or diet, nutrients, are essential for the prevention of inflammation-induced colorectal cancer from in vitro cells and in vivo animal models, and loss of nutrients can lead to more serious illness. The mediators and signaling pathways of inflammation-induced colorectal cancer have been alleviated by the interaction with bioactive food components, which play a crucial role in the development, treatment or prevention of inflammation-induced colorectal cancer.

Keywords Colorectal cancer • Chronic inflammation • Transcriptional factors • Bioactive food components • Nutrigenomics • Nutraceuticals

Y. Liu (✉)
Department of Health & Nutritional Sciences, South Dakota State University, Brookings, SD 57007, USA

Department of Cancer Biology, Mayo Clinic, Jacksonville, FL 32224, USA
e-mail: Liu.Yi1@mayo.edu

A.A. Farooqi, M. Ismail (eds.), *Molecular Oncology: Underlying Mechanisms and Translational Advancements*, DOI 10.1007/978-3-319-53082-6_14

Abbreviations

AOM/DSS	Azoxymethane/dextran sulfate sodium
AP-1	Activator protein-1
ARF	Alternate reading frame
BBR	Berberine
BFCs	Bioactive food compounds
CD	Crohn's disease
COX-2	Cyclooxygenase-2
CRC	Colorectal cancer
CVD	Cardiovascular diseases
EGCG	Epigallocatechin gallate
ERK5	Extracellular signal-regulated kinase-5
ERKs	Extracellular signal-regulated kinases
GCSF	Granulocyte stimulating factor
GI	Gastrointestinal
GLA	Gamma linolenic acid
IBD	Inflammatory bowel disease
IFN	Interferon
IL-	Interleukin-
JAK/STAT	Janus kinase/signal transducers and activators of transcription
JNKs	c-Jun NH2-terminal kinases
LPS	lipopolysaccharides
MAPK	Mitogen-activated protein kinases
MCSF	Macrophage stimulating factors
NFκB	Nuclear factor kappa B
Nrf-2	Nuclear erythroid 2-related factor 2
PEITC	Phenethyl isothiocyanate
PPARs	Peroxisome proliferator-activated receptors
PYCARD	PYD and CARD domain containing
ROS	Reactive oxygen species
SEER	Surveillance, epidemiology, and end results
SFN	Sulforaphane
TGF	Transforming growth factor
TNF	Tumor necrosis factor
UC	Ulcerative colitis

Brief Introduction

Dating back to ancient times, the Greek physician Hippocrates' quote "Let food be thy medicine and medicine be thy food" has indicated the role of nutrition in health. Despite the recognition of nutrition as bioactive nature of food, until past few decades, most of the research has demonstrated most of the diseases were caused by deficiency of macronutrients and micronutrients. With the emergence of epidemiology and the elevated risks in cardiovascular diseases (CVD), cancer, obesity, and diabetes, the focus of nutritional research has been expanded to include bioactive effects, in addition to the trophic effects of food. Colorectal cancer (CRC) is the second-leading cause of cancer-related deaths in the United States. Several factors may increase the risk of CRC, for example unhealthy diet/lifestyle, family/personal history, and inflammatory intestinal conditions. Recent findings of the potential biological effects of both nutrient and non-nutrient food ingredients warrant the use of dietary approaches to prevent or treat CRC. With new technological advancements there is a preponderance of data on the molecular mechanisms of the bioactive food compounds (BFCs). The cellular signaling pathways that lead to CRC are effectively interfered with BFCs. Although in vitro studies suggest that several BFCs can be effective and anti-cancer agents, data from clinical settings are few, inconclusive and sometimes not as encouraging as from in vitro models. Factors such as duration of intervention, failure to deliver effective concentrations at the site of action, differences in metabolism due to genetic variation and differences in the active concentration of the BFCs might be contributing to disparities in the findings from in vitro and clinical studies. Despite the increased momentum of research on BFCs, most of the clinical studies are focused on their ability to prevent cancer or other specific diseases. A major portion of in vitro studies is also designed in a disease-specific manner. In vitro and in vivo studies designed for the sole purpose of investigating the effect of BFCs on CRC, the root cause for several ailments, are not abundant. In this review we attempt to discuss inflammation-induced CRC, mediators of CRC signaling pathways, cellular mechanisms by which BFCs can interfere with intercellular signaling, evidence from human studies for the anti-cancer activity of BFCs and the effect of genetic variation among individuals on the biological action of the BFCs.

Colorectal Cancer

Colorectal cancer (CRC) is the second leading cause cancer in United States and third leading death cancer in the world. According to the data reported from Surveillance, Epidemiology, and End Results (SEER) Program, the incidence of CRC has been decreasing since the last 20 years in the United States (Fig. 1).

In brief, tumor development has three major steps that include initiation (or tumorigenesis), promotion and metastasis. Research has showed that inflammation is involved in all the steps. CRC originates from the noncancerous polyps, epithelial cells, lining the colon or rectum in the gastrointestinal (GI) tract [1]. Environmental risk factors such as air pollution, cigarette smoking, and unhealthy diet/lifestyle like over consumption of fat and high intakes of carbohydrates, are enhancing cellular mediators that promote inflammation, resulting in an upregulation of inflammatory reactions. Increased mediators such as cytokines, chemokines, and highly reactive

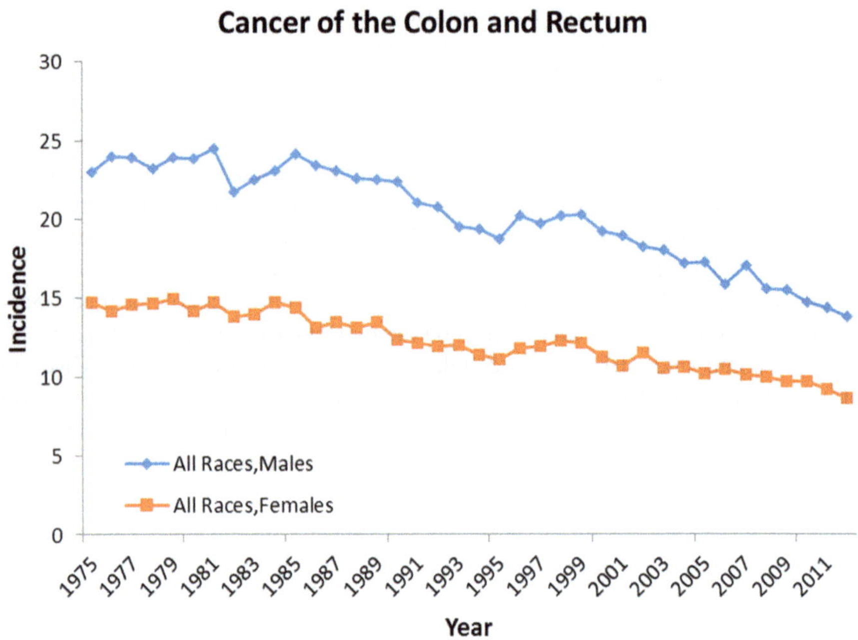

Fig. 1 Trends in colorectal cancer incidence by sex, United States, 1975–2011. Data are collected both by the National Cancer Institute's (NCI's)Surveillance, Epidemiology, and End Results (SEER) Program

oxygen species (ROS) in normal colon cells give rise to DNA mutation, genomic damage, and epigenetic alterations which may lead to initiation of CRC. Once cancerous cells form in the large intestine, they can grow through the lining and into the wall of the colon. Additional cancerous cells can also be carried in blood vessels to the liver or lungs, which cause the metastasis.

Inflammatory bowel disease (IBD) is a group of two distinct intestinal disorders with unclear etiology; Crohn's disease (CD) and ulcerative colitis (UC) [2]. UC primarily affects the mucosal lining of colon and rectum, whereas CD usually affects the whole intestinal wall and potentially may extend to any part of the gastrointestinal tract. CD and UC are at 2- to 3-fold increased risk of developing CRC and the risk factors of CRC are related with duration [3], anatomical extent [4] and severity [5] of inflammation [6]. Several factors, both environmental and genetic, have been implicated in the etiology of IBD which result in inappropriate release of the pro-inflammatory cytokines such as TNF-α, IL-6, IL-12, IL-23 and IL-17 [7]. Based on the type of disease, dietary components can either ameliorate or worsen symptoms. Western dietary pattern has been identified as a risk factor for IBD [8]. While some studies have identified nutrition as a potential etiological factor, nutrition is also important in management and remission of the disease, more so in case of CD [9]. Besides the therapeutic role played by the bioactive components of diet, nutritional intervention in IBD also works by providing optimal nutritional requirements as patients with IBD are frequently prone to malnutrition due to increased loss of fluids, avoidance of particular foods due to flares and increased nutritional needs due to systemic inflammation [10].

CRC Related Signaling Pathways

At cellular level, the pathogenesis of colorectal cancer (CRC) and inflammatory immune diseases is characterized by regulatory pathways that are complex and involves several layers of communication, cascades, crosstalk and extensive networking. This is achieved through interaction of cytokines, the chemical mediators of inflammation; cytokine receptors, present on the surface of a variety of cell types; secondary messengers which convey signals from cell surface to the interior; and transcription factors, which regulate the expression of several genes that affect CRC. A variety of cytokines, critical in regulating proliferation and differentiation of inflammatory cells are discovered and are usually named with a prefix IL (Book Multiple Sclerosis: Immunology, Pathology and Pathophysiology). For instance, from interleukin-1 (IL-1) to IL-35, interferon (IFN), transforming growth factor (TGF), tumor necrosis factor (TNF), granulocyte stimulating factor (GCSF) and macrophage stimulating factors (MCSF) etc. Cytokines communicate with cells through cytokine-receptors, which are classified into type-I family, type-II family, TNF family, TGF-β family, chemokines and immunoglobulin family receptors based on their chemical structure. Upon binding of ligands such as cytokines and natural compounds, these receptors activate secondary messengers in the cytoplasm that initiate cell signaling. The end effect of the cytoplasmic signaling by second messengers is activation of transcription factors, such as NFκB (Nuclear Factor kappa B), JAK/STAT (Janus Kinase/Signal Transducers and Activators of Transcription), MAPK (Mitogen-activated protein kinases), AP-1 (Activator protein-1) and ARF (Alternate Reading Frame), which either induce or repress the genes related to inflammation and CRC. In addition to these mechanisms, emerging literature now suggest a new mechanism called inflammasome. Several classes of proteins related to immunity such as caspase-1, PYCARD (PYD And CARD Domain Containing), NALP and sometimes caspase-5 oligomerize and form a multi-protein complex called inflammasome, dysregulation of which has been observed in a variety of CRC and inflammatory immune related disorders [11]. While this is a comparatively new area of research, some marine natural products, such as berkeleyones, meroterpenes and bromoxones, are known to modulate the secretion of IL-8 from inflammasome [12, 13].

Cytokines transduce their signal through Janus tyrosine kinases (JAK), which upon phosphorylation associate with another class of cytoplasmic proteins, signal transducers and activators of transcription (STATs). The JAK/STAT pathway plays a central role in proliferation and differentiation of cells of immune system, viral infection and tumorigenesis. Perturbations in JAK/STAT pathway are known to cause several immune related diseases [14]. Emodin, aloin and aloe-emodin obtained from rhubarb and buckthorn are known to exert anti-cancer and anti-inflammatory effects in hepatoma cells through interfering JAK/STAT pathway [15]. Quercetin and apigenin are known to have antiviral effect by modulating JAK/STAT pathway through inhibition of Hsp90 [16, 17]. These two compounds are also known to exert additive anti-proliferative effect [18]. β-escin is a triterpene extracted from horse chestnut. It is known to exert string anti-proliferative effect in A549 cells by interfering with JAK/STAT pathway [19]. Flavone, isoxanthohumol can inhibit expression of pro-inflammatory genes by blocking IFN-γ, IL-4 and IL-6 induced JAK/STAT signaling [20]. Berberine (BBR), an isoquinoline alkaloid can act on JAK/STAT pathway and inhibit differentiation of Th17 and Th1 cells [21]. JAK/STAT pathway is also a major target for the chemo-preventive activity of apigenein, a dietary flavonoid [22].

NFκB is a key rapid-acting transcription factor involved in regulation of inflammation, immunity and cancer. NFκB exists as a dimer of five different proteins. In unstimulated cells, NFκB is sequestrated in cytoplasm by IκB and activation occurs only upon uncoupling of the two. Activated NFκB moves into nucleus where it either induces or represses gene expression depending on the combinations of the subunits in the dimer. The most commonly found NFκB is the dimers of p50 and p65 which can strongly induce gene transcription in CRC [23]. NFκB can be activated by several endogenous and exogenous compounds such as bacterial lipopolysaccharides (LPS), cytokines, growth factors and viruses, and can induce pro-inflammatory genes such as chemokines; cytokines such as TNF-α, IL-1β and ILs1-6; adhesion molecules; and inflammation-related enzymes. Several classes of dietary compounds such as polyphenols, terpenes, diterpenes, sesquiterpenes, lignans, phytoestrogens are known to modulate NFκB activity and thus act as anti-inflammatory agents [24–28]. Regulation of NFκB by these compounds can occur by different means that may include degradation of IκB [29, 30], inhibition of NFκB nuclear translocation [27, 31] and affecting binding of NFκB to DNA [27, 31]. A wide variety of NFκB modulators, both natural and synthetic/semi-synthetic, have been found since their discovery. Different natural compounds can interact in modulating the activity of NFκB. For instance, a combined extract of clove, oregano, thyme, walnuts, and coffee exhibited synergism in decreasing LPS-induced NFκB activity [32]. On the other hand, a single bioactive compound may act on several signaling pathways causing multiple effects. Gamma-linolenic acid (GLA) can block MAPK (mitogen-activated protein kinases) phosphorylation, suppress the activation of the transcription factors NFκB and AP-1, lessen the oxidative stress [33] and diminish iNOS (inducible nitric oxide synthase) and pro-IL-1β expression [34]. NFκB is a master transcription factor that controls not just inflammation but also cellular proliferation, growth and apoptosis. NFκB is an excellent drug target in ailments such as cancer and inflammation related diseases and extracts from several plants and herbs are under investigation as inhibitors of NFκB [32].

Mitogen activated protein kinase (MAPK) pathway plays an important role in inflammation and immunity. There are four major groups of MAPKs in mammalian cells-the ERKs (Extracellular signal-Regulated Kinases), the p38MAPKs, the JNKs (c-JunNH2-terminalKinases)andtheERK5(Extracellularsignal-RegulatedKinase-5)or

BMK cascades [35]. MAPK activation has been associated with cardiovascular diseases, rheumatoid arthritis and pulmonary diseases [36, 37]. Several natural products such as epigallocatechin gallate (EGCG), phenethyl isothiocyanate (PEITC), sulforaphane (SFN), resveratrol, tangeretin and ligustilide are shown to exert their effects by interfering with MAPK pathway [38, 39]. Effects of these compounds vary at different doses and are also specific for the type of the kinases they modulate in the MAPK pathway. At lower concentrations, phenolic compounds and isothiocyanates activate MAPK pathway and induce the expression of pro-survival genes, but at higher concentrations, in addition to inducing these genes they also induce genes involved in apoptosis [38]. Tangeretin obtained from citrus fruit can inhibit IL-1β induced cyclooxygenase-2 (COX-2) expression by inhibiting JNK, p38 kinase and protein kinase B (PKB/Akt), but not ERK [40]. The extent of inhibition of MAPK intermediates by resveratrol varies in the order of MEK1 > ERK1/2 = JNK [37]. Ligustilide, which is isolated from Angelica sinesis reduces the symptoms of atherosclerosis and hypertension, by inhibiting JNK, ERK and p38 kinase [41].

The activator protein-1 (AP-1) family of transcription factor consists of members of Jun (cJun, JunB and JunD), Fos (cFos, FosB, Fra-1 and Fra-2), Maf (c-Maf, MafB, MafA and MafG/F/K) and Atf (Atf2, LRF1/ATF3). Ap-1 acts as a dimer formed by its family members and binds to the TPA (12-O-tetradecanoylphorbol-13-acetate) response elements present in the promoters of several inflammatory genes of cytokines and chemokines. The constituents of the dimer determine specificity towards the genes activated by AP-1. Genetic mouse models show that Jun/Ap-1 controls the expression of cytokines by transcriptional and post-transcriptional methods. Absence of JunB increases the production of GCSF and IL-6 leading to skin related inflammatory diseases such as psoriasis, systemic lupus erythematosus [42]. While AP-1 is recognized as a transcription factor involved in inflammation, it is also known to suppress inflammation under certain conditions [43–45]. Natural compounds can modulate the AP-1 activity by either reducing the expression of monomers or blocking the upstream signaling molecules that may include ERK1/2, p38, JNK and glycogen synthase kinase (GSK). Gallotannin, a natural alkaloid blocks AP-1 activity by increasing the phosphorylation of JNK and cJun [46]. Genestein decreased the phosphorylation of Akt and GSK-3 [47]. Luteolin, another flavonoid has been observed to decrease both phosphorylation of c-Jun and DNA binding activity of AP-1 [48]. On the contrary flavonoids genistein and kaempferol, at lower concentrations (20–50 μM) induced AP-1 activity by JNK and ERK pathways respectively. However, at higher concentrations (100 mM), these compounds either had no effect or slightly decreased the activity [49]. Berberine, a natural alkaloid from Berberis, inhibited AP-1 activity by decreasing the expression of cJun and cFos [50].

Peroxisome proliferator-activated receptors (PPARs) belong to a family of transcription factors called nuclear hormone receptors. After dimerization with other family members such as RXR, PPARs regulate expression of several genes involved in lipid and glucose metabolism. Recent studies show that PPARs can also play an important role in inflammation and immunity by regulating the activity of other transcription factors such as AP-1, NFκB, NFAT (Nuclear factor of activated T-cells) or STAT by different mechanisms [51]. Natural ligands that can activate PPARs include the cannabinoids [52], terpinoids such as carnosic acid and carnosol [8] and resveratol [53].

Nrf-2, nuclear erythroid 2-related factor 2, is a classical transcription factor involved in redox signaling. Nrf2 also regulates inflammation by inducing HO-1 and PrxI, which inhibits the expression of NFκB and TNF-α [54]. Several studies show that plant derived compounds such as sulforafane (from broccoli), curcumin (from *Curcuma longa* L., Zingiberaceae) and Zerumbone (from ginger) can modulate both Nrf-2 and NFκB transcription factors which forms mechanistic basis for anti-inflammatory and anti-oxidative effect of these compounds [55].

Nutrition in Colorectal Cancer Research

As we discussed from previous section, the effect of natural compounds on health and disease depends on how they interact with these signaling pathways and molecules. Substantial evidence from in vitro and animal models show that plant derived compounds such as flavonoids, lignans, terpenes and many others modulate the synthesis of cytokines in different ways [56]. Receptor up-regulation and/or down-regulation are an important mechanism of action of natural compounds [57]. Several natural compounds such as epigallocatechin gallate (EGCG), resveratrol, curcumin, lycopene, gingerol are known to modulate inflammatory signaling by binding with cell surface receptors and second messengers [58]. Our regular diet is a complex mixture of several foods. Supplementation of dietary components in clinical settings at supra-physiological concentrations as in in vitro studies is difficult. Hence, it is critical to investigate the effect of dietary patterns on inflammation rather than an individual component at defined concentrations. Such studies can be achieved by epidemiological and interventional designs. Energy density, glycemic index, fruit and vegetable intake can be said as major determinants of the effect of dietary patterns on inflammation. Several studies on obesity show that chronic inflammation could be a consequence of energy accumulation [59]. Low calorie diets are known to decrease the levels of circulating pro-inflammatory factors such as CRP (C-Reactive Protein), TNF-α, interleukins and chemokines [60]. Even among low-calorie isoenergic diets, low carbohydrate diets are shown to be better anti-inflammatory agents compared to low fat diets. Several markers of inflammation such as plasma TNF-α, IL-6, IL-8, MCP-1, E-selectin, I-CAM, and PAI-1 were lower in overweight individuals on a low carbohydrate diet compared to those on low fat diet [61]. Even the quality of carbohydrate can impact inflammation. Recent studies suggest that glycemic index is a stronger predictor of inflammation than the carbohydrate content alone [62]. Epidemiological studies such as The Harvard women's health study, The Dutch study, and others show that the blood levels of CRP were proportional to the glycemic index of the diet [63–65]. The anti-inflammatory effects of low glycemic diets were greater in individuals with high body fat percentage than those with low body fat [66]. Dietary pattern, rich in sugar-sweetened soft drinks, refined grains, diet soft drinks, and processed meat but low in wine, coffee, vegetables and fruits, typical of

Western world was associated with risk for developing type-II diabetes by causing an increased chronic inflammation [67]. While it might be difficult in the Western world to adopt low glycemic diet every day, decreasing the intake of carbohydrates and fats (high percentage of unsaturated fat) to a moderate amount, and increasing the intake of fruits and vegetables is a possible healthy alternative [68].

Such a ratio of food components is representative of Mediterranean dietary pattern and it stands as the most investigated and healthy dietary pattern to date. Several studies show that Mediterranean dietary pattern promotes various health aspects including cardiovascular diseases, Alzheimer's disease, metabolic syndrome and diabetes in addition to decreasing inflammation [69, 70]. The Mediterranean diet includes prolific use of olive oil, a rich source of not just unsaturated fatty acids but also phenolic compounds. Olive oil is also shown to down regulate several genes related to inflammatory signaling [71]. Clinical studies show that in addition to anti-inflammatory activity, protective effects olive oil could also be due to the antioxidant properties attributed to its components, such as oleic acid [72, 73]. In a clinical study, traditional Mediterranean diet and low fat diet were found to have comparable but different effects in individuals with previous coronary events. While both diets reduced body mass index, blood pressure and arginine levels, Mediterranean diet was more effective in decreasing blood leukocyte count and increasing high-density lipoprotein levels. However, low fat diet had greater reduction of low-density lipoprotein and oxidized low-density lipoprotein plasma levels [74]. While the type and amount of fats and carbohydrates are one side of the coin of Mediterranean diet, high intake of fruits and vegetables constitutes the other side. A variety of bioactive compounds such as flavonoids, terpenoids, glycosides and alkaloids, most of which have anti-inflammatory properties are an integral part of the Mediterranean diet.

Flavonoids, potent antioxidants, can also exert anti-inflammatory effect through the antioxidant response elements in the promoters of NFκB, AP-1 and other important transcription factors that regulate inflammatory gene expression. Elevated free radicals are known to trigger inflammatory mediators by up-regulating the expression of redox-sensitive transcription factors NFκB and AP-1 [75, 76]. However, there are fewer studies on their anti-inflammatory activity compared to their antioxidant activity. While there is in vitro evidence for the direct anti-inflammatory activity of flavonoids [77], it might be difficult in vivo to determine if their anti-inflammatory activity is direct or a secondary effect through reduction in oxidative stress. For instance, curcumin is shown to decrease the release of IL-8 by inducing the synthesis of glutathione, an antioxidant that scavenges reactive oxygen species and thus prevent the induction of NFκB [78]. However, curcumin also inhibits NFκB activity by preventing the degradation of the inhibitory protein IκB and nuclear translocation of p65 [79]. Regardless the mechanism, several in vivo studies, mostly animal models and some human studies associate flavonoid intake with reduction in inflammation. A 3-week supplementation of a mixture of anthocyanins (3-O-rutinosides of cyanidin and delphinidin, and 3-O-ß-galactosides, 3-O-ß-glucosides, and 3-O-ß-arabinosides of cyanidin, peonidin, delphinidin, petunidin, and malvidin) supplied as a capsule significantly reduced the blood levels of IL-4, IL-13, IL-8 and IFN-α in healthy adults [77, 80]. Consumption of a mixture of fish oil, green tea extract, vitamin E, resveratrol, vitamin C, and tomato extract for 5 weeks, has modulated the expression of several inflammation related genes to a more favorable profile (anti-inflammatory/pro-inflammatory) [81]. While it is possible in experimental set ups to supplement flavonoids at high concentrations, it is critical to know whether they exert same effects at the concentrations that prevail in a typical diet. A cross-sectional study with 8335 individuals indicates that intake of flavonoids, either a mixture or individual, is inversely associated with plasma CRP concentrations [82]. Similarly a long term and longitudinal study, Uppsala Longitudinal Study of Adult Men, followed up to 7 years shows that the dietary intake of food rich in polyphenol antioxidants was associated with lower degree of inflammation mediated by cytokines and COX [83].

Tea is a good source of flavonoids such as catechin, epicatechin and epigallocatechin. Regular tea consumption is associated with lower plasma concentration of CRP and reduced platelet activation in two epidemiological studies [84, 85]. A large cross-sectional study shows that habitual tea drinking is associated with lower levels of CRP, serum amyloid-A protein and haptoglobin [84]. Even drinking tea for a short term (6-week) lowered serum CRP and platelet activation [85]. In addition to decreasing the serum levels of inflammatory markers such as CRP, TNF-α, IL-6 and an increase in IL-1, an intervention study with Pu'er tea, a type of fermented tea, also reduced the symptoms of metabolic syndrome [86]. A double blinded clinical trial in 47 individuals indicated that chewing green tea candies might exert a positive effect on the inflammation of periodontal structures [87]. Intake of green tea (*Camellia sinensis*) contents as capsules reduced serum amyloid-alpha by 42% [88].

While the above studies support that several bioactive compounds can act as anti-inflammatory agents, there are also studies that failed to observe such an activity. Quercetin, a flavonol, occurs in abundant quantities in black tea, green tea, apples and onions. While there is ample evidence from in vitro cell lines [89, 90] and in vivo animal models [91, 92] for the anti-inflammatory activity of quercetin, human studies have rather been disappointing. While the daily intake of flavonols (including quercetin) is usually low (20–35 mg/day), quercetin supplementation, even at much higher doses (50–1000 mg/day) has failed to observe anti-inflammatory effects humans. No change in inflammatory markers hsCRP and IL-6 was observed in a tea consumption study in type-II diabetes patients [93]. A 4-week study investigating the effect of tea polyphenols on inflammation observed an inverse association with IL-6 and fibrinogen but no association with other inflammatory markers such as IL-1β, TNF-α and CRP in healthy smokers [94]. This is a short term study and smokers are known to generally have very high levels of oxidative stress and inflammation. Daily supplementary intake of 500 mg green tea polyphenols did not have any effect on blood glucose level, Hb A1c level, insulin resistance or inflammation markers [95]. In a dietary intervention study, supplementation of a mixture of resveratrol, green tea extract, α-tocopherol, vitamin C, ω-3 polyunsaturated fatty acids, and tomato extract affected overall inflammatory processes, oxidative stress, and metabolism in humans [81]. A study on the effect of consumption of black tea shows that the positive effects observed on endothelial function in patients with coronary artery diseases not attributable to catechins but the total polyphenol content of diet [96]. These studies emphasize the importance of differences in individual versus combinatorial effect of bioactive compounds. There is a critical need for small scale pilot human trials to understand the effect of natural anti-inflammatory agents both individually and in combination that would help understanding their interaction with other components of the food matrix [97]. These studies might help in resolving the differences in findings among various studies. While flavonoids have been shown to be active in vitro, studies that show their functionality in vivo are rare. This is mostly due to lack of data on clinical studies and difficulty in achieving effective doses in vivo. However, efforts to overcome these hurdles such as modification of flavonoid structures have started [98].

Nutrigenomics

Nutrigenomics and nutrigenetics are powerful tools in understanding the complex relation between dietary constituents and their biological effects. Nutrigenomics is the study of the effect of nutrients or non-nutritive bioactive compounds on gene expression and genome structure (integrity, methylation and acetylation status). A simple and elegant model for nutrient control of gene expression is up-regulation of genes involved in fat biosynthesis and down-regulation of genes involved in fat catabolism in well fed state [99]. By modulating the expression of inflammatory genes such as NFκB, PI3K/Akt, MAPK, p38 MAPK, JNK, STAT3, and AP-1, bioactive compounds in diet can play a crucial role in the development, treatment or prevention of inflammatory diseases.

For instance, a common mechanism by which flavonoids exert anti-inflammatory activity is by knocking down the transcription of pro-inflammatory genes. Flavonoids inhibit the phosphorylation of kinases involved in activating inflammatory genes. Significant evidence from in vitro studies show that flavonoids inhibit transcription of cyclooxygenase, TNF-α, NFκB, IL-1β etc. [100]. Flavonoids belong to the same class may exhibit differential activity. Luteolin and genistein have inhibited TNF-α and IL-6 expression but eriodictyol and hesperetin, belonging to the same class inhibited TNF-α expression only [101]. Flavonoids such as isoflavones, flavonols and catechins are also shown to modulate gene expression through epigenetic mechanisms such as methylation and acetylation [102]. Feeding black raspberries for 4 weeks has altered methylation status of several genes involved in Wnt pathway in colorectal cancer patients [103].

Phenylethyl isothiocyanate (PEITC), a sulfur rich component of cruciferous vegetables is known to alter gene expression in cell culture and animal models. PEITC has been shown to inhibit the expression of cyclooxygenase, nitric-oxide synthase and interleukins [104]. PEITC was able to suppress symptoms of ulcerative colitis in mice model, by modulating the expression of inflammatory genes, transcription factors and cytokines [105]. Benzylisothiocyanate, a structural analog of PEITC has also been shown to inhibit mRNA production and release of IL-1β, TNF-α, IL-6 and production of nitric oxide and PGE-2 [106]. Epigenetically, PEITC was able to induce DNA demethylation and activate the enzyme glutathione-s-transferase-π1, which is involved in development of airway inflammation [107]. In addition, PEITC modulated histone tail modifications in human colon cancer cells in a promoter-specific manner [108]. Metabolites of sulforaphane and allylisothiocyanate have been found to inhibit histone deacetylase activity in cell culture and animal models [109, 110]. In addition to the non-nutritive bioactive compounds, nutrients in diet can also modulate gene expression. Unsaturated fatty acids, are known to modulate gene expression by regulating transcription factors such as PPARs, liver X receptor and sterol regulatory binding proteins which play important role in obesity [111]. In a recent study the effect of dietary fat has been shown to be transgenerational through mechanisms such as epigenetics and imprinting. F3 generation mice from female but not male mice exposed to high fat during gestation had high body weight compared to controls [112].

Microbiota in human body plays an important role in inflammatory process especially in organ systems such as gut. For instance short chain fatty acids generated by gut microbes can modify cytokine production by T_H cells [113] and can resolve intestinal inflammation through GPCR43 [114]. Disturbances in the gut microbial profile can result in dysbiosis, which leads to several diseases including those related to immunity and inflammation [115]. Studies in mice models suggest that dietary composition can change human gut microbial profile within a day [116]. Several microbial species are involved in the metabolism of dietary fiber as well as bioactive compounds such as polyphenols. While our knowledge about the mutual effect of bioactive compounds and microbial population is still incipient, changes in the dietary concentration of polyphenols can influence the microbial profile and vice versa [117].

Owing to the genetic variation, the extent and nature of biological activity by different bioactive compounds may differ between individuals. Nutrigenetics studies how genetic variation among individuals modulates the effect of nutrients or bioactive compounds on cell metabolism. It is possible that the activity of the enzymes involved in the metabolism of a class of or a specific dietary compound is affected by variation in the nucleotide sequences such as substitution-, repeat- and insertion-deletion polymorphisms. While these polymorphisms could be specific to a race or a common ancestral lineage, they could also occur within individuals belonging to same race or lineage, and thus incite varied response to dietary intake between races or individuals. Unraveling information about the functional polymorphisms of the genes involved in nutrient metabolism will help to individually tailor dietary needs in both health and disease states. Such hypothesis has been successfully tested in a clinical study where individuals whose diets were tailored to the variants of genes involved in metabolism had better compliance and longer weight reduction than the controls [118].

Information on genetic variation among individuals can also help in individualizing the dietary requirements for treating inflammation. Genetic variation in genes involved in inflammation and adipose tissue metabolism may influence the effect of diet. Apolipoprotein is a lipoprotein involved in normal catabolism of triglyceride-rich lipoproteins. A genetic polymorphism in the gene that codes for this protein results in three different alleles 2, 3 and 4 and six different genotypes. On a low-fat/high-cholesterol diet individuals with 4/4 genotype had increased serum cholesterol levels while those with 2/2 and 3/2 had no change. However all genotypes had lower serum cholesterol on low fat/low-cholesterol diet [119]. Such a varied response can be employed in the treatment of several diseases such as metabolic syndrome [120], obesity, Alzheimer's disease [121] and cardiovascular diseases [122]. Supplementation of quercetin at 150 mg/day has lowered plasma levels of TNF-α, only in a subgroup of individuals having a particular genotype of ApoE gene polymorphism, while such effect has been nullified when the genetic polymorphism is disregarded [123]. Another study observed that the effect of green tea on hepatocellular carcinoma was dependant on the type of allele for an IL-10 polymorphism, indicating that the observed cancer preventive effects of green tea might not be same in all individuals [124]. Sulforaphane (1-isothiocyanato-4-methylsulfinyl butane), a major isothiocyanate found in brassica plants such as broccoli and watercress is known to inhibit inflammation and carcinogenesis. Once absorbed into the body, sulforaphane can be metabolized by glutathione-s-transferases (GSTM1–1 and GSTP1–1), a group of enzymes known to exhibit null mutations. Individuals without GSTM1 were observed to have slightly higher concentrations of sulforaphane metabolites in plasma and urine [125], which could be the reason for greater protection offered by crucifer consumption in null mutants than in positive subjects [126, 127]. Conversely, there are also studies that show GST positive subjects may benefit better from crucifer consumption than negative subjects, it is clear that the GST genotype affects the metabolism and therefore its biological activity in vivo [128, 129]. Similarly enzymes involved in the metabolism of polyphenols, powerful antioxidants and anti-inflammatory compounds, such as catechol-o-methyl transferases, UDP glucuronosyl transferases, cytochrome-P-450 and phenol sulfotransferases exhibit several functional polymorphisms that may affect their metabolism and purported anti-inflammatory or antioxidant activities [130–133].

References

1. Koosha S et al (2016) An association map on the effect of flavonoids on the signaling pathways in colorectal cancer. Int J Med Sci 13(5):374–385
2. Fiocchi C (1998) Inflammatory bowel disease: etiology and pathogenesis. Gastroenterology 115(1):182–205
3. Rutter MD et al (2006) Thirty-year analysis of a colonoscopic surveillance program for neoplasia in ulcerative colitis. Gastroenterology 130(4):1030–1038
4. Ekbom A et al (1991) The epidemiology of inflammatory bowel disease: a large, population-based study in Sweden. Gastroenterology 100(2):350–358
5. Rutter M et al (2004) Severity of inflammation is a risk factor for colorectal neoplasia in ulcerative colitis. Gastroenterology 126(2):451–459
6. O'Connor PM et al (2010) Mechanisms by which inflammation may increase intestinal cancer risk in inflammatory bowel disease. Inflamm Bowel Dis 16(8):1411–1420

7. Sartor RB (2003) Clinical applications of advances in the genetics of IBD. Rev Gastroenterol Disord 3(Suppl 1):S9–17
8. Rau O et al (2006) Carnosic acid and carnosol, phenolic diterpene compounds of the labiate herbs rosemary and sage, are activators of the human peroxisome proliferator-activated receptor gamma. Planta Med 72(10):881–887
9. Campos FG et al (2003) Pharmacological nutrition in inflammatory bowel diseases. Nutr Hosp 18(2):57–64
10. Bistrian BR (1999) Role of the systemic inflammatory response in the development of protein-energy malnutrition in inflammatory bowel disease. Nestle Nutr Workshop Ser Clin Perform Programme 2:1–6
11. Schroder K, Tschopp J (2010) The inflammasomes. Cell 140(6):821–832
12. Stierle DB et al (2011) Berkeleyones and related meroterpenes from a deep water acid mine waste fungus that inhibit the production of interleukin 1-beta from induced inflammasomes. J Nat Prod 74(10):2273–2277
13. Gong YN et al (2010) Chemical probing reveals insights into the signaling mechanism of inflammasome activation. Cell Res 20(12):1289–1305
14. Touw IP et al (2000) Signaling mechanisms of cytokine receptors and their perturbances in disease. Mol Cell Endocrinol 160(1–2):1–9
15. Park MY, Kwon HJ, Sung MK (2009) Evaluation of aloin and aloe-emodin as anti-inflammatory agents in aloe by using murine macrophages. Biosci Biotechnol Biochem 73(4):828–832
16. Aalinkeel R et al (2008) The dietary bioflavonoid, quercetin, selectively induces apoptosis of prostate cancer cells by down-regulating the expression of heat shock protein 90. Prostate 68(16):1773–1789
17. Proia DA et al (2011) Multifaceted intervention by the Hsp90 inhibitor ganetespib (STA-9090) in cancer cells with activated JAK/STAT signaling. PLoS One 6(4):e18552
18. Blank VC et al (2004) Antiproliferative activity of various flavonoids and related compounds: additive effect of interferon-alpha2b. Bioorg Med Chem Lett 14(1):133–136
19. Ji DB et al (2011) beta-Escin sodium inhibits inducible nitric oxide synthase expression via downregulation of the JAK/STAT pathway in A549 cells. Mol Carcinog 50(12):945–960
20. Serwe A et al (2012) Inhibition of TGF-beta signaling, vasculogenic mimicry and proinflammatory gene expression by isoxanthohumol. Invest New Drugs 30(3):898–915
21. Qin X et al (2010) Regulation of Th1 and Th17 cell differentiation and amelioration of experimental autoimmune encephalomyelitis by natural product compound berberine. J Immunol 185(3):1855–1863
22. Ruela-de-Sousa RR et al (2010) Cytotoxicity of apigenin on leukemia cell lines: implications for prevention and therapy. Cell Death Dis 1:e19
23. Grossmann M et al (2000) The anti-apoptotic activities of Rel and RelA required during B-cell maturation involve the regulation of Bcl-2 expression. EMBO J 19(23):6351–6360
24. Nam NH (2006) Naturally occurring NF-kappaB inhibitors. Mini Rev Med Chem 6(8):945–951
25. Aggarwal BB, Shishodia S (2004) Suppression of the nuclear factor-kappaB activation pathway by spice-derived phytochemicals: reasoning for seasoning. Ann N Y Acad Sci 1030:434–441
26. Gilmore TD, Herscovitch M (2006) Inhibitors of NF-kappaB signaling: 785 and counting. Oncogene 25(51):6887–6899
27. Bremner P, Heinrich M (2002) Natural products as targeted modulators of the nuclear factor-kappaB pathway. J Pharm Pharmacol 54(4):453–472
28. Salminen A et al (2008) Terpenoids: natural inhibitors of NF-kappaB signaling with anti-inflammatory and anticancer potential. Cell Mol Life Sci 65(19):2979–2999
29. Kopp E, Ghosh S (1994) Inhibition of NF-kappa B by sodium salicylate and aspirin. Science 265(5174):956–959

30. Scheinman RI et al (1995) Role of transcriptional activation of I kappa B alpha in mediation of immunosuppression by glucocorticoids. Science 270(5234):283–286
31. Straus DS et al (2000) 15-deoxy-delta 12,14-prostaglandin J2 inhibits multiple steps in the NF-kappa B signaling pathway. Proc Natl Acad Sci U S A 97(9):4844–4849
32. Paur I et al (2010) Extract of oregano, coffee, thyme, clove, and walnuts inhibits NF-kappaB in monocytes and in transgenic reporter mice. Cancer Prev Res (Phila) 3(5):653–663
33. Chang CS et al (2010) Gamma-linolenic acid inhibits inflammatory responses by regulating NF-kappaB and AP-1 activation in lipopolysaccharide-induced RAW 264.7 macrophages. Inflammation 33(1):46–57
34. Haddad JJ, Harb HL (2005) L-gamma-Glutamyl-L-cysteinyl-glycine (glutathione; GSH) and GSH-related enzymes in the regulation of pro- and anti-inflammatory cytokines: a signaling transcriptional scenario for redox(y) immunologic sensor(s)? Mol Immunol 42(9):987–1014
35. Panka DJ, Atkins MB, Mier JW (2006) Targeting the mitogen-activated protein kinase pathway in the treatment of malignant melanoma. Clin Cancer Res 12(7 Pt 2):2371s–2375s
36. Meyer LH, Pap T (2005) MAPK signalling in rheumatoid joint destruction: can we unravel the puzzle? Arthritis Res Ther 7(5):177–178
37. Kim AL et al (2006) Resveratrol inhibits proliferation of human epidermoid carcinoma A431 cells by modulating MEK1 and AP-1 signalling pathways. Exp Dermatol 15(7):538–546
38. Kong AN et al (2000) Signal transduction events elicited by natural products: role of MAPK and caspase pathways in homeostatic response and induction of apoptosis. Arch Pharm Res 23(1):1–16
39. Malemud CJ (2007) Inhibitors of stress-activated protein/mitogen-activated protein kinase pathways. Curr Opin Pharmacol 7(3):339–343
40. Chen KH, Weng MS, Lin JK (2007) Tangeretin suppresses IL-1beta-induced cyclooxygenase (COX)-2 expression through inhibition of p38 MAPK, JNK, and AKT activation in human lung carcinoma cells. Biochem Pharmacol 73(2):215–227
41. Lu Q, Qiu TQ, Yang H (2006) Ligustilide inhibits vascular smooth muscle cells proliferation. Eur J Pharmacol 542(1–3):136–140
42. Schonthaler HB, Guinea-Viniegra J, Wagner EF (2011) Targeting inflammation by modulating the Jun/AP-1 pathway. Ann Rheum Dis 70(Suppl 1):i109–i112
43. Dillon S et al (2004) A Toll-like receptor 2 ligand stimulates Th2 responses in vivo, via induction of extracellular signal-regulated kinase mitogen-activated protein kinase and c-Fos in dendritic cells. J Immunol 172(8):4733–4743
44. Mitsuhashi M et al (2004) Regulation of interleukin-12 gene expression and its anti-tumor activities by prostaglandin E2 derived from mammary carcinomas. J Leukoc Biol 76(2):322–332
45. Wagner EF, Eferl R (2005) Fos/AP-1 proteins in bone and the immune system. Immunol Rev 208:126–140
46. Erdelyi K et al (2005) Gallotannin inhibits the expression of chemokines and inflammatory cytokines in A549 cells. Mol Pharmacol 68(3):895–904
47. Park S, Choi J (2010) Inhibition of beta-catenin/Tcf signaling by flavonoids. J Cell Biochem 110(6):1376–1385
48. Hirano T et al (2006) Luteolin, a flavonoid, inhibits AP-1 activation by basophils. Biochem Biophys Res Commun 340(1):1–7
49. Gopalakrishnan A et al (2006) Modulation of activator protein-1 (AP-1) and MAPK pathway by flavonoids in human prostate cancer PC3 cells. Arch Pharm Res 29(8):633–644
50. Mahata S et al (2011) Berberine modulates AP-1 activity to suppress HPV transcription and downstream signaling to induce growth arrest and apoptosis in cervical cancer cells. Mol Cancer 10:39
51. Daynes RA, Jones DC (2002) Emerging roles of PPARs in inflammation and immunity. Nat Rev Immunol 2(10):748–759
52. Liu J et al (2003) Activation and binding of peroxisome proliferator-activated receptor gamma by synthetic cannabinoid ajulemic acid. Mol Pharmacol 63(5):983–992

53. Ulrich S et al (2006) Peroxisome proliferator-activated receptor gamma as a molecular target of resveratrol-induced modulation of polyamine metabolism. Cancer Res 66(14):7348–7354
54. Itoh K et al (2004) Transcription factor Nrf2 regulates inflammation by mediating the effect of 15-deoxy-Delta(12,14)-prostaglandin j(2). Mol Cell Biol 24(1):36–45
55. Surh YJ (2008) NF-kappa B and Nrf2 as potential chemopreventive targets of some anti-inflammatory and antioxidative phytonutrients with anti-inflammatory and antioxidative activities. Asia Pac J Clin Nutr 17(Suppl 1):269–272
56. Calixto JB et al (2004) Anti-inflammatory compounds of plant origin. Part II. modulation of pro-inflammatory cytokines, chemokines and adhesion molecules. Planta Med 70(2):93–103
57. Dvorak Z et al (2006) Differential effects of selected natural compounds with anti-inflammatory activity on the glucocorticoid receptor and NF-kappaB in HeLa cells. Chem Biol Interact 159(2):117–128
58. Aravindaram K, Yang NS (2010) Anti-inflammatory plant natural products for cancer therapy. Planta Med 76(11):1103–1117
59. Ye J, Keller JN (2010) Regulation of energy metabolism by inflammation: a feedback response in obesity and calorie restriction. Aging (Albany NY) 2(6):361–368
60. Mraz M et al (2011) The effect of very-low-calorie diet on mRNA expression of inflammation-related genes in subcutaneous adipose tissue and peripheral monocytes of obese patients with type 2 diabetes mellitus. J Clin Endocrinol Metab 96(4):E606–E613
61. Forsythe CE et al (2008) Comparison of low fat and low carbohydrate diets on circulating fatty acid composition and markers of inflammation. Lipids 43(1):65–77
62. Brand-Miller J, Buyken AE (2012) The glycemic index issue. Curr Opin Lipidol 23(1):62–67. doi:10.1097/MOL.0b013e32834ec705
63. Levitan EB et al (2008) Dietary glycemic index, dietary glycemic load, blood lipids, and C-reactive protein. Metabolism 57(3):437–443
64. Du H et al (2008) Glycemic index and glycemic load in relation to food and nutrient intake and metabolic risk factors in a Dutch population. Am J Clin Nutr 87(3):655–661
65. Pittas AG et al (2006) The effects of the dietary glycemic load on type 2 diabetes risk factors during weight loss. Obesity (Silver Spring) 14(12):2200–2209
66. Neuhouser ML et al (2012) A low-glycemic load diet reduces serum C-reactive protein and modestly increases adiponectin in overweight and obese adults. J Nutr 142(2):369–374
67. Schulze MB et al (2005) Dietary pattern, inflammation, and incidence of type 2 diabetes in women. Am J Clin Nutr 82(3):675–684. quiz 714-5
68. Djuric Z et al (2008) Design of a Mediterranean exchange list diet implemented by telephone counseling. J Am Diet Assoc 108(12):2059–2065
69. Chrysohoou C et al (2004) Adherence to the Mediterranean diet attenuates inflammation and coagulation process in healthy adults: the ATTICA study. J Am Coll Cardiol 44(1):152–158
70. Gu Y et al (2010) Mediterranean diet, inflammatory and metabolic biomarkers, and risk of Alzheimer's disease. J Alzheimers Dis 22(2):483–492
71. Camargo A et al (2010) Gene expression changes in mononuclear cells from patients with metabolic syndrome after acute intake of phenol-rich virgin olive oil. BMC Genomics 11(1):253
72. Owen RW et al (2000) Olive-oil consumption and health: the possible role of antioxidants. Lancet Oncol 1:107–112
73. Stark AH, Madar Z (2002) Olive oil as a functional food: epidemiology and nutritional approaches. Nutr Rev 60(6):170–176
74. Thomazella MC et al (2011) Effects of high adherence to mediterranean or low-fat diets in medicated secondary prevention patients. Am J Cardiol 108(11):1523–1529
75. Fan H et al (2002) Oxygen radicals trigger activation of NF-kappaB and AP-1 and upregulation of ICAM-1 in reperfused canine heart. Am J Physiol Heart Circ Physiol 282(5):H1778–H1786

76. Meyer M, Pahl HL, Baeuerle PA (1994) Regulation of the transcription factors NF-kappa B and AP-1 by redox changes. Chem Biol Interact 91(2–3):91–100
77. Gonzalez-Gallego J et al (2010) Fruit polyphenols, immunity and inflammation. Br J Nutr 104(Suppl 3):S15–S27
78. Biswas SK et al (2005) Curcumin induces glutathione biosynthesis and inhibits NF-kappaB activation and interleukin-8 release in alveolar epithelial cells: mechanism of free radical scavenging activity. Antioxid Redox Signal 7(1–2):32–41
79. Han SS et al (2002) Curcumin suppresses activation of NF-kappaB and AP-1 induced by phorbol ester in cultured human promyelocytic leukemia cells. J Biochem Mol Biol 35(3):337–342
80. Karlsen A et al (2007) Anthocyanins inhibit nuclear factor-kappaB activation in monocytes and reduce plasma concentrations of pro-inflammatory mediators in healthy adults. J Nutr 137(8):1951–1954
81. Bakker GC et al (2010) An antiinflammatory dietary mix modulates inflammation and oxidative and metabolic stress in overweight men: a nutrigenomics approach. Am J Clin Nutr 91(4):1044–1059
82. Chun OK et al (2008) Serum C-reactive protein concentrations are inversely associated with dietary flavonoid intake in U.S. adults. J Nutr 138(4):753–760
83. Helmersson J et al (2009) Low dietary intake of beta-carotene, alpha-tocopherol and ascorbic acid is associated with increased inflammatory and oxidative stress status in a Swedish cohort. Br J Nutr 101(12):1775–1782
84. De Bacquer D et al (2006) Epidemiological evidence for an association between habitual tea consumption and markers of chronic inflammation. Atherosclerosis 189(2):428–435
85. Steptoe A et al (2007) The effects of chronic tea intake on platelet activation and inflammation: a double-blind placebo controlled trial. Atherosclerosis 193(2):277–282
86. Chu SL et al (2011) A randomized double-blind placebo-controlled study of Pu'er tea extract on the regulation of metabolic syndrome. Chin J Integr Med 17(7):492–498
87. Krahwinkel T, Willershausen B (2000) The effect of sugar-free green tea chew candies on the degree of inflammation of the gingiva. Eur J Med Res 5(11):463–467
88. Nantz MP et al (2009) Standardized capsule of *Camellia sinensis* lowers cardiovascular risk factors in a randomized, double-blind, placebo-controlled study. Nutrition 25(2):147–154
89. Cho S-Y et al (2003) Quercetin suppresses proinflammatory cytokines production through MAP kinases and NF-κB pathway in lipopolysaccharide-stimulated macrophage. Mol Cell Biochem 243(1):153–160
90. Comalada M et al (2005) In vivo quercitrin anti-inflammatory effect involves release of quercetin, which inhibits inflammation through down-regulation of the NF-κB pathway. Eur J Immunol 35(2):584–592
91. Dias AS et al (2005) Quercetin decreases oxidative stress, NF-kappa B activation, and iNOS overexpression in liver of streptozotocin-induced diabetic rats. J Nutr 135(10):2299–2304
92. Stewart LK et al (2008) Quercetin transiently increases energy expenditure but persistently decreases circulating markers of inflammation in C57BL/6 J mice fed a high-fat diet. Metabolism 57(7 Suppl 1):S39–S46
93. Ryu OH et al (2006) Effects of green tea consumption on inflammation, insulin resistance and pulse wave velocity in type 2 diabetes patients. Diabetes Res Clin Pract 71(3):356–358
94. de Maat MP et al (2000) Consumption of black and green tea had no effect on inflammation, haemostasis and endothelial markers in smoking healthy individuals. Eur J Clin Nutr 54(10):757–763
95. Fukino Y et al (2005) Randomized controlled trial for an effect of green tea consumption on insulin resistance and inflammation markers. J Nutr Sci Vitaminol (Tokyo) 51(5):335–342
96. Widlansky ME et al (2005) Effects of black tea consumption on plasma catechins and markers of oxidative stress and inflammation in patients with coronary artery disease. Free Radic Biol Med 38(4):499–506

97. Dominiak K et al (2010) Critical need for clinical trials: an example of a pilot human intervention trial of a mixture of natural agents protecting lymphocytes against TNF-alpha induced activation of NF-kappaB. Pharm Res 27(6):1061–1065
98. Srinivas NR (2009) Structurally modified 'dietary flavonoids': are these viable drug candidates for chemoprevention? Curr Clin Pharmacol 4(1):67–70
99. Zinke I et al (2002) Nutrient control of gene expression in Drosophila: microarray analysis of starvation and sugar-dependent response. EMBO J 21(22):6162–6173
100. Rathee P et al (2009) Mechanism of action of flavonoids as anti-inflammatory agents: a review. Inflamm Allergy Drug Targets 8(3):229–235
101. Ueda H, Yamazaki C, Yamazaki M (2002) Luteolin as an anti-inflammatory and anti-allergic constituent of *Perilla frutescens*. Biol Pharm Bull 25(9):1197–1202
102. Gilbert ER, Liu D (2010) Flavonoids influence epigenetic-modifying enzyme activity: structure—function relationships and the therapeutic potential for cancer. Curr Med Chem 17(17):1756–1768
103. Wang LS et al (2011) Modulation of genetic and epigenetic biomarkers of colorectal cancer in humans by black raspberries: a phase I pilot study. Clin Cancer Res 17(3):598–610
104. Dey M et al (2006) In vitro and in vivo anti-inflammatory activity of a seed preparation containing phenethylisothiocyanate. J Pharmacol Exp Ther 317(1):326–333
105. Dey M et al (2010) Dietary phenethylisothiocyanate attenuates bowel inflammation in mice. BMC Chem Biol 10:4
106. Lee YM et al (2009) Benzyl isothiocyanate exhibits anti-inflammatory effects in murine macrophages and in mouse skin. J Mol Med (Berl) 87(12):1251–1261
107. Wang LG et al (2007) Dual action on promoter demethylation and chromatin by an isothiocyanate restored GSTP1 silenced in prostate cancer. Mol Carcinog 46(1):24–31
108. Liu Y, Chakravarty S, Dey M (2013) Phenethylisothiocyanate alters site- and promoter-specific histone tail modifications in cancer cells. PLoS One 8(5):e64535
109. Myzak MC et al (2004) A novel mechanism of chemoprotection by sulforaphane: inhibition of histone deacetylase. Cancer Res 64(16):5767–5774
110. Myzak MC et al (2007) Sulforaphane retards the growth of human PC-3 xenografts and inhibits HDAC activity in human subjects. Exp Biol Med (Maywood) 232(2):227–234
111. Afman LA, Muller M (2012) Human nutrigenomics of gene regulation by dietary fatty acids. Prog Lipid Res 51(1):63–70
112. Dunn GA, Bale TL (2011) Maternal high-fat diet effects on third-generation female body size via the paternal lineage. Endocrinology 152(6):2228–2236
113. Bird JJ et al (1998) Helper T cell differentiation is controlled by the cell cycle. Immunity 9(2):229–237
114. Maslowski KM et al (2009) Regulation of inflammatory responses by gut microbiota and chemoattractant receptor GPR43. Nature 461(7268):1282–1286
115. Kau AL et al (2011) Human nutrition, the gut microbiome and the immune system. Nature 474(7351):327–336
116. Turnbaugh PJ et al (2009) The effect of diet on the human gut microbiome: a metagenomic analysis in humanized gnotobiotic mice. Sci Transl Med 1(6):6ra14
117. Kemperman RA et al (2010) Novel approaches for analysing gut microbes and dietary polyphenols: challenges and opportunities. Microbiology 156(Pt 11):3224–3231
118. Arkadianos I et al (2007) Improved weight management using genetic information to personalize a calorie controlled diet. Nutr J 6:29
119. Lopez-Miranda J et al (1994) Effect of apolipoprotein E phenotype on diet-induced lowering of plasma low density lipoprotein cholesterol. J Lipid Res 35(11):1965–1975
120. Sima A, Iordan A, Stancu C (2007) Apolipoprotein E polymorphism—a risk factor for metabolic syndrome. Clin Chem Lab Med 45(9):1149–1153
121. Barberger-Gateau P et al (2011) Dietary omega 3 polyunsaturated fatty acids and Alzheimer's disease: interaction with apolipoprotein E genotype. Curr Alzheimer Res 8(5):479–491

122. Sarkkinen E et al (1998) Effect of apolipoprotein E polymorphism on serum lipid response to the separate modification of dietary fat and dietary cholesterol. Am J Clin Nutr 68(6):1215–1222
123. Egert S et al (2010) Serum lipid and blood pressure responses to quercetin vary in overweight patients by apolipoprotein E genotype. J Nutr 140(2):278–284
124. Li Y et al (2011) Green tea consumption, inflammation and the risk of primary hepatocellular carcinoma in a Chinese population. Cancer Epidemiol 35(4):362–368
125. Gasper AV et al (2005) Glutathione S-transferase M1 polymorphism and metabolism of sulforaphane from standard and high-glucosinolate broccoli. Am J Clin Nutr 82(6):1283–1291
126. Seow A et al (1998) Urinary total isothiocyanate (ITC) in a population-based sample of middle-aged and older Chinese in Singapore: relationship with dietary total ITC and glutathione S-transferase M1/T1/P1 genotypes. Cancer Epidemiol Biomarkers Prev 7(9):775–781
127. Chung FL et al (1998) A urinary biomarker for uptake of dietary isothiocyanates in humans. Cancer Epidemiol Biomarkers Prev 7(2):103–108
128. Wang LI et al (2004) Dietary intake of Cruciferous vegetables, Glutathione S-transferase (GST) polymorphisms and lung cancer risk in a Caucasian population. Cancer Causes Control 15(10):977–985
129. Joseph MA et al (2004) Cruciferous vegetables, genetic polymorphisms in glutathione S-transferases M1 and T1, and prostate cancer risk. Nutr Cancer 50(2):206–213
130. Tiihonen J et al (1999) Association between the functional variant of the catechol-O-methyltransferase (COMT) gene and type 1 alcoholism. Mol Psychiatry 4(3):286–289
131. Nielsen SE et al (1998) In vitro biotransformation of flavonoids by rat liver microsomes. Xenobiotica 28(4):389–401
132. Strassburg CP et al (1999) UDP-glucuronosyltransferase activity in human liver and colon. Gastroenterology 116(1):149–160
133. Coughtrie MW et al (1998) Biology and function of the reversible sulfation pathway catalysed by human sulfotransferases and sulfatases. Chem Biol Interact 109(1–3):3–27

Index

A.A. Farooqi, M. Ismail (eds.), *Molecular Oncology: Underlying Mechanisms and Translational Advancements*, DOI 10.1007/978-3-319-53082-6

MIX
Papier aus verantwortungsvollen Quellen
Paper from responsible sources
FSC® C105338
FSC
www.fsc.org

If you have any concerns about our products,
you can contact us on
ProductSafety@springernature.com

In case Publisher is established outside the EU,
the EU authorized representative is:
Springer Nature Customer Service Center GmbH
Europaplatz 3, 69115 Heidelberg, Germany

Printed by Libri Plureos GmbH
in Hamburg, Germany